THE
FIX

MICHAEL MASSING

UNIVERSITY OF CALIFORNIA PRESS

Berkeley · Los Angeles · London

University of California Press
Berkeley and Los Angeles, California

University of California Press, Ltd.
London, England

First Paperback Printing 2000

Published by arrangement with
Simon & Schuster

Designed by Edith Fowler

Library of Congress Cataloging-in-Publication Data

Massing, Michael.
    The fix / Michael Massing.
      p.   cm.
    Includes bibliographical references and index.
    ISBN 0-520-22335-7
     1. Drug abuse—United States.   2. Drug abuse—
Government policy—United States.   3. Drug traffic—
United States.   4. Narcotics, Control of—United States.
I. Title.
HV5825.M255   2000
362.29′18′0973—dc21   99-045376
                                      CIP

Manufactured in the United States of America
10 9 8 7 6 5 4 3 2 1

The paper used in this publication is both acid-free and
totally chlorine-free (TCF). It meets the minimum
requirements of ANSI/NISO Z39.48-1992 (R 1997)
(*Permanence of Paper*). ∞

To my parents, Emanuel and Marjorie,
and my sister, Jo Ann

Contents

PREFACE TO THE PAPERBACK EDITION

OF THE MANY PUBLIC exchanges I've had since the *The Fix* first appeared, the one that said the most about why the drug war persists came on "Talk Back Live," a daily talk show on CNN. "Has the Drug War Failed?" was the day's theme, and the peg was a new Justice Department report showing that the number of inmates in state and federal prisons had hit 1.8 million—many of them drug offenders. Appearing along with me were Darrell Gilliard, a Justice Department analyst, and Richard "Bo" Dietl, a former New York homicide detective and the author of a tell-all book about his career called *One Tough Cop*. The show was broadcast from Atlanta before a live audience. Gilliard was patched in from Washington and Dietl and I participated from Manhattan. I was already at my desk in the studio when Dietl was ushered in and seated at a desk fifteen feet away. After the technicians fitted us for mikes, we were left alone in the darkened studio to await the start of the show. Dietl, who had blow-dried gray hair, a neatly trimmed mustache, and a thick build that filled his dark double-breasted suit, sat stiffly at his desk, seemingly determined to avoid conversation.

When the show started, host Bobbie Battista went first to Gilliard in Washington for a quick summary of the report. When he was done, she turned to Dietl for a reaction. Did he think the drop in crime nationwide was linked to the rise in the prison population? Of course, Dietl said. He recalled how, when making homicide arrests in New York, he constantly encountered repeat offenders who had been released. "If they keep getting out of jail," Dietl gruffly remarked, "they're going to keep committing crimes." "What rights," he went on, "does the person walking down the streets have when a guy's going to walk up to them with a gun, or a knife, and robs them, or kills them, or maims them?" Dietl added: "Let's build more jails . . . because the good people in America . . . don't want to be victims of crime."

When it was my turn, I said that, for the most part, the nation's prisons were being filled not by violent felons but by non-violent drug offenders. Those who had violent records, I said, should be put away. "For those who don't," I added, "I think we need to stress rehabilitation. That way we can break the cycle of their constantly going in and coming out and crowding our prisons."

It was time for a commercial. With the cameras off, Dietl and I sat awkwardly at our desks. Deciding to make some small talk, I asked Dietl how long he'd been with the NYPD. In a clipped tone he noted the years he'd been on the force and the neighborhoods he'd been assigned to. He paused. "You know, I don't really disagree with you," he said. Surprised, I asked what he meant. Dietl said that he, too, felt that the nation's drug laws were too harsh and that they were filling our prisons with low-level offenders. He began describing the case of a childhood friend who in the mid-1980s had been arrested for attempting to sell three ounces of cocaine to an undercover cop. Under New York's Rockefeller drug laws, his friend had gotten twenty-five-years-to-life; more than twelve years later, he was still serving them. While the man had made a mistake, Dietl said, he was having to pay an absurdly high price. He had been so troubled by the case, he added, that he had written Governor George Pataki, a personal acquaintance, to plead for executive clemency. But Pataki had rejected the plea. Getting worked up, Dietl said he planned to mention the case when the show resumed.

When it did resume, however, Dietl said nothing about the case. Instead, he lashed out at drug users and the many horrible crimes they commit. "In my experience, from locking up several thousand people," Dietl thundered, "most of the time they were under the influence of either alcohol or drugs when they were committing the crimes." Dietl said he favored taking children to morgues to see the bodies of people who had died from drug overdoses. "I hate to scare little children," he said, "but I want them to be afraid. I want them to, if somebody asked them about using drugs, to say, 'Oh, no, I don't want that. I saw a dead person in a refrigerator.'"

When Dietl was finished, Battista called on a defense attorney in the audience. Of the hundreds of clients he had represented, the man said, most had been under the influence of drugs or alcohol. And the "most frustrating" thing, he added, was how hard it was for them to get help. For low-level nonviolent offenders, he said, "it is almost impossible in today's climate to get treatment."

"You know, there is one thing that I would just like to say," Dietl interjected. He began talking about a 1984 case in which a man had broken into a house in New York and killed ten people, eight of them children. "We went to trial with it," Dietl declared. In testimony, he said, it came out that the man had been under the influence of cocaine while committing the crime; as a result, the jury had convicted him only of manslaughter. "Now, if that's an excuse, I have a problem with that," he said.

Asked by Battista to comment, I momentarily considered exposing Dietl, but, instead, I again stressed the importance of distinguishing between violent thugs, who deserved to be put away, and small-time drug offenders whose misconduct sprung from their drug use. The key was to break these users of their habits, and the most cost-effective way of doing that, I said, was treatment.

The show ended a few minutes later, and, as our mikes were being removed, Dietl expressed regret at not having found the time to mention his friend's case. I said that I would be interested in seeing a copy of the letter he had written to Pataki. Dietl asked for my address and promised to send it.

It arrived a few weeks later. In it, Dietl described his long-time friendship with the offender, Michael La Marca. During his twelve-plus years in prison,

Dietl wrote, La Marca had "conducted himself in the most exemplary manner." In "my many years in law enforcement," he added, "I have seen many miscarriages of justice. This case truly cries out for your consideration of Executive Clemency."

Included with Dietl's letter was a copy of La Marca's own six-page petition to the governor. Quoting Emerson, Psalms, and the Roman philosopher Boethius, it was full of reflection and remorse. At the time of his arrest, La Marca wrote, he was a happily married thirty-seven-year-old with three daughters aged one to eight; now, the oldest of them was in college and the other two were in high school. For five years, he went on, he had served as the personal secretary to the Catholic chaplain. He had counseled fellow inmates in finding jobs, organized a weekly class for the physically disabled, completed a course on substance abuse, and been elected the prison's Man of the Year. Included with La Marca's petition was a letter from the prison's Catholic chaplain, who attested to "the depth of his remorse and his eagerness to correct the wrongs which have brought suffering to so many." "As a Catholic priest and a trained Social Worker," the chaplain wrote, "I have no hesitation whatsoever in recommending Michael for Executive Clemency."

Despite it all, Governor Pataki had rejected La Marca's plea. Clearly, given his political ambitions, Pataki did not want to risk a Willie Horton, releasing someone who might go out and commit a heinous crime and thus unleash an outcry from all those tough guys who have built their careers on exploiting the public's fears about drugs and crime. The type of alarmist statements Bo Dietl made on CNN—so at odds with his own private views—shows the extent to which public posturing on the drug issue continues to impede the progress toward reform.

Still, the fact that even a former cop like Dietl has come to recognize the punitive nature of our current policy shows the extent to which the public mood is changing. The ongoing excesses of the drug war, and its continuing failure to reduce the incidence of drug abuse, have produced a growing backlash. Already, voters in a half-dozen states and the District of Columbia have approved measures to make marijuana available to individuals who need it for medical purposes. In Arizona—one of the nation's most conservative states— voters by a two-to-one margin approved a measure requiring that low-level drug offenders be mandated to treatment rather than prison. Since then, hundreds of drug offenders have been diverted from prison to programs, saving the state millions of dollars in prison costs.

In New York, Judith Kaye, the state's top judge, used her 1999 state of the judiciary address to call for an overhaul of the Rockefeller drug laws. Among the groups endorsing such a move was the New York State Catholic Conference, representing the state's Catholic bishops. And, in Connecticut, the state legislature—building on the work of a blue-ribbon task force appointed by

Governor John Rowland—voted to expand needle-exchange programs and increase insurance coverage for substance abuse.

Particularly dramatic was the turnaround of John J. DiIulio, Jr. A professor of public policy at Princeton University and a senior fellow at the conservative Manhattan Institute, DiIulio was for years an influential advocate for tougher sentences and expanded prisons. In his 1996 book *Body Count*, co-written with former drug czar William Bennett and John Walters, DiIulio ridiculed those who raised questions about the relentless expansion in the nation's prisons. "It is simply a (deadly) myth that our prison cells are filled with people who don't belong there, or that we would somehow be safer if fewer people were in prison," DiIulio and his colleagues wrote. By March 1999, however, DiIulio, in a *Wall Street Journal* article titled "Two Million Prisoners Are Enough," was arguing that the sharp rise in the prison population was producing "rapidly diminishing returns." "Current laws," he added, "put too many nonviolent drug offenders in prison." Calling for a policy of "zero prison growth," DiIulio advocated the repeal of mandatory-minimum drug laws, the release of drug-only offenders, and the mandating of more drug treatment. All in all, it would be hard to imagine a more radical change of heart.

At the federal level, drug czar Barry McCaffrey himself seemed at times to have undergone a conversion. At every opportunity, the retired four-star general was speaking out about the need to reduce the demand for drugs and about the role treatment should play in that. When, in June 1998, New York Mayor Rudolph Giuliani announced his intention to phase out the use of methadone as a treatment for heroin addiction, McCaffrey boldly challenged him. Visiting New York City in September 1998, the drug czar spent an afternoon at a methadone clinic in lower Manhattan, listening to clients describe how methadone had helped save their lives. And, in a talk to 1,000 cheering members of the American Methadone Treatment Association, McCaffrey decried the "stigma and fear" surrounding methadone. "The good you do," he declared, "is incredible."

In the end, McCaffrey's efforts paid off. In January 1999, Giuliani publicly acknowledged that he had been wrong about methadone—a rare admission of error from the stiff-necked mayor. Over subsequent months, McCaffrey worked to liberalize federal methadone guidelines so that the medication could be dispensed not only in clinics but also in hospitals and doctors' offices—something that had been prohibited since the early 1970s.

Yet, aside from that, progress at the federal level has been minimal. Certainly the new rhetoric about the importance of drug treatment has not been reflected in the federal drug budget. Of the $18 billion Washington was committed to spending on drug control in 1999, two-thirds was earmarked for law enforcement and interdiction and just one-third for treatment and prevention—the same skewed proportion as in the past. As a result, the nation's treatment centers remained severely underfunded.

To the extent that the government was willing to undertake a new initiative in the drug field, it was not in America's cities, but in Latin America. Alarmed by the growing instability in Colombia, Barry McCaffrey—the same Barry McCaffrey who had spoken so eloquently about the need to treat hardcore addicts—proposed spending an additional $1.3 billion on U.S. drug-control efforts in the Andean region. Most of that money would go for military assistance and training in Colombia, as well as high-tech interdiction programs by Customs and the Coast Guard. This was on top of the $289 million in security assistance Colombia was already receiving from the United States—more than any other country except Israel and Egypt.

In offering such aid, the Clinton Administration seemed determined to repeat past U.S. failures in the region. Both the Reagan and Bush administrations had made disruption of the Colombian cocaine trade a top priority. For more than a decade the DEA, CIA, FBI, and the Pentagon had worked together to dismantle the Medellin and Cali cartels. And, by the mid-1990s, they had largely succeeded, with most of the top drug lords dead or in jail. And the result? Cocaine continued to flow into the United States unabated. Indeed, even as the cartels were crumbling, Colombian traffickers succeeded in creating a thriving new heroin industry, and today that drug is available in the United States at record high purities. Despite this history of futility, Washington is preparing to sink even more money into the Colombian drug war. It is this stubborn unwillingness to learn from the past that has fed the growing interest in change. And, increasingly, the type of public-health approach outlined in *The Fix* seems to be gaining favor. At this point, the most pressing challenge seems to be figuring out a way to get that approach adopted.

Having had the chance, since my book appeared, to observe the policy-making process up close, my thinking on this point has evolved. Initially, I felt that any movement toward reform would have to come from the grassroots. Only by mobilizing Americans at the community level to pressure their elected officials, I thought, could real progress be made.

It was thus with great interest that I watched "Close To Home," Bill Moyers's five-and-a-half-hour series on drug addiction, broadcast on public television in March 1998. The series—inspired by Moyers's efforts to deal with the addiction of his own son, William Cope Moyers—made a strong pitch for treating drugs as a public-health, rather than criminal-justice, problem. In an effort to generate support for such a change, the series made a point of showing how addiction strikes at all sectors of American society; one full hour was devoted to interviews with nine recovering addicts of varying hues and backgrounds. Another hour, on the value of treatment, provided an inside look at two treatment centers that had helped Moyers's son. The final installment—on the politics of the drug issue—urged the government to invest more heavily in treatment and prevention.

To help magnify the series' impact, the Robert Wood Johnson Foundation put up $2 million to organize related events around the country. Town hall meetings were held to discuss the broadcast, and live call-in shows with experts were aired to coincide with it. Channel 13/WNET in New York published six companion guides to help stimulate discussion, and PBS set up a Website to coordinate community-based efforts to combat addiction.

In the end, thousands of people participated in events linked to the broadcast. Yet, from a political standpoint, the impact was limited. Unlike alcoholism, drug addiction remains highly stigmatized in this country, and getting middle-class families affected by it to speak out will take more than a documentary on public TV. In recognition of this, William Cope Moyers has helped set up the Alliance Project, designed to develop grassroots support for drug reform. Its coordinator, Jeffrey Blodgett, helped organize Paul Wellstone's first campaign for the U.S. Senate, and one can only hope that this effort will be equally successful. Clearly, though, that could take years.

In the meantime, what might be done? Having seen the obstacles to bringing about change at the grassroots, I began to mull the possibility of sparking it at the top. In *The Fix*, I attempt to show how, in the early 1970s, the government made treatment its top weapon in fighting drug abuse. It did so because the Nixon White House became convinced that such an approach could actually work, and because, as a staunch law-and-order advocate, Richard Nixon knew he would not be accused of being soft on drugs. Given the Democrats' continued timidity on the issue, I began to wonder if a Nixon-style Republican might be able to carry out a similar reform today.

Two candidates came to mind: George W. Bush and George Pataki. Soon after becoming governor of New York, in 1994, Pataki—concerned about the continuing flow of drug offenders into New York's prisons—had expressed support for modifying the Rockefeller drug laws. And Governor Bush had made "compassionate conservatism" his ideological touchstone; certainly providing more money for drug treatment would seem to qualify for such a designation.

Alas, over time, it became increasingly hard to conceive of either man as a drug reformer. The more Pataki came under consideration as a candidate for higher office, the less willing he was to speak out in favor of reform. And, whatever George W.'s own personal experience with cocaine, as governor of Texas he tightened the state's penalties for drug possession, and he showed little interest in providing more services for addicts. Indeed, one of the most interesting aspects of the whole did-he-or-didn't-he-use-cocaine flap was all the attention it focused on Texas's draconian drug policy. All in all, the Republican Party today is very different from what it was twenty-five years ago, and the policies Nixon pursued on drugs seem far too radical for current-day politicians, Republican or Democrat.

So, if reform seems as unlikely to come from on high as it does from below, what's the alternative? A possible one began to take shape in my mind during a visit to Albany, New York, on March 1, 1999. This was "lobby day," when various interest groups descend on the New York State Legislature to press for the inclusion of specific items in the state budget. Some treatment providers from New York City—seeking more money for rehab—had set up meetings with several legislators and their aides, and they had asked me to sit in to talk about my research. Watching the treatment providers in action, I felt that, while well-motivated, they were not effective advocates for their cause. Rather than make a general case for the value of drug treatment, each lobbied for his own particular type of program. One methadone provider implored a state legislator to come up with new ideas for increasing public acceptance of methadone. Another pressed a legislative aide on an arcane state regulation that he wanted changed; as he rambled on, I saw the eyes of the staffer glaze over.

To make matters worse, most of the legislators being lobbied were liberal Democrats already inclined to support treatment. "We're not the ones you need to convince," a blunt, bearded staff member observed. The ones who needed convincing, he said, were the Republicans who controlled the State Senate, many of whom came from conservative districts that liked the idea of building more prisons. It was also important, he said, to get to George Pataki, who was likely to veto any increases in treatment the legislature might approve. We began talking about how this might be done. "You have to get to the right people," the staffer said—people who knew the governor and the Republican legislators and who could impress them with the need for more funds for treatment. "Could such an approach really work?" I asked. "Absolutely," the aide said—"if you get the right people."

Intrigued, I raised this idea with others experienced in the drug policy field, and they, too, said they thought it could work. Putting it into practice, one would begin by selecting a particular state or city to focus on. One would then recruit a group of prominent individuals willing to speak out on, and meet with officials about, the need for more treatment dollars. Such a coalition might include corporate executives, doctors, professors, clergy, teachers, union leaders, and representatives of law enforcement and criminal justice.

This last group is particularly important, for the participation of cops, prosecutors, and judges in the reform effort could provide cover to politicians worried about looking soft on drugs. And, based on my own conversations, there seem to be growing numbers of officials who—exasperated by the endless flow of petty drug offenders into the criminal justice system—would be willing to advocate more treatment.

The broader the coalition, however, the narrower its objectives will probably have to be. Prosecutors and police officials willing to support more funds for treatment, for instance, might shy away from endorsing reform of the drug laws. The extent of political sensitivity on this issue became apparent to me at a conference held in Aspen, Colorado, by the Physicians Leadership Network for Drug Reform, a bipartisan group of doctors committed to treating drug abuse as a public-health issue. While united over the need for more treatment, the physicians clashed over a host of other key reform goals, such as expanding needle-exchange programs and eliminating mandatory-minimum sentences. In the end, the group—regarding these items as too controversial—decided to limit itself to the most basic goal of seeking more money for treatment. As this suggests, the process of building a reform coalition can be slow and laborious. All marches, however, must begin with the first step.

The value of coalition-building on the drug issue has already become apparent in one city. Baltimore has long had one of the nation's worst drug problems. And, like most other cities, it traditionally relied on law enforcement to deal with it. But that did little more than fill the city's jails, and local officials began seeking a different way. Back in the late 1980s, Mayor Kurt Schmoke had made national headlines by calling for the decriminalization of drugs, but as mayor he lacked the authority to achieve that. Looking for a more practical approach, in 1993 he named Peter Beilensen—then completing a residency at the Johns Hopkins Medical School—to be his new health commissioner, with the goal of treating addiction as a public-health problem.

To accomplish that, they needed backing from the community, and over time they got it from a wide array of groups, including public-health specialists at the Johns Hopkins University; the Greater Baltimore Committee, a group of leading businessmen; the Abell Foundation, an influential local philanthropy; the Baltimore Neighborhood Collaborative, a coalition of community groups; and, finally, Thomas Frazier, the police commissioner, who had concluded that the city could not arrest its way out of its drug problem. Also lending support was George Soros's Open Society Institute, which has an office in Baltimore. Together, these groups helped procure millions of extra dollars (both public and private) for drug treatment, and the number of available slots in the city soon doubled. Eventually, the city hopes to make treatment available on request.

The city is also trying out a number of innovative programs to help addicts, such as simplifying the treatment admissions process, sending outreach teams into troubled neighborhoods, and providing vocational and other ancillary services—all ideas advanced in this book. What's more, Peter Beilenson is being advised by a Scientific Advisory Committee whose thirteen members include several addiction specialists who had worked on Richard Nixon's drug program. Among them is Dr. Jerome Jaffe, who served as Nixon's drug czar, and who is a central character in this book. In the coming months, the Baltimore experiment will provide a real-life test of the policy prescriptions advocated in *The Fix*.

INTRODUCTION

The Problem

IT WOULD BE HARD to think of an area of U.S. social policy that has failed more completely than the war on drugs. Since 1981, the federal drug budget has soared from about $1.5 billion a year to more than $17 billion. The United States has sent spy planes over the Caribbean, built a paramilitary base in Peru, financed coca-eradication programs in Bolivia, and set up giant radar-bearing balloons on the Mexican border. From the South Bronx and South-Central Los Angeles to Fort Wayne, Indiana, and Yakima, Washington, narcotics agents have conducted stings, infiltrated drug gangs, hired confidential informants, and busted drug dealers. In 1996, more than 1.5 million people were arrested for drug offenses. The nation's state and federal prisons, which in 1980 housed fewer than 30,000 drug offenders, today harbor nearly 300,000. Despite it all, cocaine is cheaper than ever before, and heroin is being sold at purity levels six times those of the early 1980s. And the abuse of these drugs remains rampant. In 1996, the number of cocaine-related visits to hospital emergency rooms topped 144,000—an all-time high.

In trying to explain the drug war's failure, politicians and journalists have cited a gallery of foreign culprits—the president of Colombia, the Mexican police, the Nicaraguan contras. If only we could clean house in Bogotá, or root out corruption in Mexico, or rein in the CIA, we're told, the flow of drugs into the United States would abate. If only it were so. After years of relentless war making, it should by now be apparent that, no matter how many labs we smash, no matter how many shipments we seize, no matter how many drug lords we nab, cocaine and heroin are going to keep pouring in. As long as the nation's appetite for drugs remains strong, the traffickers are going to find a way to supply it. Any progress made in tackling the drug problem, then, is going to have to come at home.

Here the most commonly discussed alternative to the drug war is legalization. Legalize drugs, it's said, and the vast criminal networks that traffic in
them, and that commit so much violence, would suddenly disappear. As evidence, the legalizers commonly cite Prohibition. The outlawing of alcohol in
1919 gave rise to speakeasies, bathtub gin, and Al Capone. Once Prohibition
ended, so did most of these ill effects. Why not do the same with heroin and
cocaine?

Unfortunately, the end of Prohibition was also accompanied by a sharp
rise in alcohol use. Between 1934 and 1944, per capita consumption in the
United States jumped from 0.97 to 2.07 gallons. If illicit drugs were suddenly
legalized, might not consumption similarly increase? History is full of cautionary examples. In the early 1970s, for instance, doctors routinely began prescribing Valium (a minor tranquilizer) for everyday cases of anxiety. As the number
of prescriptions increased, so did the incidence of abuse; by the late 1970s,
Valium was sending more people to hospital emergency rooms than any other
drug, heroin and cocaine included. As physicians became aware of Valium's
dangers, they began writing fewer prescriptions for it, and the number of
emergency cases began dropping as well. Clearly, making drugs easier to get
can increase the extent to which they are abused, and one can only imagine
what would happen if such potent intoxicants as heroin and crack suddenly
became available by prescription, or were sold openly in shopping malls.

By now, the risks of legalization have become so evident that even one-
time advocates no longer talk about it. Instead, they have flocked to a new
standard: harm reduction. Developed in Western Europe in the late 1970s,
this school has recently gained much attention in the United States, due in
part to the decision by financier George Soros to back such organizations
as the Lindesmith Center in New York and the Drug Policy Foundation in
Washington, both of which are dedicated to this approach. Drugs, the harm
reductionists argue, are here to stay, and we have no choice but to learn how
to live with them. Rather than legalize drugs, they say, we should attempt to
reduce the harm drugs cause. To that end, they advocate a variety of reforms,
such as making methadone more available, expanding needle-exchange programs, and creating "safe injection rooms" as alternatives to shooting galleries.
The harm reductionists would also like to replicate the heroin-maintenance
experiments now taking place in Switzerland, in which addicts are given daily
doses of the narcotic so that they won't have to buy it on the street.

Some of these ideas clearly make sense. Needle-exchange programs, for
instance, have repeatedly been shown to be an effective hedge against HIV
transmission, and it's time they were expanded. The same is true of methadone
programs; over and over, they have demonstrated their ability to help heroin
addicts regain some normalcy in their lives. More generally, harm reduction,
by stressing the importance of helping addicts cope with the ill effects of their
dependence, offers a welcome corrective to the intolerance that has for so

long dominated the public's attitudes toward drugs and those who abuse them.

Sometimes, however, harm reductionists take tolerance too far. In their eagerness to condemn the excesses of the drug war, they are often reluctant to speak frankly about the dangers associated with drug addiction itself, and to intervene to stop it. The problem is most apparent at needle-exchange programs. With heroin users docilely lining up to get new syringes, such sites would seem an excellent place to work with addicts and encourage them to address their problem. And, at some exchanges, the counselors do this, working over time to gain the trust of their clients and, ultimately, raising with them the possibility of reducing or stopping their drug use. Too often, though, these exchanges— resolutely determined not to judge users—blithely hand out needles to all comers. Even women who are visibly pregnant will be handed new syringes, no questions asked. Certainly, if a pregnant woman is going to shoot up, she should be able to do so with sterile needles. At the same time, every opportunity should be taken to urge her to deal with her habit so as not to endanger her baby. To do this, however, would be to express a judgment that addiction is an abnormal state, and this some harm reductionists cannot bring themselves to do.

Likewise troubling is the growing tendency in the substance-abuse field to "medicalize" addiction and cast it as a purely physiological condition that is beyond the individual's power to control. Addiction, it is said, is a "brain disease" that alters the actual chemistry of the brain and, in the process, eliminates the possibility of individual volition. Leading the way in popularizing this notion has been the National Institute on Drug Abuse, which in recent years has doled out hundreds of millions of dollars to researchers to study the effects of addiction on the brain. Alan Leshner, the institute's director, has tirelessly toured the country, giving slide shows demonstrating how the chronic use of, and craving for, drugs "lights up" portions of the brain. Proponents of the brain-disease model go so far as to maintain that drug addiction is no different from diabetes or hypertension; all are chronic medical conditions that can be controlled through the use of pharmacological agents like methadone, insulin, or blood-pressure medications.

In showing that the craving for drugs has a strong physiological dimension, the brain-disease approach has helped dramatize the compulsive nature of addiction. Yet, in denying that addicts have *any* control over their behavior, proponents of this model are contradicting abundant evidence to the contrary, not to mention common sense. If addiction is an exclusively physiological disorder that permanently alters the brain, how have so many addicts managed to break their habits? When we hold up as role models people who have succeeded in overcoming their dependency on alcohol or illicit drugs, aren't we applauding their strength of character? Without stigmatizing addiction, we should be willing to acknowledge that, when addicts steal to support their habit or neglect to feed their children, they are at least partly responsible for their

deeds. While well-intentioned, adherents of the brain-disease model, by denying the role of volition in addiction, feed the public's suspicions that drug re-
formers are trying to sell them a bill of goods.

THE KEY, THEN, is to find an alternative to the drug war that does not flinch in
acknowledging that drugs themselves, when used to excess, often cause harm.
And, with their emphasis on addiction, both harm reduction and the brain-
disease model can help point the way toward a more effective policy. From the
debate in Washington, one might logically conclude that the main threat drugs
pose to the nation consists of teenage drug use. Every time a new survey appears showing a small upturn in high school drug use, Democrats and Republicans rush to proclaim a national emergency. In fact, teenage drug use, while up
some in recent years, remains well below the peak levels of the late 1970s.
What's more, most of that increase consists of marijuana use. And, while pot is
not harmless, it is not the problem heroin and cocaine are. And, fortunately,
the use of these drugs among young people remains negligible. According to
the University of Michigan's annual Monitoring the Future study, for instance,
only 2.3 percent of all high school seniors in 1997 used cocaine in the prior
thirty days; a mere 0.5 percent used heroin.

In contrast to teenage pot smokers, adults who regularly use heroin, cocaine, and crack do pose problems. They commit muggings, abuse children,
suffer overdoses, and transmit diseases. They engage in unsafe sex, use welfare
checks to buy drugs, and prey on family members. In all, drug researchers estimate, there are about 4 million hard-core users in the United States. While
these addicts constitute only 20 percent of all drug users in the United States
(most of the rest being casual, or occasional, users), they consume about three-
fourths of all cocaine and heroin used here. They are also responsible for most
of the pathological behavior associated with drugs.

Who are these hard-core users? From news accounts, one might conclude
that they are mainly members of the privileged classes. Every time a stock-
broker or lawyer suffers a drug overdose, it seems to make headlines. Certainly,
plenty of affluent Americans are addicted to drugs. Yet the attention they
receive is out of all proportion to their number. The government's annual
National Household Survey on Drug Abuse, for instance, reveals no great
epidemic of chronic drug use among the middle class. The situation is very
different in the inner city. The research data consistently show that hard-core
users are disproportionately poor, unemployed, and members of minority
groups. They tend to be found not in swank condominiums or suburban split-
levels but in the tenements and housing projects of urban America. Even
among whites, the typical addict is not a model or musician but a truck driver,
construction worker, or other member of the working class—a group often invisible to the celebrity-hungry media. Any effort to alleviate the nation's drug
crisis must confront the problem of these down-and-out addicts.

In undertaking this book, I set out to find people who were doing interesting work with such users. For several weeks, I hung out at a Daytop adolescent treatment center in Brooklyn, talking with its clients. Each had an interesting story to tell, but the director seemed reluctant to let me attend counseling sessions, and I eventually gave up in frustration. Next, I began spending time at a courthouse in Brooklyn, sitting next to a state judge as he disposed of drug cases. For an outsider, seeing the wheels of justice turn is always fascinating, but, as I watched the pathetic procession of sad-sack defendants through the court, I came to feel that I needed to learn more about their lives on the street, before they entered the criminal justice system.

I thus eagerly accepted an offer from Richard Curtis, a street ethnographer at the John Jay College of Criminal Justice, to take me to a shooting gallery. What better window could I hope to find into the world of hard-core drug users? The gallery was located in an apartment on the top floor of a moldering tenement in the Bushwick section of Brooklyn. The tenant—himself a heroin addict—charged his fellow users a few dollars to use the place to inject. The apartment was surprisingly neat, and Curtis and I were invited to sit at a round table in the kitchen. Two users joined us, and I eagerly began asking them about their drug-taking careers. Meanwhile, the lean Latino man on my left prepared to shoot up. Out of the corner of my eye, I watched as he tapped some grains of dope from a glassine envelope into a metal bottle cap. He added some water, then warmed the bottom of the cap with a Bic lighter. When the mixture had turned viscous, he wrapped a belt around his left arm and inspected it for a usable vein. He then took a syringe and drew up the liquid from the bottle cap. Throughout, I had continued to chatter away, but at the moment he plunged the needle into his arm, I turned to watch—and suddenly passed out. A few seconds later I came to to find myself drenched in sweat. The other junkie at the table was yelling at Curtis, angrily demanding to know who I was. "No journalist would do that, man!" he shouted. He was so agitated that I feared he might turn violent, but he then slinked off into the bathroom to shoot up, and when he came out he had a goofy, contented smile on his face. Curtis and I quickly left, however, and when we got outside I decided that I would not use a shooting gallery as my main research venue.

I began to wonder if I would ever find one. Then, during an interview, a counselor at a detox center mentioned to me a dogged street worker named Raphael Flores who ran a drop-in center in Spanish Harlem. When I expressed interest in meeting him, he gave me his number. I called and arranged to stop by. On my initial visit, in January 1992, Raphael invited me to sit in on a conversation he was having with a seventeen-year-old girl from a nearby housing project. Of mixed Puerto Rican and Greek descent, the girl was clearly bright—she loved the plays of Tennessee Williams—but she was getting so high on beer and pot that she was on the verge of dropping out of school. Watching Raphael talk with her, I sensed that he had a special ability to work with inner-city drug users, and, with his permission, I began visiting his center on a regular basis. My time there provided me an inside look at the drug world of Spanish Harlem and the hard-core users who populated it. And, the more I saw of Raphael in action, the more I became convinced that he had developed a unique system for getting those users off the street.

While spending time with Raphael in Spanish Harlem, I was also researching the history of U.S. drug policy. I did not expect to find much of interest. As far as I knew, the nation had been fighting, and losing, the war on drugs for the last twenty-five years. In the course of my interviews, however, several drug-policy veterans urged me to take a closer look at the Nixon years. Nixon? Hadn't he actually *launched* the war on drugs? In fact, he had, but, as I began delving into that period, I found that there was much more to the story. When Nixon became president, in 1969, the nation was in the grip of a raging heroin epidemic. In response, his administration created a national network of treatment facilities that offered help to all those who wanted it. In short order, the epidemic was brought under control. The more I learned about the Nixon Administration's policy, the more it seemed to mirror the work Raphael Flores was doing in Spanish Harlem, and the more I felt that it could serve as a model for the nation today.

And we are desperately in need of such a model. On few issues have politicians been more oblivious to the lessons of history, or the hard results of research. The clamps of ideology have taken hold of the drug issue and won't let go. As a result, the policies being formulated in Washington today bear little relation to what is taking place on the street. This book attempts to bridge that gap. It depicts two very different worlds—that of drug addicts in Spanish Harlem, and of drug policymakers in Washington—with the aim of showing how they might be brought closer together. In Part One, I describe Raphael Flores's work with the chronic drug users of Spanish Harlem. I also look closely at the life of one of those users in an effort to better understand the nature of addiction. In addition, I assess the efforts of the local police precinct to clean up Spanish Harlem's most drug-ridden intersection. In Part Two, I recount how the Nixon Administration succeeded in stanching the heroin epidemic of the early 1970s, and how its policy subsequently fell victim to budget cuts and changing views of addiction. In Part Three, I return to Spanish Harlem to describe the dramatic events that engulfed Raphael and his center, and to assess the impact of Rudolph Giuliani's campaigning to rid the city of drug dealers. In the concluding chapter, I attempt to outline a new public-health approach to the nation's drug problem, one based not on the punitive powers of the law but on the healing powers of medicine.

PART ONE

THE STREET
1992

1

The Street Worker

"I NEED HELP," announced a slender dark-eyed woman as she trudged into the office of Hot Line Cares on a frigid afternoon in early 1992. "I'm tired of getting high." Slickly dressed in a leather jacket, black jeans, and dark purple shirt, the woman was accompanied by her two daughters, cute round-eyed toddlers who were so padded against the cold that they looked like midget snowmen.

Apologizing for the lack of heat in the office—ice wouldn't melt in it Raphael Flores motioned the woman into a seat in front of his bulky desk, one of four in the cramped, scruffy office. A lumbering walrus of a man in his mid-forties, Raphael had a large fleshy face, a shock of unruly hair combed back from his forehead, and a gap-toothed smile that he flashed like a company trademark. Dressed in his usual thrown-together fashion—green Army jacket, faded jeans, and plaid vest—he wore no watch, and his glasses were missing an earpiece. On his desk were a few scraps of paper, a half-empty cup of coffee, and a Bible so worn it looked like it had been through the Crusades. Ralph, as friends called him, had been working with the addicts and alcoholics of Spanish Harlem since 1970, when he founded Hot Line Cares. Located on the second floor of an otherwise abandoned tenement, Hot Line was one of the few places in the area where addicts could simply walk in off the street and get immediate help.

Lydia Botero lived two blocks away in the James Weldon Johnson housing project. As she took off her daughters' coats and helped them into some chairs, she explained that she was into speedballing, injecting a mixture of heroin and cocaine. "I see things in my house and use that as an excuse to get high," she said wearily. "My mother sniffs coke on weekends. My sister is eight months pregnant and sniffs coke every day. I'm banging. They say I'm a junkie." Lydia wanted a detox, a short-term process in which drugs are flushed from the body.

"How soon do you want to go in?" Raphael asked, the words coming out slowly but orderly, like soldiers marching in file.

"Tomorrow," Lydia said. Fortunately, she had Medicaid, and her mother would be able to look after her kids.

"Do you want a *real* program, one lasting seven to twelve months?" Raphael asked.

Lydia nodded yes. Raphael was pleased. By itself, he knew, detox was rarely enough to break a drug habit. Only by following up with a longer, more intensive program could most addicts get clean. Many, however, had no intention of doing so. Some simply wanted to lower their tolerance so as to get a bigger kick from their drugs. Others wanted a break from the street—"three hots and a cot," in dope slang. Raphael would work only with those addicts who indicated some willingness to get clean. And Lydia seemed to be one.

As they talked, Lydia's daughters, who had been merrily munching Gold-fish crackers, began to grow restless. Taking a box of Pampers from her bag, Lydia excused herself and led the two girls into the bathroom. When they emerged a few minutes later, one of the girls was crying. Raphael picked her up in his large hands and, cradling her, asked Lydia how much she'd been doing.

"The past week, I've been doing just heroin—one or two bags a day, sometimes three," she said, adding morosely, "I'm twenty-five years old and going nowhere."

Raphael asked if she could afford a bus ride out of the city. The fare would be $42 round-trip. Lydia said she could.

Luckily, it was a Monday, a good day to get people into detox, since many patients were discharged over the weekend. Picking up the phone on his desk, Raphael squinted through his glasses at the exposed-brick wall across the room. On it hung a large bulletin board covered with index cards, each bearing the name and number of a program, arranged by category. There were detoxes and rehabs, shelters and food pantries, hospital emergency rooms and suicide hot lines. This was Hot Line's directory, an invaluable network of programs and contacts that Raphael had built up over the years.

Given the late hour—the light was already fading outside the soot-covered windows that lined Hot Line's back wall—Raphael knew the chances of getting a bed in the city were nil. Altogether, New York had just 500 drug detox beds (plus another 400 for alcohol). The city's largest provider, the Beth Israel Medical Center on lower First Avenue, had more than 100 beds, but the demand for them was so great that addicts would begin lining up at six in the morning in anticipation of the seven-thirty opening; within two hours, all the beds would be gone, and those turned away would have to return the next morning. Hospitals outside the city, while also crowded, tended to be less overwhelmed, and Raphael, scanning his directory, found the number of one north of the city and dialed it. "We'd like a bed in detox," he said, his tone quietly urgent. "Yes," he said after a pause, "she has Medicaid." Another silence. "You won't take her until Friday? That's too long a wait."

Just by looking at Lydia—her face was ashen and glistening with sweat—Raphael could see that her last bag of dope was wearing off. At this rate, she would barely last four hours, let alone four days. Peering at the bulletin board, he found the number of another hospital and dialed it. It, too, was full. While he continued calling around, Lydia gathered up her kids and took them down the short corridor that led to Hot Line's dingy back room. She placed the girls on opposite ends of a tattered couch, and they quickly fell asleep. When she returned to the front, Raphael was still on the phone, and the sight made her slump. "This girl is literally sick," he observed, shaking his head. "We don't want to lose her."

Finally, after nearly an hour of calls, he located a hospital in Westchester County that said it would probably have a bed the next day. Before committing it, though, the intake worker had to check with the hospital's insurance unit to make sure Lydia qualified. Since it was nearly five o'clock, he said, he would have to call back the next morning.

Lydia was dejected. "I'm going to drop off my kids and then go outside for a bit," she said, sheepishly referring to her hunger. "I'm sorry, I have to."

Raphael did not try to dissuade her. Withdrawing from heroin was like having a bad case of the flu, and Raphael could hardly blame her for wanting relief. Lydia went into the back room and woke her kids, then helped them on with their coats. Offering to walk her back to her apartment, Raphael picked up one of the girls, and the group headed off into the arctic afternoon. Crossing Third Avenue and continuing along 112th Street, they came upon a group of police officers who were handcuffing two crack sellers in front of a bodega. One of the sellers, a young Hispanic man, was mouthing off, and the cops, angry at his insolence, nervously fingered their nightsticks as they yelled at him to shut up. Raphael and Lydia scurried past. A block on, they arrived at the Johnson Houses, a jumble of squat maroon-colored apartment blocks. They took the elevator to Lydia's apartment, a spotless place with plastic coverings on the sofas and an enamel portrait of the Last Supper on the wall. Lydia's mother and sister came out to greet Raphael and take the children. He urged them to make sure Lydia returned to Hot Line the next day, and they said they would.

Raphael was nonetheless worried, for, as soon as he left, he knew, Lydia would head out onto the street to "cop," or buy drugs. And, in the process, he might lose her. Over the years, he had seen it happen time and again—addicts sucked back into the street for want of a bed. Sometimes, Raphael would actually stay overnight in a client's apartment, sleeping on a couch or cot, to make sure she did not wander. In this case, however, he was willing to rely on

Lydia's mother (even though she used drugs herself). Heading down Lexington Avenue, he turned left onto 111th Street and, coming to a tenement at the end of the block, rang the bell to the apartment of Sister Leontine O'Gorman. Sister, as everyone called her, was an elderly nun who for years had been dispensing good works in Spanish Harlem; in the process, she had referred many people to Hot Line. Earlier in the day, she had promised Raphael some food, and he was now going to collect it.

For Raphael, as usual, was short of cash. Hot Line Cares led a Perils-of-Pauline-like existence, forever being pulled back from the tracks by an emergency fundraiser or sudden act of philanthropy. Constantly behind on its rent, the center had to go to court every few months to avoid eviction. Its three telephones were half the number it needed, and when a document had to be copied, staff members would have to carry it down the street to an employment office that let Hot Line use its machine. In summer, the sole source of relief was a dust-encrusted fan; in winter, the only heat came from an anemic portable radiator. Overall, the center got by on a budget of about $70,000 a year, from which Raphael drew a salary of $13,000.

His assistants got by on even less. In its diversity, Hot Line's staff resembled the cast of *Taxi*. Ethel Curtis was a hard-bitten, tough-talking Polish-American resident of Spanish Harlem. She had first met Raphael when one of her sons had gotten into trouble with the law; Raphael had housed him at Hot Line until he could get back on his feet. A former alcoholic, Ethel had never done any type of community work, but, seeing the success Raphael had in getting people into treatment, she had volunteered to help, and she was now working to get some of her own neighbors into programs.

Alain Bigot, a Frenchman in his early forties, had worked as an executive chef in an Italian restaurant in midtown until a heavy cocaine habit led him to crack and the street. He had met Raphael one day while waiting to enter a detox, and, at his invitation, had stopped by Hot Line after finishing it. Entering an outpatient program, Alain began volunteering at Hot Line while seeking a full-time job. With his stylishly cut hair, formal Gallic manner, and heavy French accent, Alain seemed far from his normal milieu, but he found working with other addicts an aid to his own recovery.

Raphael's top assistant was Marvin Yates, a chubby, voluble African-American from Bedford-Stuyvesant. After graduating from high school, Marvin —also in his forties—had spent twelve years working for a cleaning company before succumbing to a long-term drinking problem. After several cycles of programs and relapses, including four years spent drinking in parks and shelters, Marvin had ended up in East Harlem. Going by Hot Line for a detox referral, he had returned to the center after completing it. Volunteering, Marvin proved so adept with clients that Raphael asked him to stay on full-time. In lieu of a salary, Raphael let him sleep in Hot Line's back room. Every night after work, Marvin would unfold a cot, drawing the portable radiator near for heat. Marvin, who favored T-shirts with in-your-face expressions like, "I'm not opinionated, I just have strong opinions," frequently clashed with his no-less-headstrong boss, but together they made a good team, with Marvin generally tending to Hot Line's black clients and Raphael to its Hispanic ones.

In the office, Raphael seemed a cross between a supply officer and an air-traffic controller, juggling calls while scheming to obtain that scarcest of resources, a bed. On the phone, he would alternately plead, cajole, joke, flatter, and scold as the situation demanded. "You've been in this business how long and you've never heard of Medicaid paying for a car service?" he would growl. If a client came in late on a Friday—usually the hardest time to make a placement—Raphael would take it as a personal test. "If you can't get someone in on a Friday afternoon," he liked to say, "you're not a real Hot Line."

He was a familiar presence in the neighborhood, barreling purposefully down the street, his shirttail flapping out behind him. Often, he would be off on a "home visit," meeting with family members worried about a loved one. Sometimes, he would be accompanying a client to a hospital to be detoxed. En route, he would frequently run into people he'd helped over the years. Often, he'd not remember their names—Raphael had no head for them—but he could usually recall their cases to the last detail, and he would listen intently as he was updated. If he saw a junkie on the street, Raphael could not resist approaching him and describing his ability to get people into detox. If the addict expressed interest, Raphael would jot down Hot Line's address and urge him to visit. Even late at night, Raphael, returning to his apartment on 105th Street after a long day of work, would stop to chat with a nodding junkie or shuffling wino, hoping to gain one last recruit before turning in.

HE CERTAINLY had a large pool to draw on. Hot Line was located in the heart of Spanish Harlem, a vibrant section of East Harlem bounded by 125th Street on the north and 96th Street on the south, by Fifth Avenue on the west and First Avenue on the east. While many blacks lived here, it was the Puerto Ricans who predominated. Since World War II, they had been pouring in, displacing the Irish and Italians who had long lived there. With its bodegas selling mangoes and yucca, its *pastelerias* serving sugary pastries and *café con leche,* its *botánicas* dispensing scents and statues for use in religious ceremonies, El Barrio, as it was called, still had a touch of San Juan about it. But it also had the unmistakable feel of the ghetto. On almost every social index, from unemployment and single-parent families to HIV transmission and infant mortality, Spanish Harlem ranked near the bottom of New York neighborhoods, and the level of drug abuse was correspondingly high.

Indeed, two blocks south of Hot Line Cares, on 110th Street, was one of the city's largest open-air drug markets. Here, on the block between Lexington and Third—a bustling crossroads that included a U.S. post office, a public library, a supermarket, a bodega, a bakery, and a Chinese carryout—two or three dozen dealers would always be out: flush-faced, glassy-eyed men offering Elavil and Xanax, Valium and methadone, cocaine and, especially, heroin. The dope sold on 110th Street was among the best in the city, and people would come from as far away as Connecticut and Pennsylvania to buy it. Every day, an estimated 5,000 to 7,000 bags of heroin were sold here, generating revenues of up to $25 million a year. The dealers were so brazen that they would actually shout out brand names, the labels proudly advertising the toxic nature of their product: Poison, Tyson, DOA, Hot City, Natural Born Killers.

The action was especially thick at the intersection of 110th and Lex. The No. 6 subway train stopped here, disgorging a new batch of customers every few minutes. On three of the corners stood grubby convenience stores, which did an around-the-clock business in soda, beer, and cigarettes. On the remaining corner rose the DeWitt Clinton Houses—four eighteen-story red-brick towers that looked like the legs of a giant coffee table turned upside down. More than 2,000 people lived in the project, and, with few recreational areas around, they used 110th Street as a sort of front yard, swelling the crowds that hung out on the southeast corner, by the stairs leading down into the subway station. Sometimes, the crush got so great that pedestrians had to cross to the other side of the street to get by.

Whenever he found himself passing through the area, Raphael liked to stop at La Segunda Reyna, a grimy, thimble-sized bakery on Lexington that sold stale Cuban sandwiches and fifty-cent cups of coffee. The place was usually full of junkies exchanging tips about quality and brand strength. The "stock market," Raphael called it, and, sipping his coffee, he would unobtrusively listen in, trying to find out the latest on the street.

With the exception of a three-year stint in the Army, Raphael had spent all of his forty-five years in Spanish Harlem. And, during them, he had learned as much about drug addicts as anyone in the city. He knew where they went to cop, when they liked to get high, what it was like to go through withdrawal. He also knew addicts' cons and scams, their ability to wheedle money and manipulate emotions. Yet he never lost sight of the broken humanity beneath the soiled exterior. And he was intensely aware of how many addicts wanted help. He could see it in their receptivity when he went up to them on the street. And he could see it in the forty to fifty people who visited or called Hot Line every week for referrals.

Of course, those addicts did not want help all the time, or even most of it. For many, taking drugs was a source of intense pleasure, an activity they would no sooner renounce than eating or screwing. Drugs also helped them cope with the stresses in their lives, from being unemployed to losing a loved one. Yet the point often came where the drugs themselves began causing serious problems, from physical ailments to family disputes to trouble with the law. And, when that happened, addicts were often open to help. That openness, however, could be quite fleeting, and, if help was not available immediately, they would usually end up back on the street.

Unfortunately, help was rarely available immediately. In New York, as in most U.S. cities, the demand for drug treatment far outstripped the supply. According to official estimates, New York in the early 1990s had more than a half-million drug and alcohol abusers. To serve them, the city had some 55,000 publicly funded slots. Of these, about 35,000 were in methadone-maintenance programs—outpatient clinics that provided patients a daily dose of the synthetic narcotic. These slots were reserved exclusively for heroin addicts; even so, they could accommodate less than 20 percent of the city's estimated 200,000 IV users. Most of the remaining slots were in drug-free (i.e., nonmethadone) outpatient clinics, which provided counseling and drug tests once or twice a week. For addicts in need of intensive care, the city had just 5,800 residential beds. At any one time, about 3,500 people were on waiting lists for drug or alcohol treatment.

Scarcity was just the start of the problem, however. For, in the world of New York health care, drug treatment was the Balkans, a chaotic, contentious region full of internal strife and rivalries. Each program featured a different regimen, served distinct populations, had special admissions criteria. Not every program was right for every individual. Yet the city had no central intake unit, no place where addicts could go to apply for admission. There was not even a registry that listed openings. If a Holiday Inn is full, it will at least call the Ramada down the street to see if it has a vacancy. Not so two treatment programs. Methadone clinics and therapeutic communities regarded each other as apostates, and detox units would no sooner cooperate with one another than Ford with GM. Even when there were openings, the onerous paperwork requirements could be a major deterrent. "The system is not set up so that people who want help can get it immediately," Raphael observed. "As a matter of fact, it's set up to be the opposite."

Hot Line Cares sought to remedy this. Raphael had no formal training, but, through two decades of trial and error, he had developed his own system for dealing with addicts. From nine to six, an addict could stop by at any time and speak with the first available counselor. Taking an intake form, the counselor would find out what the client was using and for how long, what special problems he had, and what (if any) insurance he had. (Alcohol was treated like any other drug.) The counselor would then lay out the available options—a detox in the city, say, or a long-term program upstate—and the client would indicate his preference. Getting on the phone, the counselor would begin calling around to programs, keeping at it until a slot was found. At a time when getting a bed could take weeks, Hot Line could usually locate one within forty-eight hours.

After a client was accepted into a program, Hot Line would arrange for him to be transported to it. To make sure the person got there, Hot Line would send along an escort. Staff members had accompanied clients as far away as Buffalo, an eleven-hour bus ride from the city. While a client was in a program, Hot Line would try to monitor his progress, and, when he was ready to be discharged, Hot Line would arrange to meet him. By thus tracking clients through the system, Hot Line tried to make sure they didn't get lost.

THE BARRIERS the system posed to addicts seeking help were so intricate and baroque, so lacking in reason and common sense, that only by seeing someone like Raphael in action could one truly appreciate them. One afternoon, for instance, Sister summoned him to talk with a heroin addict who had taken refuge in her apartment. Hurrying over, Raphael found a slender white woman with shoulder-length bleached-blond hair and limpid green eyes. Carol Ann Sanders was a single mother who came from a blue-collar town outside Wilkes-Barre, Pennsylvania. She had become hooked on heroin a few years earlier, after a car accident had left her in great pain. Even in Pennsylvania, Carol had heard about 110th Street, and she began traveling there to cop. Tiring of the commute, she eventually decided to remain full-time. For a white woman to live on 110th Street was not easy, but Carol, who was in her early forties, somehow managed to get by, sleeping in a partly abandoned tenement and turning tricks to support her habit. Having developed some nagging medical problems, however, she now wanted help.

Even in her grimy, emaciated state, Carol remained an attractive woman, with the type of cheekbones that were normally a ticket out of hick Pennsylvania towns. After hearing her story, Raphael felt she was a good candidate for detox. Unfortunately, she had no Medicaid. That automatically ruled out most of the hospitals in the city, which followed a strict policy of no insurance, no detox. The handful of hospitals that did accept uninsured individuals required two forms of official ID, such as a birth certificate or Social Security card, plus an apartment lease or other proof of residence. Street-level addicts were no more likely to have such documents than they were mutual funds. Certainly, Carol had no address, and she had long ago lost or sold off whatever ID she had once had.

Warming to the challenge, Raphael found out Carol's place of birth and, calling up the records bureau there, persuaded a clerk to Fed Ex him a copy of her birth certificate. He also got Sister to write a letter stating that Carol was staying with her—a commonly accepted ploy. When all was in order, Carol presented herself at Sister's, ready to go. Since it was already midmorning, Raphael decided to take her directly to North General, a hospital at Madison and 122nd. Carol, who wore a baggy GEORGETOWN T-shirt and steel-tipped red-leather boots, complained nonstop on the way over. "I'm sick as a dog," she moaned between puffs on a cigarette. "I need five dollars. C'mon, Ralph, I'm going to throw up." Raphael, who was wearing a rumpled green jacket and carrying a Guinness tote bag, told her that he could not support her habit but that the hospital might give her some methadone to hold her.

Arriving at North General, a modern, understated red-brick facility, Raphael escorted Carol to the detox intake unit on the ground floor. A man in a white coat directed them to Mrs. Williams, a large woman with short hair seated at a nearby desk. "This is my client Carol Ann," Raphael said, flashing a copy of her birth certificate as if it were a winning lottery ticket. "I know it's late, but this girl is dying out there."

"We have only one female bed, and that's for a woman in crisis," Mrs. Williams said curtly.

"What about tomorrow?" Raphael asked.

"We don't have any females scheduled to leave tomorrow," she said.

"*Please* help me," cried Carol, who was nearly in tears.

"Sweetheart," the woman said, "there's nothing I can do with no beds."

Curious, Raphael asked how many beds there were for women. Five, Mrs. Williams said. For men, there were thirty-one.

"What about St. Luke's?" the woman said, softening slightly. She picked up the phone and called the hospital. She got a taped message.

"Thank you, Mrs. Williams," Raphael said, genuinely appreciative. Carol, who was sweating and complaining of cramps, continued to badger him for money.

"You've got to stop that," Raphael said. "I know you're hurting, but I can't put out no funds."

Since no one was answering the phone at St. Luke's, Raphael decided to go there in person. In the cab ride over, he railed at the setup at North General: "Five beds for women! They expect you to come every day and wait. What a waste of time." Arriving at St. Luke's, a chaotic jumble of buildings near Columbia University, Raphael led Carol up to the detox unit. As she slipped into a plastic bucket chair in the drab waiting room, Raphael went up to the intake window and asked for the person in charge.

"They're not here," the man said with a frown. "That's number one. There are no beds—that's number two. And it's too late—that's number three. Come back tomorrow morning at seven-thirty."

Struggling to stay cool, Raphael said, "Can you tell me if there'll be any beds tomorrow?" With a sigh, the man disappeared, returning a minute later with the woman in charge. Raphael asked if anyone was scheduled to be discharged the next day.

"We don't give out that information," she snapped. "Come back tomorrow." She paused. "Does she have Medicaid?"

"No," Raphael replied hopefully, "but we have all the appropriate documents."

Relenting slightly, the woman said, "I know there'll be four beds. If she's here at seven o'clock and she's one of the first four, she'll be admitted—as long as she has the documents."

Raphael was excited, but, wanting no surprises, he took Carol down to the Medicaid office on the first floor. Going up to a strongly built man seated at a desk, Raphael explained that he wanted to make sure he had everything he needed to get his client into detox. When he mentioned that Carol had been living in an abandoned building but staying with a nun, the man, whose name was Patterson and whose title was "Medicaid expediter," asked if he had a letter from the nun. Raphael quickly produced it. When informed that Carol had not worked in years, Patterson starchily said that she had to go to the state office building on 125th Street both to get proof that she was not employed and to apply for work.

Raphael had not anticipated that one. "Is there any way we can waive that?" he asked deferentially.

"We have to confirm she's not working," Patterson said matter-of-factly. He then gathered up Carol's documents and excused himself.

"I'm *dying*," Carol said when he had gone. "Look at me. I hate looking at myself." She had dark circles under her eyes, cuts on her cheeks, and an angry sore on her mouth.

"You just have to live twenty-four hours more," Raphael said, trying to comfort her. "If you leave now, you're dead."

"I can't go twenty-four hours," she moaned. "I'll kill myself. I'll walk in front of a car."

"Let it be a slow-moving vehicle," Raphael said with a grin. "I did that once—I got a guy admitted with a broken leg."

"I'm not playing," Carol protested.

"*I'm* not playing," he said sharply.

When Patterson returned, he gave Raphael one form for the Department of Labor and another for Sister, who was to acknowledge that she provided Carol shelter and food.

By this point, Carol could barely move, but Raphael somehow managed to get her outside and into a cab. Ten minutes later, they pulled up in front of the state office building, a somber monolith on 125th Street. At the employment office on the second floor, Raphael went up to a booth in the middle of the room and got a form to apply for work, then helped Carol fill it out. After returning it to the booth, he led her back downstairs and out the main door to the Department of Labor office, whose entrance was on the street.

"Now that we've registered with the employment office, we have to go to unemployment to make sure you're not employed," he explained. Thinking out loud, he added, "For an addict to walk through this—it's unbelievable. There has to be a system that's better than this."

Finding twenty people in line, Raphael took a place in it while Carol collapsed into a chair. When Raphael's turn came, he called her over. "Have you worked in the last year?" the woman asked. Carol shook her head. The woman filled out a form and handed it to her.

As they were leaving, a woman in line with braided hair and a pin in her nose waved to Raphael. "Sir, don't I know you?" she said, smiling.

"Yeah, girl, give me a kiss!" Raphael said. "How's she doing?" A few months earlier, Raphael had helped a friend of the woman's get into a treatment program in Buffalo. She was still there and doing well, the woman said.

Rejoining Carol, who was standing by the door, Raphael was vibrating with excitement. "This kind of shit turns me on!" he cried.

The only remaining variable was Carol. Walking with Raphael east along 125th Street, Harlem's central commercial artery, Carol stopped in front of a Body Shop. Either Raphael was going to help her out, she said, or she was going to have to take care of business. Explaining yet again that he could not do anything for her, Raphael admonished her to be at Sister's by six the next morning. Carol promised she would, then disappeared into the swirl of pedestrians on the street.

Keyed up over her situation, Raphael awoke at three the next morning, and by six he was at Sister's. Carol had not shown. Raphael walked around the corner to the tenement where she had been crashing and, climbing the stairs, called her name, but there was no response. He went back to Sister's to wait, and at six-thirty the buzzer rang. It was Carol, looking much calmer than the day before. A client had been good to her, and the bag she'd bought was still holding her. Sister produced a ten-dollar bill, and with it the two took a cab to St. Luke's, arriving at seven-fifteen. No other women were present, and, with all her documents in order, Carol was admitted without hassle.

"She never would have made it on her own," Raphael said with considerable understatement after she'd been admitted. "She'd still be out there—subject to arrest or an OD." Ecstatic, he added, "I'm on a high."

There was not much time to celebrate, however. For getting Carol into St. Luke's was only the first step toward getting her well. The next was seeing her through detox. In the detox unit—a secured ward with common rooms for eating and counseling plus smaller two-person bedrooms—Carol would receive a daily dose of methadone to relieve her withdrawal symptoms. Each day, the dose would be reduced, until at the end Carol would be free of drugs.

That, at least, was how it was supposed to work. In reality, Carol was in for a rough time. In the past, hospitals would keep heroin patients up to fifteen days—the amount of time thought necessary for a thorough detox. With the rise of managed care, however, hospitals had begun reducing the number of days they would keep patients in detox. At St. Luke's, the process was down to seven days. "People who sniff heroin might do well with a seven-day detox," Raphael observed, "but people who've been IV-ing for years need more time. You can be sure that when they leave, they're hungry for drugs."

To get around this, Raphael had developed his own system, called "piggy-back" detox. After a person was discharged from one detox, he would immediately arrange for her to enter another. Whenever possible, he would use the community hospital in Ellenville, a blue-collar town about ninety minutes north of the city. Rather than use methadone, like most hospitals, Ellenville used clonidine, a blood-pressure medication that, while helping to calm clients, had none of methadone's addictive properties. (Medical studies have found clonidine to be a highly effective detox agent; nonetheless, few of the detoxes in New York City use it, since doing so would require monitoring patients' blood pressure, a chore that hospitals are loath to take on.) By the end of this second detox, most of Raphael's clients felt much less of an urge to get high.

Even then, the probability of relapse was strong, for detox by itself is rarely sufficient to eliminate the craving for drugs. That's why longer-term programs are so important. "The primary focus of detox should be getting people into a program," Raphael noted. "Unless a counselor raises the possibility, most clients don't realize there's another way." Yet, at most hospitals, this was not a priority. One study, in fact, found that only 14 percent of detox clients were referred to longer-term programs. It's not hard to see why. In New York, hospitals are reimbursed up to $1,000 a day for each day a patient remains in detox. If patients relapse, their eventual return is almost guaranteed. In Raphael's view, detox was nothing more than a "racket" designed to fill beds.

Raphael hoped to avoid all this in Carol's case. As her methadone was cut back, however, she began feeling restless and experiencing hot flashes; by her fifth day, her discomfort had become so great that she signed herself out of the ward. Like a homing pigeon she made straight for 110th Street, where she immediately got high.

As with many of his clients, Raphael could not tell whether Carol's relapse was due more to the program's weaknesses, or her own. Whichever the case, he was not discouraged. Often, it took two, three, or more exposures to treatment before the process took hold. The key was to keep at it. By working with drug users over time and gaining their trust, Raphael and his staff found they could help even the hardest of the hard-core.

2

Hard Core

ONE EVENING in January 1992, Marvin Yates, having finished his day's work at Hot Line, was on his way out to get some carryout food when, in the ground-floor corridor leading to the street, he saw a tall black woman struggling to catch her breath. "Sister told me to come here," sputtered the woman, who was wearing a cap and dungarees and appeared to be in her late thirties. Marvin, who could pick a con artist out of a police line, stiffly informed her that Hot Line was closed for the day but that he could refer her to a shelter for the night. The woman said she wasn't interested and split.

The next day, however, Sister Leontine called Marvin to say that the woman's mother wanted to see him. Nancy Hamilton lived at 110th and Park, in one of the Clinton Houses' four towers. Marvin, who was still struggling to stay sober, normally avoided 110th Street and its many temptations, but, with Sister making a special appeal, he agreed to pay a visit. Grabbing an intake form, he walked down Third Avenue and turned right onto 110th. Hurrying past the swarms of junkies and hustlers there, he walked the two blocks to Park and turned left, then left again into Clinton Building Number One. Taking a graffiti-scarred elevator to the fourth floor, he walked down the dimly lit corridor until he found 4H, then knocked.

The door opened to reveal a frail figure in a wheelchair. "Praise the Lord, someone's come to help my child!" Nancy Hamilton cried. Her daughter Yvonne, whom he'd encountered at Hot Line, was also there. Getting a better look at her, Marvin could see that she was a big woman, about five-ten and 170 pounds, with broad shoulders and large hands. Her round face was framed by a mop of short, straight hair and creased by narrow, piercing eyes that seemed to be sizing up the world around her. Nancy tearfully explained how drugs had turned her beloved daughter into a raging terror and how no one had been able to do anything about it.

Looking around, Marvin could see the toll Yvonne's drug addiction had taken. Everything in the three-bedroom apartment was faded and covered with dust. Most of the lightbulbs were bare, and some of the doors were missing knobs. Beneath the grime, however, Marvin could detect the signs of a once-thriving family. In the living room were track trophies and yellowing photos of smiling young girls. To one side was a piano, and on a table sat a two-foot-high plastic penny jar. Scattered everywhere were Bibles and hymnals, all of them well thumbed.

As he began talking with Nancy, Marvin felt an immediate bond. Like his own parents, Nancy had been raised in South Carolina, and she radiated a similar air of courtliness and spirituality. Promising to do whatever he could, Marvin took an intake form and began asking Yvonne about her drug habit. She said that she had been using crack for about seven years, smoking as much as two hundred dollars' worth a day. She had two children, but for the time being they were being looked after by others. She had Medicaid and was willing to enter a detox.

Returning to Hot Line, Marvin began making the usual round of calls, and in short order he managed to locate a bed in a hospital in Manhattan. Yvonne entered without protest. Because crack and cocaine do not cause physical withdrawal, the detox process for them rarely lasts more than four or five days. For addicts accustomed to sleeping in the street, the experience could be quite relaxing, and so it was for Yvonne. The ward had a TV with HBO and a rec room where patients could play cards. The only requirement was that they attend daily group sessions. By the end of the process, Yvonne felt more rested than she had in years.

She had no intention of quitting, however. And so, even as Marvin was trying to find a residential bed, Yvonne was back on crack. Frustrated, Marvin nonetheless wanted to keep working with her, for, having spent so much time on the street, Yvonne seemed—in the twelve-step lingo Marvin liked—"sick and tired of being sick and tired." While waiting for her to come around, Marvin kept in touch with her mother. By coordinating his efforts with Nancy, he knew, he had a much better chance of getting Yvonne off the street. Finding in Nancy a sort of surrogate mother, Marvin began stopping by 4H at the end of the workday. Often, Nancy would give Marvin money to buy some Chinese food and, munching on dumplings and lo mein, she would talk about her family and the woes that had befallen it. "I have no peace, Marvin," Nancy would say, and, hanging out at her apartment, Marvin could see why.

Aside from Yvonne, Nancy had to contend with another daughter, Anne, who, nearing fifty, had been on heroin since her teens. When young, Anne looked like Diana Ross, but decades of mainlining had left her gaunt, gray, and hobbled. Even so, she remained an engaging and gregarious person who, when not out hustling, liked to read biographies and the *Daily News*. Anne spent much of her time in Apartment 17E, a putrid drug den where addicts from 110th Street went to get high. Whenever she grew tired of the tumult there, however, she would come stay at her mother's, using the bathroom to shoot up.

Over the years, Anne had had five children by three different men, and Nancy had had to take them all in at one time or another. Two remained with her. Paul, laconic and sluggish, was not much trouble, but Shondelle was showing every sign of following in her mother's footsteps. Not quite thirteen, she was hanging out with boys until the wee hours, drinking "forties" (forty-ounce bottles) of malt liquor. When she needed money, Shondelle would seek out her mother in 17E, nonchalantly sidestepping the junkies on the floor.

Fortunately, two of Nancy's children had turned out better. James, a tall, handsome man who wore dark suits and drove a Jaguar XJ6, was the pastor at a Pentecostal church in Queens. For years, Nancy had been a regular at his services—long, emotional affairs at which elderly women whirled in the aisles and spoke in tongues. A talented piano player, Nancy had been director of the gospel choir. Of late, her failing health had cut into her attendance, but she made sure to be present on the day James was ordained a bishop—the proudest in her life. (Marvin, who often went with Mary to church, accompanied her to the ceremony.)

Nancy's eldest daughter, Joyce, lived with her husband in a middle-class section of the Bronx. A heavyset, oval-faced woman, Joyce taught at a high school in East Harlem, and after classes she would frequently drop by 4H. Seeing the chaos in the place, Joyce was always urging her to move, but Nancy had lived in Clinton for more than twenty-five years and had no intention of leaving now. To help out, Joyce frequently gave her mother gifts, but on each visit she would notice that some of them were missing. When she asked why, the answer would always be the same: Yvonne.

To feed her drug habit, Yvonne was taking everything from the apartment that wasn't nailed down—TVs, radios, cameras, fur coats, watches, a VCR, even her mother's wedding ring—and peddling it on the street. With the proceeds, she would rush to 109th and Madison, her favorite crack spot. Often, while sitting with her mother, Joyce would hear Yvonne banging on the door, demanding to be let in. At Joyce's insistence, Nancy would refuse, but once Joyce left, she always relented, and more of her possessions would end up on the street.

Of the many troubles in her life, none tormented Nancy as much as her youngest daughter's drug habit. Yvonne was her baby. Growing up, she had always been a dutiful daughter. And she was so smart. At one point, however, crack had simply taken over her life, and Nancy, talking with Marvin into the night, would try to figure out where she'd gone wrong.

IF ONE WERE to draw up a profile of a typical crack addict, it would look a lot like Yvonne Hamilton. From the start, crack found a special foothold among African-Americans, particularly those living in the inner city. Within the inner city, housing-project residents seemed especially susceptible to the drug. And, within the projects, women seemed most vulnerable. Far more than heroin or any other illicit drug, crack snared women, especially single ones. Yvonne fell into all these categories. As such, she can help clear up some of the misconceptions that have developed over the nature of hard-core drug users in the United States.

Over the last decade, the image of those users has fluctuated wildly. In the initial phase of the crack epidemic, they were seen as deranged individuals belonging to some subhuman species. The early tone was set by *Newsweek,* which in 1986 ran three cover stories on crack and cocaine, each more breathless than the last. In one, Arnold Washton, a specialist in cocaine treatment, was quoted as saying that "crack is the most addictive drug known to man right now. It is almost instantaneous addiction, whereas if you snort coke it can take two to five years before addiction sets in." To illustrate the point, *Newsweek* offered a series of cautionary vignettes: "Art F. was a fortyish San Francisco lawyer when cocaine took over his life. He was both a dealer and an addict. At the peak of his addiction, he smoked $1,000 worth of [crack] a day. Somewhere along the way he lost his wife, his two children and his Marin County home."

Over the next several years, the press would routinely run garish accounts of crack-crazed behavior, from mothers leaving their children unattended for days at a time, to men and women performing depraved sex acts in moldering crackhouses, to a teenager so hooked on the drug that her parents had her chained to a radiator. (BEHIND GIRL'S CHAINING, SIREN CALL OF THE STREETS, the headline in the *New York Times* declared.) The image of the unregenerate crackhead reached its apogee with Spike Lee's 1991 movie *Jungle Fever,* in which Samuel L. Jackson played a shiftless Harlem man who rips off his parents, mooches off his brother, and smokes away his days in the "Taj Mahal," a warehouse-sized crackhouse teeming with glassy-eyed zombies beyond all hope of redemption or recovery.

Around the same time as *Jungle Fever* appeared, a group of scholars and civil libertarians, concerned about such lurid depictions, began meeting regularly in Princeton, New Jersey, under the direction of Ethan Nadelmann, an assistant professor of politics at the Woodrow Wilson School. (In 1994, Nadelmann would move to New York to set up the Lindesmith Center under the sponsorship of George Soros.) The Princeton Working Group on the Future of Drug Policy viewed all the hand-wringing over crack as just another eruption of American drug hysteria, akin to the "Reefer Madness" scares of an earlier era. Gradually, the group developed a revisionist view of the crack phenomenon, and of drug addiction generally, which it disseminated in a series of articles and essays. Eventually, these writings were collected by the

University of California Press in a volume titled *Crack in America: Demon Drugs and Social Justice.*

Typical is "The Social Pharmacology of Smokeable Cocaine: Not All It's Cracked Up to Be," by John Morgan, a pharmacologist at the City University of New York Medical School, and Lynn Zimmer, a sociologist at Queens College. The crack story, they write, is "simply the most recent installment in a series of morality tales that simultaneously construct and confirm Americans' belief in the power of drugs to disinhibit and harm users." Challenging Arnold Washton, Morgan and Zimmer write that "many crack users take the drug occasionally, do not engage in prolonged binges, and do not become dysfunctional." They add: "Although there *are* risks involved in using crack, they have been consistently exaggerated. . . . most of the problems associated with crack are products of the social context in which it arose and is used, not its pharmacological powers. . . ."

Dan Baum, a former reporter for the *Wall Street Journal,* takes the revisionist view a step further in his book *Smoke and Mirrors: The War on Drugs and the Politics of Failure.* An account of how politicians over the years have exploited the drug issue, the book belittles the notion that drugs are at all dangerous and that addicts lead lives that are at all abnormal. In discussing whether heroin addicts commit crime, for instance, Baum writes that

> almost all addicts commit *some* crime to get by. Most of that crime, though, is selling heroin to other addicts. Innocent citizens are not, by and large, hit over the head by heroin addicts. In fact, if drugs were legal, most addicts would be leading largely law-abiding lives. Many hold jobs, or do legitimate spot work, to earn most of their money. Moreover, most who steal were thieves *before* becoming addicted, so the theory that addiction leads to crime is dubious.

As this passage makes clear, the revisionists generally belong to the legalization/harm-reduction camp. If addicts were left alone, they argue, they would cause little harm to themselves or others. By contrast, the drug alarmists, viewing hard-core users as hopelessly hooked, tend to support cracking down on them.

AS THE CASE of Yvonne Hamilton shows, neither side has it quite right. Yvonne first tried crack in 1985, in the early stages of the epidemic. Outwardly, she did not seem a good candidate for addiction. At the time, she was working full-time as a van driver for United Cerebral Palsy (UCP). Every morning, she would pick up wheelchair-bound kids in Brooklyn and Queens and take them to the UCP rehab center in Manhattan. In the afternoon, she would drive them back. Her pay, though hardly bountiful ($350 a week after taxes), allowed her to go out with friends to restaurants, the movies, and nightclubs. Yvonne was so fond of doing the hustle that her friends called her the Disco Queen.

Beneath the surface, however, Yvonne's life was anything but placid. For seven years, she had been working for UCP, and the task of driving her handicapped charges back and forth had long since settled into a routine. And, once the day was over, she would invariably find herself back on 110th Street. The sight of its boarded-up buildings, littered sidewalks, and corner drunks always depressed her. The Clinton Houses themselves were full of low-income families struggling to get by at a time when Washington had turned its back on urban America. Apartment 4H was especially chaotic, with Anne forever running off on drug missions, her son Henry in and out of trouble, and several younger children always in need of attention. At one point, nine people from three generations were living in the three-bedroom suite.

It was hardly what one would have expected, given Nancy Hamilton's upbringing. As a young girl in South Carolina, she had been raised by an evangelical mother who frowned on smoking, drinking, and even lipstick. After the family migrated to New York in the 1920s, Nancy's mother—horrified at the fleshpots of Harlem—had kept her busy with piano lessons and Sunday school. On graduating from high school, Nancy married a merchant seaman, and together they had three children—James, Frank, and Joyce.

She had planned to raise them according to the same strict standard as her mother, but in the end it was she who strayed. On her own for the first time, Nancy got sucked up into Harlem's rollicking nightlife, sampling its bars and after-hours clubs. Like many members of her generation, she became overly fond of alcohol, and in its corrosive acid her marriage quickly crumbled. Her husband fled to Middletown, New York, a small town north of the city, and took Joyce with him. (James would later escape by joining the Army.)

With World War II opening up new opportunities for blacks, Nancy went to work for the railroads. She also stepped up her carousing. Taking up with a pimp named Pretty Boy Floyd, she had Anne, who, born into turmoil, would begin hustling before she was out of grade school. Nancy was not inclined to remarry, but after the war she met a fun-loving Baptist preacher named Carl Hamilton, and, after an extended courtship, the two exchanged vows. Carl moved in with Nancy and Anne at their tenement on 129th Street, and, on March 23, 1955, Yvonne joined them.

From the start, Yvonne was well provided for, but her parents, engrossed in their own lives, had little time for her, and even before she could walk, Yvonne was throwing tantrums. Her fits grew worse when, in 1960, her parents separated. Carl moved into an apartment in Central Harlem, and Yvonne, at five, began dividing her time between the two residences. In 1965, when she was ten, she moved with her mother into the newly opened Clinton Houses. With Nancy away working most of the days, Yvonne began hanging out in the Puerto Rican social clubs that lined 110th Street. Taking up pool, she was soon beating opponents twice her age, but, falling in with an older crowd, she got a quick education in the neighborhood's seamy side. Tall and ungainly for her age, Yvonne was the butt of frequent jokes, and in reaction she became a bit of a bully.

It was around this time that Yvonne had her first brush with drugs. Tellingly, it came at home. Her mother, who was prone to headaches and anxiety attacks, had a medicine cabinet full of tranquilizers and sleeping pills, and one day Yvonne decided to try one. She felt pleasantly drowsy. By twelve, she was nipping from the bottles of liquor her mother kept in the apartment. Alcohol, she found, took the edge off her loneliness, and before turning thirteen she got drunk for the first time.

In junior high, Yvonne began attending wild "hooky parties" at which students would make out and get high. Limiting herself at first to Boone's Farm and other cheap brands of wine, she quickly branched out into marijuana. Her intake of both increased in high school. Her school—Julia Richmond, on East 67th Street—had 4,500 students, and Yvonne, like so many others, quickly got lost in it. Showing up for school in the morning, she would hang out on the steps, smoking joints and joking with her friends. When truancy notices were sent home to her mother, Yvonne would wait around in the lobby of her building and intercept them. By the tenth grade, she had fallen so far behind that she decided to drop out of school altogether.

Fearing that Yvonne would follow in Anne's footsteps, her mother, who was now working as a home attendant on the Upper East Side, pressed her to look for work. It was the early 1970s, the peak years of the Great Society, and Yvonne, stopping by a manpower training office on 107th Street, learned of the Job Corps. A program that sought to get young people out of the ghetto and into a trade, the corps operated some seventy centers across the country, and Yvonne soon found herself headed to one of them, in Astoria, Oregon. Yvonne liked the setting—a spit of land jutting spectacularly into the Columbia River—and her courses, which covered general subjects like math and social studies as well as her chosen field (food studies).

But the center was no less vast than her high school, and Yvonne, exposed to hundreds of girls like herself, began experimenting further. At a cast party for a play she was in, she was offered LSD for the first time, and, washing it down with a glass of vodka, had to be restrained from jumping into the Columbia River. Alcohol was her main escape, though. One evening, Yvonne got so smashed in town that the police had to drive her back to the center. She was grounded for two months. Otherwise, though, the Job Corps did not intervene, for it had no program to treat substance abuse, and after Yvonne completed her course, she was sent to Seattle to prepare meals in a veterans hospital. She continued to drink and pop pills, however, and, a few months before her job was scheduled to end, Yvonne, feeling lonely and depressed, returned to East Harlem.

For a while, Yvonne straightened out. Prodded by her mother, she enrolled in a G.E.D. course and eventually got her certificate. Again dropping by the manpower office on 107th Street, she learned of a new federal program, called CETA (after the Comprehensive Employment and Training Act), which provided menial jobs to hard-to-employ teens and adults. Yvonne got one as a librarian's assistant in an elementary school. Though paying only $70 a week, the position kept her off the streets for the next several years.

When the funding for it ran out, in 1978, Yvonne, feeling discouraged, stationed herself in front of the TV in 4H, where she downed beers and watched soaps. Her mother was beside herself. Having already lost her son Frank to a shoot-out and her daughter Anne to the streets, she did not relish the idea of losing Yvonne, too. By now, Nancy had been born again and was regularly visiting her son James's church in Queens. She relied on Yvonne to drive her there, and, on arriving, would always try to coax her inside. But Yvonne resisted. The services could last for hours, and she had little patience for all the holy-rolling and hallelujah-ing that took place at them. Failing at that, her mother pressed her to find work. One day, Yvonne, hearing of an opening at United Cerebral Palsy, stopped by its offices on 23rd Street to apply. To her surprise, she got it. For the first time in her life, she had a real job.

At first, Yvonne liked the work, and the opportunity it provided to be around kids. As tedium set in, however, Yvonne, facing several hours in the middle of the day with little to do, began visiting the Irish pubs in the area. At first, she limited herself to a beer with lunch, but her consumption gradually increased, until eventually she was drinking nonstop from midmorning until midafternoon. After work, she would hole up in her mother's apartment and drink Buds and Ballantines. If she wanted company, she would head upstairs to Apartment 9D to chug vodka with her friends Louise and Sonya. Often, she would drink all night, then have a beer before going to work in the morning. Though she wouldn't admit it, she was an alcoholic.

One day in 1985, Yvonne, stopping by 9D, found her friends getting high as usual, but not on vodka. Instead, they were smoking "base" (from "free-base"), a form of purified cocaine. Marveling over its kick, they urged Yvonne to join them. She declined. She had tried cocaine a few times and not enjoyed it. This was different, her friends assured her, and so Yvonne reluctantly put the pipe to her lips. At once, she felt a burst of pleasure go off in her brain. It quickly surged down her body, tingling her skin, roiling her stomach, grabbing her groin. "I'll do this drug until the day I die," she told herself.

The next day at work, she could think of nothing else, and in the evening she went back to 9D to smoke with Louise and Sonya. Drawing on the pipe, Yvonne felt all the burdens in her life—the turmoil in her family, the grimness of the projects, the dead-end nature of her job, the sense of being trapped in the ghetto—suddenly lift. Night after night, she would return to 9D, getting high with her friends. Once she learned how to prepare base herself, she would smoke alone in her mother's apartment while Nancy was away at church.

Before long, dealers were selling ready-made nuggets on the street, and Yvonne would make frequent detours in her van to pick some up. And, once it was in her possession, she could not resist using it. Becoming stuck in traffic in the Queens Midtown Tunnel, for instance, she would roll down the window and light up, knowing that her mute passengers could not protest.

Within six months of her first toke, Yvonne was spending virtually her entire paycheck on crack, and when that ran out, she began going through her bank account. After several minor accidents at work, she realized that it was only a matter of time before she would be found out. Feeling edgy and exhausted, Yvonne asked for, and was granted, a leave of absence. She took her last paycheck, for more than $800, and went on a wild crack binge that lasted several days. She never would return to work.

ACCORDING TO the revisionists, crack is not nearly as addictive as it's been made out to be. "Today, many doubt that crack causes instant addiction," John Morgan and Lynn Zimmer write in "The Social Pharmacology of Smokeable Cocaine." Narrowly speaking, they are correct. Yvonne did not become an addict the moment she put the crack pipe to her lips. Yet, from the very start, the drug exerted a remarkable pull on her, transforming her in a matter of months from a dutiful worker to a full-blown addict. And her experience was hardly unique. One of the most thorough analyses of cocaine and crack addiction is *Cocaine Changes: The Experience of Using and Quitting,* a study of 267 heavy cocaine users, 53 of them crack users or freebasers. Interestingly, all three authors (Dan Waldorf, Craig Reinarman, and Sheigla Murphy) came to the project with revisionist views, traces of which remain in their book. "Treatment clinicians routinely claim, and the media routinely echo them, that crack is instantly addicting, and that once users get that first good hit they will stop at nothing to get another and another until their very lives are destroyed," they write. Such views are "overly simple," they add, noting that many of their subjects smoked cocaine "for months without getting into a pattern that could be called seriously abusive or compulsive."

"That said, however," they go on, "we must report that a clear majority of our freebasers offered compelling testimony on the extraordinary hold this form of cocaine use can have over those who indulge in it more than a few times. For many, relationships were ruined, families neglected, jobs lost, savings accounts emptied, and health imperiled because they found freebasing simply overpowering." Even in the face of "overwhelming evidence of harm," the authors write, these users continued to smoke, "taking hit after hit until they felt their lungs would collapse or until heart palpitations forced them to stop." These effects were found to be especially acute among the disadvantaged. Affluent users, fearful of losing jobs and homes, had many reasons to quit; poorer ones had few. In Yvonne's case, the many strains in her life all made her easy prey for a drug promising instant relief.

And the consequences would prove devastating. Yvonne's behavior on crack offers a real-life rebuttal to the rosy accounts of addiction offered by the revisionists. Like many users, Yvonne initially exploited those closest to her— in this case, her mother. Approaching seventy and in failing health, Nancy was largely dependent on her Social Security checks. Yvonne knew when they arrived, however, and, intercepting them, would rush out to cash them. Sometimes, she would volunteer to buy things for her mother, then disappear with the money and return hours later, looking dazed. To make matters worse, Anne's son Henry had also become hooked on crack, and he and Yvonne would fight over the few scraps Nancy had to offer. In 1986 alone, the police were summoned to 4H fifteen times, and their reports offer a chilling look at the effect crack was having on the Hamilton household:

June 19, 1986: Yvonne and Henry fight, throw clothes around house.
August 3, 1986: Anne says Yvonne banged on her door demanding money, then grabbed her and began choking and smacking her in hallways. No injuries.
November 9, 1986: Nancy reports $60 missing—thinks Henry took it.
November 30, 1986: Anne complains that Yvonne dragged her from kitchen into a back bedroom and removed [$20] from victim pants pocket, then fled apt in unknown direction. Victim appeared intoxed and refused to go to 23 [Precinct]. No injuries.

By the spring of 1987, Yvonne—having exhausted her mother's resources —began preying on the community at large. An expert at shoplifting, or "boosting," she relentlessly worked the aisles of Bloomingdale's and Alexander's, Lord & Taylor and the Gap, stuffing dresses, shirts, and sweaters under her coat and walking cold-bloodedly from the store, returning again and again until recognized by security. Hitting local supermarkets, she would grab steaks (a practice known as "cattle rustling"), cans of tuna fish, and packets of Combat roach control, then sell them on 110th Street. Casing bars, Yvonne would sidle up to tipsy patrons at the counter and lift their wallets. Using the credit cards inside, she would order furniture from department stores and have it delivered to the lobby of her building, then sell it off in an impromptu auction. "I was a thief every day," she said, looking back on her drug career.

She did not limit herself to property crimes. Taking advantage of her size, Yvonne would approach meek-looking men on the street and begin sweet-talking them; once their guard was down, she would grab them in a choke hold with one arm while emptying their pockets with the other. She robbed widows and pensioners, the sick and disabled. She even went after "Blind Lee," an elderly blind man who lived in her building, shaking him down several times in the elevator.

The revisionists have a ready explanation for such behavior: the illegal status of drugs. Whatever crime and violence drugs generate, they assert, drug prohibition is responsible. As evidence, they invariably cite one study: "Crack and Homicide in New York City, 1988: A Conceptually Based Event Analysis," by Paul Goldstein and three other researchers. Goldstein examined 414 homicides committed in an eight-month period. Of these, the police classified 218 as drug-related. Examining these homicides more closely, Goldstein divided them into three categories: *psychopharmacological,* i.e., homicides caused by the effects of the drugs themselves; *economic compulsive,* caused by the need to finance a drug habit, and *systemic,* caused by the black-market nature of drug distribution. Of the 218 drug-related murders, Goldstein found only 31 to be psychopharmacological in nature, with alcohol the culprit in most. Another 8 qualified as economic compulsive. Most of the rest—three-quarters of the total—were found to be systemic in nature, involving territorial disputes, the robbing of dealers, and the like. From this, the revisionists have concluded that most drug-related violence is the consequence of drug prohibition.

On closer inspection, however, the Goldstein study does not lend itself to such a sweeping conclusion. For one thing, it was conducted in a single city over a narrow period of time—one in which turf battles over drugs were raging. For another, the study focused solely on homicide, a relatively rare form of violence. Goldstein himself noted in his article that recent studies of drug users and sellers "revealed greater proportions of psychopharmacological violence when all violence, and not just homicide, is examined." Drug-related homicidal violence, he explained, "is most likely to be systemic because of the powerful weaponry typically carried by drug traffickers"—weaponry not commonly found on drug users.

Goldstein's work on drugs and violence has been carried on by, among others, Barry Spunt, an associate professor of sociology at the John Jay College of Criminal Justice in New York. After analyzing hundreds of interviews with violent drug users, Spunt concluded that their actions are due far more to psychopharmacological factors than to economic or systemic ones. "People coming down from crack or withdrawing from heroin feel so shitty," he observed. "The frustration, the anxiety, the tension, can make them do really weird things. They're street people, and the desire for drugs becomes so strong that they'll do anything to get it. People with a history of violence may become more inclined to do violent things. Even those without such a background can flip out and engage in violence."

These tendencies should not be exaggerated. As Goldstein noted in one study, "most crimes committed by most drug users are of the nonviolent variety —for example, shoplifting, prostitution, and drug selling." Still, it would be foolish to airbrush the activities of addicts—especially where crack is concerned.

Before trying crack, Yvonne Hamilton was no angel; nonetheless, the drug unhinged her in a way even drinking had not. "Alcohol is a depressant," she observed. "You're down. Drinking allowed me to open up to other people, to venture into new things. Drinking, I never would have thought of robbing people. Crack gave me the confidence to do that. I was very self-centered and selfish, and drugs intensified that. It made me feel smarter than the rest of the world. It made me become very physically aggressive. I did a lot of things under the influence of crack that I otherwise would not have."

BY THE SUMMER of 1987, Yvonne was spending most of her time in Apartment 9D. It had become a popular gathering spot for crack users in and around the project, and as the traffic into it increased, Yvonne—showing new entrepreneurial savvy—proposed charging admission. Louise, the tenant, was vehemently opposed, but one week while she was away on vacation, Yvonne declared the apartment open for business. Anyone willing to pay the $2 entry fee could come and get high. By the time Louise returned, her apartment had become a full-fledged crackhouse. She was livid, but Yvonne threatened to beat her up if she didn't go along, and before long two hundred users a day were snaking in and out of the apartment.

One day, Anne knocked on the door and asked Yvonne if she could spend the night there. Yvonne was reluctant; once Anne got her foot in the door, she knew, there was no telling how long she might stay. But Anne had nowhere else to go, and so Yvonne relented. Sure enough, within days Anne was bringing up dope fiends from 110th Street, and the crackhouse was soon doubling as a shooting gallery. This did not please the crackheads, who looked down on the junkies, and Yvonne and Anne did their best to keep the two groups in separate rooms, but they were always spilling out, and eventually the apartment became an all-purpose drug den. Putting aside their usual rivalry, the sisters agreed on a rough division of labor: Yvonne would keep the books, recording entry times and payments, while Anne would be the "works lady," supplying syringes and other paraphernalia.

With so many addled individuals packed into such tight quarters, all clamoring for money and sex and attention, 9D became a blight on the entire building. The management file on the apartment soon bulged with eviction notices, court documents, and police reports recording everything from shootings to medical emergencies. In one episode, Yvonne was arrested after stabbing Louise three times with a penknife. "Apt. said to be crack house—under investigation," the police report noted.

With the police aware of the goings-on in 9D, closing it down would have seemed a straightforward matter. And it would have been had drugs actually been sold there, for the law made it easy to evict tenants for dealing drugs. Where simple use was involved, however, the city had to go through a long series of hearings and notices. Such safeguards had been put in place to prevent such unwelcome outcomes as, say, the eviction of an elderly tenant for a grandchild's use of drugs. As a result, though, the Housing Authority had a hard time shutting down even Wal-Mart–sized drug dens. Yvonne knew this. Even in her intoxicated state, she had mastered the city's housing code and so made sure that no drugs were sold in 9D. And the authorities were stymied.

In other ways, too, Yvonne was able to foil the system. Like most hard-core users, she showed remarkable ingenuity in averting anything that might get in the way of her habit. Overall, her behavior, while demonstrating the horrors of addiction, also showed how ill equipped the city was to deal with it.

A chilling example of both occurred in the fall of 1987, when Yvonne discovered she was pregnant. Though barely acquainted with the father (a fellow Clinton resident), she hoped that having a child might somehow turn her life around, and she enrolled in a prenatal program at Metropolitan Hospital on East 97th Street. When asked if she used drugs or alcohol, she admitted only to smoking cigarettes; in fact, she continued to use crack throughout her pregnancy. Admitted to the hospital in late December, she snuck in a half-dozen vials of crack and smoked them in the bathroom.

On Christmas Eve 1987, Yvonne gave birth by cesarean section. Gerald Hamilton weighed only six pounds, and hospital workers—sensing that something was amiss—decided to test his urine. It came back positive for cocaine. Gerald was, in short, a "crack baby."

The revisionists have taken great exception to this term, and to the dire pronouncements associated with it. For instance, George Soros's Lindesmith Center, in a fact sheet called "Cocaine and Pregnancy," maintains that, while cocaine (and crack) use during pregnancy is "certainly inadvisable," initial reports about the problems associated with it, such as low birth weight and physical defects, have not been supported by later studies. In most cases, the paper asserts, the real problem is not cocaine use but poor prenatal care and the use of alcohol and tobacco. "Addressing risk factors beyond cocaine use—including inadequate nutrition and health care and the use of legal drugs—increases the likelihood of a healthy mother and child," the paper states. All in all, it claims, the "pharmacological impact of cocaine" on the fetus "has been greatly exaggerated."

To an extent, this assessment is correct. The idea that babies exposed to crack *in utero* are irreparably damaged has been contradicted by recent studies showing that, with the proper nurturing, many of these children can develop normally. Typically, however, the revisionists, in minimizing the harm caused by crack and cocaine, go too far. For the reality is that crack—more than almost any other factor—nullifies a woman's maternal instincts, causing her to neglect the most basic needs of her children, in both the prenatal and postnatal stages. In New York, for instance, the introduction of crack set off a horrifying epidemic of child abuse and neglect, with the number of reported cases soaring from 36,305 in 1985 to 59,353 in 1989.

Yvonne's case would vividly illustrate the toll crack has taken on the inner-city family. With the results of Gerald's urine test in, a caseworker was summoned to the hospital and, determining him to be at risk, informed Yvonne that, to leave the hospital with him, she would first have to enroll in a program for drug-using mothers. Such a program was offered at a nonprofit health-care center down the street, and Yvonne agreed to sign up. She was also assigned a counselor from the city's child welfare bureau who was to check on her regularly.

Such safeguards would prove no match for Yvonne, however. While she would duly attend classes at the health-care center, she would sit mutely during the group sessions on drugs, waiting patiently for them to end. When it came time for her weekly drug test, she would sneak in a substitute specimen; the supervision was so lax that she never got caught.

As a new mother, Yvonne qualified for a biweekly welfare check for $238; as soon as it arrived, she would rush out to the Western Union office on Lexington to cash it, then head to the crack dealers on Madison. She did the same with the money she got from WIC (Women, Infants, and Children)—a federal program set up to feed young children. Neither welfare nor WIC had any procedures to make sure their money was used properly. When her checks ran out, Yvonne would take Gerald around to various apartments in the building, claiming tearfully that he was hungry. Donations in hand, she would dump Gerald off with whomever she could find, then rush back to 9D.

By any standard, Yvonne's behavior constituted child neglect, and had the city discovered it, it could have taken Gerald from her. But Yvonne was determined to prevent this. Once a month, her caseworker would make a site visit, and, though it was unannounced, the woman always came on a weekday between nine and five. Yvonne would watch for her out the window of 9D. If Yvonne saw her approaching, she would quickly bolt. On the rare occasions when she was trapped inside, she would simply ignore the woman's knocking until she left.

In early February 1988, Yvonne's neglect of Gerald became so glaring that Anne's son Paul—now ten years old—called the Housing Police. According to its report, Yvonne "repeatedly leaves Gerald with numerous unknown persons —known crack users." Child welfare, the document added, had sent a caseworker to investigate but had found "no need" for a report, for "child and apt appeared normal." For child welfare to declare things normal when Gerald was being passed around among strangers shows how derelict it was in protecting the city's children. "Child welfare was very negligent," Yvonne would later observe. "The caseworker was OK, but for her it was just a nine-to-five job. Most people such as myself have little trouble beating the system. Children are subject to abuse by people like myself, and the city is very lax about it." (That would prove no less true in the case of Yvonne's second child, a daughter named Nancy Lee, who was born out of wedlock in 1989.)

On June 7, 1990, Yvonne's luck finally seemed to run out. That afternoon, she stopped by 9D to get high. Just as she was smoking her last rock, there was a commotion at the door. "Don't move!" a man shouted at her, pushing a gun in her face. When he identified himself as a cop, Yvonne was actually relieved—she thought she was being robbed. Someone in the apartment, it seemed, had sold drugs to an undercover. Yvonne, who had several crack stems in her bra and a handful of vials in her pocket, managed to shake them out before the cops got around to searching and handcuffing her.

The group was herded downstairs and driven to a holding pen at 115th and Fifth. After the arrests were processed, they were driven downtown to Central Booking, in the basement of police headquarters. After posing for a mug shot and having her fingerprints taken, Yvonne was driven around the corner to the women's detention area, a grim holding pen crowded with prostitutes and drug addicts. Several hours later, her name was called and she was led to an arraignment court on the ground floor of the Criminal Courts Building. There, in a stark chamber that had all the charm of a Greyhound bus terminal, an assistant district attorney read out the charges against her: the criminal sale of a controlled substance in the third degree, a Class B felony.

It was a serious charge. New York State's drug laws are among the toughest in the country. Originally passed in 1973 at the instigation of Governor Nelson Rockefeller, the Rockefeller Laws, as they have come to be known, are most notorious for the harsh sentences they mandate for those caught trafficking in small quantities of heroin or cocaine. The mandatory minimum penalty for selling two ounces of cocaine, for instance, is fifteen years to life. Yet such cases, while dramatic, are relatively few in number. Far more common, and more insidious in some ways, are the lengthy sentences doled out to run-of-the-mill street-level dealers. In New York, the sale of even a single vial of crack or bag of heroin is considered a B felony, the second highest of the state's five felony classes (A being the highest). Other B offenses include armed robbery, first-degree rape, and first-degree manslaughter. Assault with the intent to cause serious physical injury is a lesser C felony. In other words, selling a vial of crack is considered more serious in New York than slashing someone's face with a razor (as happened in the case of the model Marla Hanson). If convicted, Yvonne faced a year or more in prison.

Yet the criminal justice system would prove no more adept at dealing with her than would any other part of the bureaucracy. For there was simply nowhere to put her. In the previous seven years, New York State, in a massive prison-building boom, had increased the number of beds in the system from 25,000 to 46,000. Over the same period, however, the number of inmates had kept pace, rising from 30,500 to 55,000. So, despite a near-doubling in size, the prison system was still 20 percent over capacity. And drug cases were largely responsible. By 1990, nearly one of every two new inmates in the state was a drug offender. And judges in the city were tired of dealing with them.

"To sentence a low-level guy to two to four years for a two-bag transaction is an exercise in futility," said Manhattan Judge Herbert Adlerberg in his cluttered chambers. A tough-talking, chain-smoking jurist, Adlerberg had presided over thousands of drug cases since joining the bench in 1983, and they had left him deeply critical of the way the system worked. "For every drug offender who is locked up, there are five to take his place," he noted between puffs of a Lucky Strike. "I've seen it happen over and over again. And do you know how much it costs to keep a prisoner upstate for a year? It's a telephone number." Prisons, Adlerberg added, "should be reserved for really bad guys. Instead, they've been crammed with low-level offenders."

For all the havoc Yvonne had wreaked in Spanish Harlem, no one would consider her a career criminal; whatever crimes she had committed, they were mostly a by-product of her habit. That was certainly apparent to the arraignment judge, who, looking at her rap sheet, saw a single misdemeanor arrest for assault, and so he ordered her released on her own recognizance, with an order to return in a few weeks for the final disposition of her case.

Yvonne was a free woman. Exultant, she hopped on the No. 6 train and headed back to 110th Street. During the booking process, Anne had slipped her some food stamps, and Yvonne, arriving in Spanish Harlem, stopped by a grocery store to cash them. She then hurried to a nearby crack seller. Back at the Clinton Houses, she found to her disgust that the door to 9D had been padlocked. Cursing, she ducked into a nearby stairwell and, barely twenty-four hours after her arrest, she was again getting high.

She did not have to resort to the stairwell for long. Within days, the regulars from 9D had managed to pry the lock off the door, and, to the dismay of police, management, and tenants, the flow into the apartment quickly resumed. Stepping up its efforts to close the place down, the Housing Authority continued to encounter procedural obstacles. Eventually, though, it would receive an assist from the tenant herself. Under a program designed to prevent homelessness, the state was sending Louise checks to help with her rent. In effect, the state was subsidizing the operations of the drug den. With all the recent commotion, however, Louise had failed to make several payments, and on December 12, 1990, city marshals arrived to board the place up. At long last, the drug den was out of business.

It was only a matter of days, however, before a new one opened up. Apartment 17E had long been a gathering spot for Clinton House druggies, and the regulars from 9D quickly moved there. The new operation would prove even more disruptive than the old one, with police officers, paramedics, and social-service workers constantly being summoned there. Many of the visits concerned the apartment's legal tenant, a frail woman in her late sixties named Sally who was thought to be suffering from elder abuse—another malevolent by-product of crack. After visiting the apartment in February 1992, two social workers sent a memo to the building manager that captured the lurid climate inside:

> It was unbelievable the amount of "traffic" coming in and out of [17E]. There were about ten other people in Sally's three room apartment. There were three "bodies" laying on [her] bed at 3:00 p.m. We asked her to come with us into the kitchen to conduct our interview. . . . When I checked the refrigerator to see if she had food, one of the women became very menacing to us.
>
> [We] both felt endangered in an extremely hostile environment. We also saw two people who were involved in "strange" activities in the bathroom.

The social workers recommended that the city's Protective Services for Adults unit intervene, but it never did. Once again, the system had failed.

Yvonne was now into her seventh year of crack use, and, increasingly on edge, she was getting into more and more fights. On one occasion, two customers in 17E gave her $45 worth of crack to find them a hooker. Yvonne went off and smoked up the stuff herself. After waiting a decent interval, she returned to the drug den, only to find the two men waiting for her. They beat her so badly that she had to spend eight days in the hospital. After her release, she immediately went back to 17E, but her crack cronies had grown so tired of her antics that they would not let her in.

Feeling isolated and despondent, Yvonne turned to her one remaining refuge—her mother. By now, however, Nancy had little to offer her. Suffering from emphysema, asthma, and a heart condition, she had taken to a wheelchair, and even going to church had become an ordeal. Meanwhile, her family was continuing to unravel. Anne's son Henry, who had remained with her all these years and who had survived countless arrests and fights, was hunted down by a gang to which he owed money and shot dead in the street; to send a message, his executioners cut off his penis. Anne's daughter Shondelle had discovered "blunts," a high-octane joint in which marijuana is wrapped in the brown outer leaf of a Phillies Blunt cigar. Combined with malt liquor, blunts could be quite debilitating, especially for a girl not yet thirteen. In July 1991, Shondelle showed up for the first time in the police reports on 4H, listed as a "chronic runaway."

Now Yvonne was again coming around and demanding money. Her sister Joyce urged Nancy to change the lock on the door. Several times, Nancy agreed to do so, only to buckle under Yvonne's pleading and give her a key. In late 1991, however, Nancy, her patience exhausted, put her daughter out for good.

And so, in early 1992, Yvonne found herself out on the street, battling the cold, loneliness, and the relentless siren call of drugs. One evening, after ripping off a fellow user, Yvonne was racing up Third Avenue, looking for a place to hide, when she remembered having heard of a drop-in center on Third Avenue. Two blocks north of 110th Street, she found it. Ducking inside, she encountered a pudgy black man in the corridor. Where the housing authority, child welfare bureau, and police department had failed to contain Yvonne's habit, Hot Line Cares was now going to get a shot.

3

Priorities

BY MARCH 1992, Yvonne was ready for another detox. This time, Marvin found a bed in a hospital in Beacon, a town about an hour north of the city. In addition to its detox ward, the hospital ran a thirty-day residential program, and Marvin hoped to get Yvonne into it. Before leaving, Yvonne took the spending money her mother had given her and bought some angel dust, weed, and crack, then smoked it on the way up. By the time she reached the hospital, she was completely wasted. Nonetheless, she was admitted to the detox and managed to complete it without incident. Unfortunately, the residential program had no beds, and so Yvonne returned to 110th Street, where she again relapsed.

Though frustrated, Marvin blamed the system in this case as much as Yvonne and so was willing to work with her one more time. In April, he arranged for her to enter another detox. At the appointed hour, however, Yvonne did not show. Furious, Marvin was ready to cut her off, but then Nancy called to say that Yvonne was in the hospital; while smoking crack, she had been attacked by a man with a bat who had knocked out all her teeth. After being discharged from the hospital, Yvonne stopped by Hot Line. Still severely bruised, she had the look of a beaten animal about her, and Marvin, reluctantly agreeing to give her one last chance, proposed that she come stay at Hot Line while he sought a bed for her. Yvonne agreed and, getting some clothes from 4H, she took up residence at the office, sharing the back room with Marvin.

Over the next week, Marvin would not let Yvonne out of his sight. All the while, he was trying to place her in the community hospital in Ellenville, New York. The detox ward there had only twelve beds, allowing counselors to develop a good rapport with clients. And the setting, amid the Shawangunk Mountains, a rugged arm of the Catskills, seemed to have a calming effect on patients. If any place could succeed with Yvonne, Marvin felt, it would be Ellenville. And a bed there soon became available.

On the morning Yvonne was scheduled to leave, Marvin let her go to 4H to say goodbye to her mother. While there, Yvonne saw $50 in cash and food stamps lying around and reflexively swiped it. Sensing that this would be her last chance for a while to get high, she hurried outside and bought a dozen vials of crack and two forties of malt liquor, then consumed it all on the street. Edgy and agitated, she returned to Hot Line.

Seeing her condition, Marvin slipped a sharp letter opener into his bag as he prepared to accompany her to the Port Authority Bus Terminal. The subway ride there went smoothly enough, but once they reached the terminal—a crumbling, malodorous maze of ticket windows and boarding ramps—Yvonne began to get jumpy. She asked if she could hold the bus ticket, but Marvin, sensing a ruse, refused. She then asked if she could get some food, but Marvin again said no. When the time to board finally arrived, Marvin, seeing Yvonne hesitate, grabbed the letter opener and pointed it at her.

"Get on the bus!" he ordered.

"I guess I'll have to take the bus just to get away from you," Yvonne said with a bitter laugh, and with that she stepped on to the bus and handed the driver her ticket.

Two hours later, an intake worker from Ellenville called to say that Yvonne had arrived safely. Still worked up from all the crack and booze in her system, Yvonne was lashing out at everyone on the ward. As the days passed, however, she began to settle down. Marvin, meanwhile, was rushing to find a residential bed for her. Knowing Yvonne, he felt it would be best to avoid a coed facility, with all the distractions male clients could pose. Unfortunately, in all of New York State, there was no more than a handful of all-women programs—another glaring gap in the treatment system. Recently, Marvin had read a brochure about New Hope Manor, an all-women center in Barryville, not far from Ellenville. Marvin knew little about the program, aside from the fact that it stressed education and was run by nuns. Given Yvonne's religious upbringing, Marvin felt she would thrive in such a setting. Phoning the facility, he found it would have an opening the day Yvonne was due to be discharged.

With her options dwindling, Yvonne reluctantly agreed to go along, and, when her detox was complete, she boarded a bus for Monticello, a town near Barryville, and a representative from New Hope was there to pick her up. The program was housed in a cluster of wooden buildings on a bucolic estate set in the wild, wooded Delaware Water Gap on the New York–Pennsylvania border. Yvonne had no intention of staying. Hoping to persuade her mother to send her bus fare to return home, she asked for permission to call her. The nuns refused, explaining that new clients could not make outside calls. Yvonne next thought of hitchhiking, but the nearest highway was miles away, and, as a tall black woman in the backwoods of New York, she had visions of being stranded on some roadside. So, with a sigh, she grabbed her bag and, climbing the stairs to the second-floor bedroom she'd been assigned, tossed it onto one of the bunk beds. Yvonne Hamilton was about to get her first real dose of drug treatment.

MOST AMERICANS regard drug treatment as physicists do cold fusion—a wonderful idea, if only it worked. Even many liberals, while supporting more money for treatment, have serious doubts about its effectiveness. Their skepticism is understandable, given how frequently relapse occurs. Relapse is so common that experts have incorporated it into the very definition of drug addiction. A "chronic relapsing disorder," they call it. Even so, the research data on treatment's effectiveness are striking.

The most comprehensive assessment of drug treatment ever conducted in the United States is the Treatment Outcome Prospective Study (TOPS), a long-term study underwritten by the U.S. National Institute on Drug Abuse. A team of investigators from the Research Triangle Institute in North Carolina interviewed more than 11,000 drug users entering forty-one programs between 1979 and 1981. The programs included residential facilities, methadone centers, and drug-free outpatient clinics. The clients were interviewed upon entering the programs, then at varying intervals for up to five years.

The final report, published in 1989, noted that few of the clients remained completely drug-free for the full five years; outright "cures," it stated, "were extremely difficult to achieve." Overall consumption rates, however, declined sharply. Of clients in methadone programs, for instance, 63.5 percent said they were heavy heroin users in the year prior to treatment; three to five years later, only 17.5 percent were. In residential programs, the number of heavy users dropped from 30.9 percent prior to treatment to 11.8 percent three to five years later. The reductions in criminal activity were equally dramatic, with clients committing crimes at one-third to one-half the pretreatment rate in each of the three types of programs.

There was an important qualification to these findings: For programs to have any lasting impact, clients had to remain in them for some time. For those dropping out after a few weeks, the posttreatment rates of drug use and crime showed little improvement. After three months, however, outcomes improved with the amount of time in treatment. "Our most dramatic finding," TOPS reported, "is that drug abuse treatment has been notably effective in reducing drug abuse up to five years after a single treatment episode."

TOPS was conducted prior to the explosion in cocaine and crack use. Given the special problems involved in treating these drugs (for instance, the ineffectiveness of methadone), the TOPS findings cannot be automatically applied to them. An effort to fill this gap was undertaken by the RAND Corporation. In 1992, researchers C. Peter Rydell and Susan S. Everingham, in a study funded in part by the U.S. Army, set out to compare the effectiveness of treatment with that of three other types of programs: source-country efforts (attacking drug production abroad), interdiction (seizing drugs on their way to the United States), and domestic law enforcement (arresting and incarcerating sellers and buyers). How much additional money, they asked, would the government have to spend on each approach to reduce national cocaine consumption by 1 percent? Applying the same systems-based approach RAND used during the Vietnam War, Rydell and Everingham devised a model of national cocaine consumption and fed into it more than 150 variables, ranging from seizure data and price trends to household-survey results and budget figures. For each of the four approaches, Rydell and Everingham punched in different resource allocations, then projected national consumption rates over a fifteen-year period.

They were amazed at the results. Relying solely on source-country programs, the government would have to spend an additional $783 million to reduce U.S. cocaine consumption by 1 percent. Relying on interdiction, it would have to spend $366 million more, and on domestic law enforcement, $246 million. If it relied solely on treatment, however, the government would have to spend just $34 million more. In other words, treatment was seven times more cost-effective than domestic law enforcement, ten times more effective than interdiction, and twenty-three times more effective than attacking drugs at their source.

"One might wonder how this squares with the (dubious) conventional wisdom that, with treatment, 'nothing works,' " Rydell and Everingham wrote in their final report, published in 1994. They offered two explanations:

First, evaluations of treatment typically measure the proportion of people who no longer use drugs at some point after completing treatment; they tend to underappreciate the benefits of keeping people off drugs while they are in treatment—roughly one-fifth of the consumption reduction generated by treatment accrues during treatment. Second, about three-fifths of the users who start treatment stay in their program less than three months. Because such incomplete treatments do not substantially reduce consumption, they make treatment look weak by traditional criteria. However, they do not cost much, so they do not dilute the cost-effectiveness of completed treatments.

Treatment is so effective, Rydell and Everingham found, that even if one discounts all posttreatment effects and takes into account only those effects registered while addicts are actually in programs, treatment still outperformed the three other approaches.

Rydell and Everingham's findings on treatment are all the more striking in that they deliberately used a very low figure (13 percent) for the proportion of heavy users who do not return to heavy use after treatment. A more recent study by the U.S. Substance Abuse and Mental Health Services Administration indicates that the figure may be much higher. More than 4,400 clients entering treatment between July 1993 and October 1995 were interviewed at the time they entered treatment, at the time they left, and a year later; the accuracy of their responses was checked by random drug tests. Seeking to study the most hard-core cases, the researchers concentrated on programs serving people in public housing, on welfare, and in the criminal justice system. The results, released in September 1996, showed sharp declines in use for every drug studied. The number of clients saying they used crack, for instance, dropped from 39.5 percent prior to treatment to 17.8 percent a year later; for heroin, the number went from 23.6 percent to 12.6 percent. Overall, drug consumption decreased by roughly 50 percent.

EVERY STUDY of drug treatment has arrived at the same conclusion: whatever the type of program or the drug involved, treatment produces impressive reductions in both drug consumption and criminal activity, at a relatively low cost. Unfortunately, the lack of programs, and the barriers to entering them, means that only a fraction of those who might benefit actually do.

No one knows exactly how much unmet demand there is for drug treatment in the New York area, but a bit of arithmetic shows that it is enormous. According to the New York State Office of Alcoholism and Substance Abuse Services, an estimated 1.6 million of the state's 14.1 million residents have alcohol and/or drug problems serious enough to need treatment. Applying a common rule of thumb, treatment providers estimate that 25 percent of that number, or 400,000, will seek treatment in a given year. To serve them, the state has approximately 121,000 slots. With those slots turning over an average of once every six months, the system registers nearly 300,000 admissions a year. That leaves more than 100,000 unable to get help.

That number no doubt understates the gap, since many people, aware of the lack of slots, don't even bother to apply. The system is so overburdened that few publicly funded programs engage in advertising. If they did post phone numbers and encourage people to call, one can only guess at the response.

The number seeking help could be boosted further if providers, becoming more active still, went out on the street and sought people in need. "Outreach," this practice is called. Unfortunately, few people in New York City engaged in it. Raphael Flores, however, was an exception. Rather than simply sit back and wait for clients to appear at Hot Line, he liked to go out and corral them. His walks around the neighborhood provided daily demonstrations of outreach's ability to recruit people into treatment.

One day, for instance, while walking along Lexington Avenue near 110th Street, Raphael ran into a short, dumpy woman he'd counseled several years earlier. "When you coming in, girl?" he said, giving her a bear hug. "You still there?" she asked, embarrassed at her slovenly appearance. "Yeah, we're still there," Raphael warmly replied. "Come by Friday. I could get you into a three-month program." The woman said she'd think about it, then moved off.

"Hot Line needs to be open twenty-four hours," Raphael said after she'd gone. "We'd probably see a lot of people like her if we did outreach at night. You get a different, tougher population then. And they'd respond. A lot are craving when the sun comes up. At four or five in the morning, when they're coming down—that's the time to get them." Raphael wished he had a detox van that he could send into copping zones to sign up addicts on the spot. "I'd put it right there on 110th Street," he said. "And not one of the addicts there would mess with us."

A detox van was only one of several ideas Raphael had to improve his operation. Another was hiring someone to handle clients' paperwork. He also wanted to take on a legal counselor to help clients caught up in the criminal justice system. More ambitiously, Raphael wanted to take over the empty floor above Hot Line's office and convert it into a sort of halfway house for addicts waiting to enter treatment. Such a facility would enable Hot Line not only to keep watch over clients but also to prepare them psychologically for the world they were about to enter. Raphael already had a name for it—Hot Line House —and Marvin, who had had such success housing Yvonne, had adopted the idea as his own personal project.

Given Hot Line's financial problems, however, none of this was imminent. Every day, Raphael had to take time out from his work to call potential funders. He did not have much to show for it. As with many grassroots workers, his talent for working with people was matched by his ineptitude in running an office. He was so bad with money that, the one time he tried to keep a checking account, he gave up in frustration after three months. He found grant applications even more perplexing, approaching them as if they were bar exams.

In the summer of 1992, for instance, Raphael was struggling to renew a $25,000 grant he had received the previous year from the New York State AIDS Institute. To evaluate Hot Line's work, the institute sent an auditor down from Albany. Charles Silberman spent a full day with Raphael, and he came away amazed. "He went right up to people on the street," he recalled. "He approached one woman who was bathing in a hydrant and urged her to come with him. He was putting his life on the line, talking with a whole lot of folk who weren't all there. It was like seeing Mother Teresa in action." And Marvin, he said, was like an "angel of mercy—sleeping there in the office, working with very little money." Silberman was further struck by Hot Line's ability to track people through the system. "I'd never seen anyone else who made such an effort to do that," he said.

Back in Albany, Silberman spent hours on the phone with Raphael, coaching him on the grant renewal. Eventually, Raphael managed to complete it. To be approved, though, the application needed the blessing of Angelo Del Toro, East Harlem's representative in the New York State Assembly. Together with his brother William, Del Toro ran a political machine in East Harlem that controlled most of the state funds entering the district. Raphael regarded the brothers as little more than poverty pimps, but, swallowing his reservations, he went by Del Toro's office to plead his case. The assemblyman remained noncommittal, however. Drug addicts did not vote, and so Hot Line's work was not high on his list of priorities.

And so it went generally. Whatever Raphael's personal limitations as a fundraiser, he operated in a political climate that was inhospitable to the type of street work he was doing. Despite having the nation's worst drug problem, New York City invested few funds in drug treatment, leaving the responsibility for this to the state. The great bulk of its antidrug resources went into law enforcement. When crack hit the city in the mid-1980s, for instance, the Koch administration created few new treatment slots, despite the soaring demand for help. Instead, it formed tactical narcotics teams (TNTs), large squads of undercover cops whose mission it was to occupy drug-infested neighborhoods for two or three months at a time, scooping up every dealer in sight, then move on to the next neighborhood in need. In 1989, the number of drug arrests in the city would hit a record 94,887; nonetheless, the demand for drugs would not diminish.

When David Dinkins became mayor, in 1990, he decided it was time for a new approach. To develop it, he appointed a thirteen-person panel under the direction of former U.S. Attorney General Nicholas Katzenbach. The group's report, submitted in May 1990, decried the shortage of drug treatment in the city. Overall, it noted, residential treatment was available for only 2 percent of the city's cocaine and heroin addicts. For the city's 125,000 teenage addicts, only 2,100 slots were available. As for pregnant women addicted to cocaine, 87 percent of the city's treatment programs would not accept them, even when they had Medicaid.

To rectify this, the Katzenbach Report urged immediate action. To help drug-using pregnant women, it recommended creating several thousand new slots reserved exclusively for them. To help at-risk teens, it recommended transforming schools into community centers that would remain open sixteen hours a day, offering recreational programs, education courses, and social services. And, to make treatment more accessible, the study group called on the city to develop a network of "intake, assessment and referral centers." Since resources were limited, the report suggested starting with a single pilot center. Addicts appearing at it "could get immediate attention," the report stated. "The environment would be comfortable and welcoming; light snacks would be provided. Services would include crisis intervention (using acupuncture, among other methods), assessment, counseling, 12-step programs, medical care, daycare, and referral for treatment." If an addict wanted treatment, the counselor would help locate a vacancy and assist him in collecting documents and setting up appointments. A recovering addict, the report stated, would accompany the client "to be sure that he or she reaches the treatment site and was accepted into the program."

In short, the Katzenbach Report proposed setting up a center very much like Hot Line Cares. Certainly, the projected cost—$1 million—was paltry. Yet no such center would get created. For, soon after the report was issued, New York was convulsed by a vicious crime wave, punctuated by a rash of high-profile killings. DAVE, DO SOMETHING, the *New York Post* implored, capturing the city's mood. Forced to respond, Dinkins introduced a $1.8 billion, four-year program called "Safe Streets, Safe City." While some of that money would go for social services, most would be earmarked for a massive expansion of the city's police department. For all intents and purposes, the Katzenbach Report was dead, and along with it any chance of improving services for addicts. Instead, the city was going to throw even more troops at its drug problem. And Spanish Harlem was going to be a major battleground.

4

The Police

FOR THE RESIDENTS of Spanish Harlem, the drug trade on 110th Street was a source of unending grievance. Well-dressed men and women on their way to work in the morning would have to weave their way past a gauntlet of importunate dealers. Young mothers out to buy milk would have to steer their strollers around drunks passed out on the sidewalk, and senior citizens visiting the post office would have to squeeze past dealers just to get inside the door.

No one was more exercised about this than Miriam Lopez-Falcon. A forty-two-year-old woman with a round face, dark, flashing eyes, and a plow-ahead style, Lopez worked for Congressman Charles Rangel. Rangel's main district office was on 125th Street, but to serve Spanish Harlem he maintained a satellite office at 108th and First, and for the last several years Lopez had run it. And, during that time, she had heard more complaints about 110th Street than about anywhere else.

The last straw came on April 22, 1992, when the CBS News show *48 Hours* aired a program on the sudden resurgence of heroin in the United States. The show traced the flow of the narcotic from the lush highlands of Southeast Asia, where it originated in the form of bright red opium poppies, to the gritty cores of urban America, where it was hawked in open-air markets. Of all the markets in the country, CBS chose to focus on 110th Street. Tracked by a hidden camera, correspondent Erin Moriarty mixed with grubby-looking dealers who shouted out brand names in what she called a "virtual outdoor shopping mall of heroin."

"I can't tell you how many people came up to me and said, 'Did you see that about 110th Street?' " recalled Lopez, who had actually been born on the street. "I was embarrassed. This is my neighborhood, and here it had received national exposure for having one of the worst blocks in the country. It reflected badly on the community, especially the Latinos living here. It had a tremendous impact on our pride as a people." It was time to act, Lopez decided.

Among those she approached was Christiana Pinto, the head of the Aguilar Library. A stately turn-of-the-century building with a cast-iron facade framed by monumental classical columns, the library sat in the thick of the dealing on 110th Street, and Pinto, a stout native of Argentina, had waged a long and determined battle against it. Seeing the dealers mill about out front as young schoolchildren sought to enter, she would intrepidly rush outside to shoo them. Always, though, they would return, and the street's reputation was getting so bad that Pinto was having trouble recruiting staff.

Sylvia Velazquez, the president of the Clinton Houses tenants association, was similarly vexed. Junkies had turned the project's stairwells into shooting galleries and its courtyard into a commodity exchange, and Velazquez, a soft-spoken but determined woman with a hard mouth and hooded eyes, had worked tirelessly to mobilize her fellow tenants. Whether out of fear or apathy, however, they refused to get involved. Now, with Miriam Lopez proposing a community-wide effort, both she and Pinto expressed their readiness to help.

In the end, though, Lopez's main ally would be her boss. Since arriving in Congress in 1970, Charles Rangel had been a relentless crusader against drugs. As chairman of the House Select Committee on Narcotics Abuse and Control, he was forever decrying the toll drugs were taking on the nation and the government's failure to do anything about it. His message was unvarying: the country was relying too heavily on law enforcement in its battle against drugs. "We can build all the jails and prisons we want," he had declared at a 1991 hearing.

> We can hire all the police we want. We can double and triple the checkpoints along the U.S.-Mexico and the U.S.-Canadian border. We can seize more drugs from boats, cars, and airplanes. We can give people stiffer sentences and we can do more undercover operations and street sweeps. But the fact of the matter is that none of this is going to make a whole lot of difference in the overall scheme of things unless we address the environmental factors that lead some people to drug abuse.

At every opportunity, Rangel would hammer away at the need to combat the "root causes" of drug abuse, such as unemployment, homelessness, and illiteracy. He was particularly insistent on the need for more treatment. During the Reagan-Bush years, Rangel would repeatedly haul administration officials before his committee to lambaste them for putting too much money into prisons and not enough into programs.

Yet, when it came to practical efforts to help addicts, Rangel always seemed to be AWOL. Methadone was a good example. The number of methadone slots in New York fell far short of the demand, and for years providers had been crying for relief. With his repeated calls for more treatment, Rangel would have seemed a natural supporter. But many of his constituents disliked methadone, feeling it substituted one addiction for another, and Rangel faithfully went along. From his earliest days in Congress, he had harassed methadone providers, going so far in the late 1980s as to order the General Accounting Office to investigate them. Partly as a result, the availability of methadone in New York had remained frozen. More generally, Rangel's district —one of the most drug-ridden in the country—was among the most underserved by treatment, and as a result he was widely scorned by local providers (Raphael Flores among them).

On the subject of street-level drug dealing, Rangel was outspoken on the futility of police action. "I'm the best mover of drug pushers in the whole country," he observed sardonically in his seventh-floor office on 125th Street. "I can go to any town hall meeting—they tell me where the drugs are, and I can promise they won't be doing drugs there. Because I get that response from the police. They work on the case, and—Boom! But I can't say I'm eliminating the drug problem—I'm pushing it around. The drug dealers don't go away— they go to another place."

When it came to 110th Street, however, politics again intervened. While his seat was one of the safest in Congress, Spanish Harlem had long been its soft underbelly, for its residents always suspected that Rangel neglected their interests in favor of his black constituents. And, for the first time, those residents had a powerful advocate, in the person of their city councilman, Adam Clayton Powell IV. Powell's father, the legendary Adam Clayton Powell, Jr., had represented Harlem in Congress until 1970, when Charles Rangel, then an insurgent young lawyer, narrowly beat him. Young Adam was now eager to avenge his father's defeat, and, with a Puerto Rican mother and fluency in Spanish, he was a rising star in Spanish Harlem. And Rangel was eager to head him off.

And so, when Miriam Lopez approached him about the drug dealing on 110th Street, Rangel did not talk about the inadequacy of law enforcement, or the tragedy of sending young black men to prison, or the need for more drug treatment. Instead, he decided to call in the cops. In June 1992, letters under his name went out to One Police Plaza, the headquarters of the police department; the 23rd Precinct, which covered 110th Street; the Housing Police and Transit Police; and the Drug Enforcement Administration, asking them "to plan a strategy that would rid 110th Street of drugs and crime once and for all." A meeting was called for July 27, 1992, at Rangel's Spanish Harlem office, and showing up for it were about two dozen police chiefs, inspectors, captains, sergeants, and DEA agents, plus representatives from the Manhattan D.A.'s office, inspectors from the U.S. Postal Service, and several community leaders. "I never saw so much brass in my entire life," Miriam Lopez exulted.

Rangel's most famous attribute was his voice—a nasal, gravel-filled bull-horn—and at the meeting he used it to inveigh against the dealers on 110th Street. The hardworking citizens of Spanish Harlem deserved better, he said, and he was determined to provide it. First, though, he would need the cooperation of the police officials in the room. Rangel asked for assurances that they would put aside the bureaucratic rivalries and jurisdictional disputes for which New York law enforcement was famous. One by one, the officials in the room stood up and pledged their support.

To succeed, Rangel went on, the campaign would have to address quality-of-life concerns in the area. One Hundred Tenth Street needed new street-lights. Service at the post office had to be improved. The vacant lot next to the post office had to be put to productive use. Still, it was agreed, the police would take the lead. Captain John Stoker, the commanding officer of the 23rd Precinct, promised to use all the resources at his disposal to force the dealers off the street. As his day-to-day liaison, Stoker said, he was naming one of his sergeants, Steven Ringe. In closing, the participants agreed to meet on a monthly basis to assess the campaign's progress. The Sunshine Project, as it was named, would test the ability of the nation's largest police force, backed by Congress's foremost antidrug activist, to suppress the drug trade on a single city block.

OUTWARDLY, Steve Ringe seemed a fairly typical cop. A large man with a soft, pale face set off by a shock of spiky black hair, he was white (like three-quarters of the force), had no more than a high school education, and suffered from that common cop affliction, an expanding waistline. In some key respects, though, the thirty-three-year-old sergeant stood out. On a force known for its swagger, he was polite and easygoing. And, whereas many cops in poor neighborhoods saw local residents as potential "perps," Ringe saw people not unlike himself. Raised in working-class Brooklyn, he had dropped out of school in the ninth grade and for a time run with a Spanish gang. Eventually, he learned to do electrical work and earned a G.E.D. Joining the NYPD in 1983, he was assigned first to Bedford-Stuyvesant and then to downtown Brooklyn. Though it was not common at the time, Ringe would frequently park his squad car and walk the streets in an effort to get to know local residents.

Arriving in East Harlem in 1991, he found drugs preoccupying him like nothing else. In his office at the station house—a cubist cement fortress located on 102nd Street—Ringe kept a map on which he plotted the shifting fortunes of the local drug trade. Each sales spot was marked by a dot, color-coordinated by drug: red for heroin, light blue for crack, yellow for angel dust, and so on. Every time a spot closed down, Ringe took down a dot; every time a new spot opened, he put one up. The pattern was always changing, but the overall number of dots—about one hundred—never seemed to go down. And, always, 110th Street had the largest cluster.

Now Ringe was going to get the resources he needed to attack the problem there. As part of Mayor Dinkins's Safe Streets, Safe City program, the Two-Three was in the process of getting nearly seventy new cops. Most were to be assigned to foot patrol—part of the department's more general shift toward community policing. In contrast to traditional policing, in which cops rode around in squad cars, responding to 911 calls, community policing encouraged them to get out into the street and mix with local residents. Becoming acquainted with neighborhood problems, officers were to work with those residents to address them.

Community policing seemed especially well suited to the drug trade. Under the old system, TNT units would move into a designated neighborhood and remain until it was clear of dealers. Once the teams moved on, however, the dealers would quickly reappear. Under community policing, the precinct would work with local residents to address the conditions that allowed the drug trade to flourish. If heroin addicts were shooting up in an abandoned building, for instance, the police could have it sealed. If dealers were operating in a housing project, the tenants could help identify them.

A fervent supporter of community policing, David Dinkins named one of its top practitioners to be his police commissioner. Lee Brown had just completed eight years as the police chief in Houston. Taking over a force notorious for brutality and racism, Brown had aggressively recruited minorities, assigned cops to foot patrol, and opened police substations in high-crime districts. By the end of his term, the police department had become one of the city's most respected institutions, and Brown one of the nation's most celebrated cops. In New York, he hoped to carry out a similar transformation.

It would not be easy. Community policing was disdained by many New York cops, who saw it as little more than social work. Steve Ringe was not among them. Ever since his days in Brooklyn, he had believed in the power of community outreach —especially where drugs were concerned. "Drugs are a community problem," Ringe noted, "so the only way to deal with them is through community policing." The Sunshine Project would provide an excellent laboratory for the new approach.

THE PROJECT officially got under way on September 11, 1992, with a noontime meeting at the Aguilar Library. Several rows of folding chairs had been set up inside the library, a cavernous place with square pillars topped by sculpted flowers. The participants—largely the same as had met at Rangel's office in July—agreed that Sunshine would have two phases. In the first, the police would hit 110th Street with everything they had, weeding out dealers in order to restore a semblance of order to the block. In phase two, the community would be mobilized to make sure the dealers stayed away.

Steve Ringe was responsible for phase one. Together with his counterparts at Housing, Transit, and Manhattan North Narcotics (a unit of the Narcotics

Division), he devised a battle plan for a six-block target area around 110th and Lexington. Normally, two beat cops patrolled the intersection; now four would. At the Clinton Houses, the Housing Police would increase the frequency of their vertical (roof-to-lobby) patrols, while the Transit Police would monitor the 110th Street subway station. At all hours, squad cars would cruise the intersection.

Most important, the police would mount regular buy-and-bust operations —the bread-and-butter of street-level drug enforcement. A trial run was organized for mid-September. At Manhattan North's command post on 143d Street, undercover cops photocopied stacks of $5 and $10 bills to be used as "buy" money. Around noon, the agents piled into unmarked cars and headed south toward 110th Street, parking out of the sight of the dealers. Working in two-man teams, the agents filtered onto the street and mingled with the crowd there. While one cop looked on to make sure nothing went awry, the other approached a dealer and made a buy. The agents then left the area and radioed a description of the seller to a team of cops waiting around the corner. Speeding to 110th Street, the officers jumped out and nabbed their quarry. In all, four sellers were picked up that day—not a bad haul for one block on a single afternoon.

Soon the raids were taking place twice a week. Overall, in September, 116 narcotics arrests would be made in the target area. To make sure they did not get lost in the system, two assistant D.A.'s were assigned to track them.

It was not just street-level sellers who were being hit. To make a real dent on 110th Street, the police knew, they would also have to dismantle the drug organizations that operated there. The main focus was Hot City heroin, the most popular brand on the street. For intelligence, the police relied heavily on confidential informants—mostly small-time dealers agreeing to cooperate in return for leniency or money. In a matter of weeks, they were able to trace the source of Hot City to an apartment building in the South Bronx. Staking it out, they waited for the right moment to strike, and in late October they arrested a young Hispanic man believed to control the brand. Almost overnight, Hot City disappeared from the street.

By early November, the constant raids, arrests, and patrols were clearly having an effect. The crowds hovering by the uptown subway entrance were thinning out, and for the first time in years people could walk from Lexington to Third without being accosted by a dealer. Senior citizens were able to visit the post office without being harassed, and children could enter the library without having brand names shouted in their face.

The change was apparent to everyone arriving for the November 5, 1992, meeting of the Sunshine Project. The area in front of the library, which in September had been so clogged with dealers, was now free of them, and even the used-clothes vendors normally stationed by the entrance were gone. Inside, bulky cops wearing navy windbreakers mixed with city housing officials and community board members. Shortly after noon, the doors of the library opened and in strode Charles Rangel. Two days earlier, Rangel had been easily re-elected to a twelfth term in Congress (and Bill Clinton had defeated George Bush). Wearing a sharply tailored brown suit, Rangel vigorously pumped hands and slapped backs as he made his way to a table in front, where he joined Captain Stoker, Miriam Lopez, and Chris Pinto.

"I want to thank all of you for this special effort," Rangel boomed. "We wanted to see whether you in law enforcement could test a system—whether, if the necessary services and resources were brought in in a very limited way, we might have a pilot project, the type of thing we could apply in other parts of the city." It was not going to be easy, he went on. "We've picked one of the roughest areas in the city. But if we can bring in some resources and get some money for scholarship programs or recreational facilities, or perhaps a playground—it can't just be law enforcement. If you have some ideas, let me know."

There was, however, little talk of scholarships or playgrounds during the meeting. Instead, the focus remained squarely on law enforcement. In October, it was announced, the police had made 130 drug arrests in the target area. Some 2,000 glassines of heroin had been seized in one operation and 300 vials of crack in another. It was the news about Hot City, though, that stirred the loudest response. "The guy who runs it, we found, lives in the Bronx and brings it into Manhattan," said Sergeant Ronald Mejia of Manhattan North Narcotics. "We got him. He's about to be indicted. Last week, there was little Hot City being sold on the block." The applause was vigorous.

After a representative from the D.A.'s office described the priority being given 110th Street, Rangel, growing restless, again took the floor. Noting that "people in the community might not know what's going on," he said he'd be happy to talk with local groups to spread the word. Unfortunately, he added, his presence was required elsewhere. "Let me thank all of you for the spirit that exists here," he said. "As a little lady told me yesterday, 'I voted for you and Clinton, so there are no excuses now.' " Rangel acknowledged the applause as he left the meeting. He went no farther than the other side of the library, however, where a reporter for New York 1, a local news station, was waiting to interview him.

The Sunshine discussion lasted another hour. The local community board, it was noted, had asked the city to install new lights on 110th Street, but the order would take more than a year to fill. The vacant lots across the street, it was found, had private owners and would have to be investigated further. Overall, though, the tone was upbeat. "The feedback of the last two weeks has been tremendous," said Chris Pinto, her normally stern face aglow. "Not only people who come into the library, but merchants and people who use the street can see the impact. I've been here about nine years, and this is the first time I've said anything positive about 110th Street. Thank you from the bottom of my heart."

It was left to Sergeant Ringe to offer a warning. The narcotics arrests

made on 110th Street in October had accounted for 25 percent of all such
arrests in the precinct, he said, down from 32 percent in September. "That's a
good sign," he noted in his usual level tone. "It means the dealers are moving
to other places. Now it's time for the next phase—getting the community
involved. We talked about getting merchants involved, about getting people to
write letters to the D.A.'s office, about signing up people from the Clinton
Houses." Ringe expressed disappointment at the low turnout by local residents;
only a half-dozen had bothered to attend.

In an effort to change that, Chris Pinto approached several of the merchants in the area about getting involved. None wanted to. Some, like the
owners of the three convenience stores at 110th and Lex, derived so much of
their revenue from the area's junkies that they had little interest in banishing
them. Sylvia Velazquez was faring no better at the Clinton Houses. As everyone
there knew, the dealers had a network of informants inside the project, and
cooperating with the police could bring immediate reprisal. Consequently, only
one of Clinton's four buildings had mustered a patrol, and even it was too
feeble to have much effect.

And Steve Ringe's worst fears were beginning to materialize. At the precinct house, he was getting reports of new dealer sightings—on 109th Street,
one block to the south of 110th; on Madison Avenue, two blocks to the west,
and on Third Avenue, a commercial strip where drug activity was previously
unknown. The principal of P.S. 108, an elementary school at 109th and Madison, called to say that she had noticed a sharp increase in the dealing around
the school since the start of Sunshine. If the police didn't act, she said, somebody was going to get hurt.

Sensing an opportunity, Ringe arranged to come speak. About thirty-five
parents showed up for the meeting, held in the school's auditorium. After
some welcoming remarks by the principal, Ringe stood up in the well of the
auditorium and launched into a discussion of his favorite topic. "All the resources we have can't help if the community is not involved," he said. "The
fact that you came to this meeting shows you care about your community. You
have so much ability to help us. You become our eyes and ears." Ringe urged
people to join the NYPD's Drugbusters program, which took anonymous tips
over a twenty-four-hour hot line. Because the dealers undoubtedly had their
own eyes and ears present, he hastened to add, volunteers should wait until
the end of the meeting to sign up.

In the end, just one person did. "People in this neighborhood are not
even willing to drop a dime," Ringe wearily observed in his office a few days
later. "It's very hard to light a spark here. We'll continue to do our share, but
the community phase does not seem to be working."

The dealers themselves seemed to sense this. Week by week, more and
more of them were filtering back into the intersection. Rather than take up
their old posts on 110th Street, they were setting up shop around the corner,

on Lexington between 109th and 110th. This block had no library or post office, only a liquor store, a pawn shop, two convenience stores, and the Segunda Reyna bakery. With so many junkies passing in and out of the bakery, the dealers blended in nicely in front. Whenever police cars approached, lookouts would yell *"Bajando"* (they're coming), and the dealers would quickly scatter; after the cars passed, they would quickly return. As it became clear that they had the police outnumbered, the dealers grew more and more brazen, so that even when a cop stood at 110th and Lexington, they would continue selling on Lex, a hundred feet away. If the cops walked toward them, the dealers would simply move farther down the street, keeping a hundred-foot gap at all times in a comic but chilling game of cat and mouse.

THE JANUARY 1993 meeting of the Sunshine Project took place on a raw winter day, with wet snow changing to rain and back again. The mood inside the library was similarly glum. The number of community participants was down to three; just about everyone else was a cop. In 1992, it was announced, the police had made a stunning 2,700 narcotics arrests in the precinct—more than 1,000 of them in the six-block target zone. Yet, as everyone agreed, conditions were as bad as ever. Captain James Tuller of the Housing Police said that, as a result of the crackdown on 110th Street, he was receiving more complaints from the Johnson Houses, two blocks to the north, and so was planning to reassign some of the officers currently at Clinton.

That brought a sharp protest from Sylvia Velazquez. "Johnson doesn't have the concentrations of dealers we have on Lexington Avenue," she complained. "Our front doors get broken, and they're not fixed for three, four, or five days—sometimes even two weeks. People come in, they do drugs, leave needles all around, urinate, and defecate. We need three or four officers to constantly walk the project."

"A uniformed presence is not the answer," Sergeant Ringe put in. "If I stand in the lobby, nobody would do anything while I'm around, but they'll go around the corner and do it. We need to train tenants so that if they see somebody loitering or urinating, they call us. If people call, you'll get the attention you need."

"Sylvia's problem is aggravated by the enormous numbers of people we're seeing on the corner," said Chris Pinto, her face grim once again. "Maybe two hundred people have been arrested in the last month, but another three hundred totally new ones have taken their place. Two days ago, they were out here like barflies. At night, it's almost impassable. You have to use your elbows to get the pack out of your way." Expressing gratitude to the police for all their work, Pinto said, "Now it's a question of convincing people to participate. Sylvia, where are the rest of the tenants? They've put the whole responsibility on you."

"A lot of people who live in the projects are afraid," Velazquez replied. "If you talk to an officer, they think you're snitching. And then you're gone. They'll put a dead rat in front of your door."

The discussion continued in the same dark vein for another half-hour. Adding to the gloom was the knowledge that the library—one of the street's few remaining anchors—was about to close for repairs. As the meeting was ending, an officer rushed in to tell Sergeant Ringe that a young man had just been shot in front of the junior high school at 108th and Third. Ringe hurried out of the library and climbed into a police van, which sped off toward the hospital where the wounded man had been taken.

Captain Tuller, meanwhile, was summoned to 109th and Lexington, where a SWAT team conducting a drug raid in the Clinton Houses had discovered a hand grenade. A bomb squad had been called out, and emergency police vans clogged the street in front of the building. Standing on the sidewalk in the rain, Tuller conferred with several of his men, then headed in to investigate.

Across the street, meanwhile, on Lexington between 109th and 110th, the drug trade was booming. Despite the rain and flurries, the bomb squad and police cars, a hundred or so people were surging up and down the street, looking to cop. At one point, a crowd of junkies rushed up to a tall, haggard man wearing a navy woolen cap and a beige parka. At first, it looked as if a fight was breaking out, but in fact the man had a fresh supply of Tombstone dope—the most sought-after brand now that Hot City was gone. Frantically waving their arms, the customers tried to outshout one another as they placed their orders. Within minutes, the stock was gone.

Amid the chaos, an ambulance pulled up in front of one of the convenience stores at 110th and Lex. A crowd was gathered around a middle-aged black man sprawled on the pavement—the apparent victim of a drug overdose. Two paramedics jumped out and checked his vital signs, then placed him on a stretcher and slid it into the van. They quickly got in and took off for nearby Metropolitan Hospital.

Back in his office a few days later, Steve Ringe could not hide his disappointment. "We're losing the block," he said with a sigh. "We're just pushing the dealers around." He pointed to the map on the wall. There, the red dots that had once lined 110th Street were now clustered along Lexington. After making a thousand arrests in a single year, the police had succeeded mainly in pushing the dealers off one block and onto another.

5

Buyers and Sellers

THAT THE POLICE were having such trouble cleaning up 110th Street was no accident. However chaotic the dealing there might have seemed to outsiders, it was in fact highly organized, with a half-dozen or so groups controlling the area. Like most drug organizations in New York, they were not large, having a few dozen members at most, but they were tightly structured. Usually, a single family was in charge, with employees drawn from the same ethnic group. And they were rigidly hierarchical, with four or five layers separating the general at the top from the sellers at the bottom. The higher-ranking the individual, the less contact he had with the merchandise and the more insulation he had from the police.

Charlie, a lieutenant in one 110th Street organization, was a good example. A black man in his late thirties, Charlie had spent twenty years in the drug underworld, most of them with his current employer. Based in the South Bronx, the group employed about fifty people and ran a half-dozen spots. Meticulously groomed, with short curly hair and a neatly trimmed goatee, Charlie stood five-eight but seemed taller because of his muscular build. His specialty was transportation. Once a day, he drove to a "mill house" in the South Bronx, an apartment where the day's supplies of heroin and cocaine were readied for distribution. The drugs had been procured by the organization's general, a middle-aged Puerto Rican whose street name was Macho. If the heroin was of high purity—80 or 90 percent—it could be cut fifteen or twenty times with additives like lactose (milk sugar) or mannite (a baby laxative); low-grade heroin could be stepped on only five or six times. Once it was cut, the heroin was sifted through a fine mesh screen, then tapped out into small glassine envelopes that were stamped with the brand's logo. The envelopes were then taped and counted out into piles of ten (called bundles), which in turn were gathered into bunches of several hundred and placed into brown paper bags for delivery to the street.

East Harlem was Charlie's domain. The distance from the mill house to 110th Street was not great, but police surveillance was always a threat, and so Charlie frequently varied his route, gliding through the back streets of the Bronx, then alternating among the various bridges that spanned the Harlem River. In Manhattan, he would head for 110th Street but stop several blocks short, parking near the apartment building that was serving as the organization's "stash house." Inside was a sergeant, or manager, with whom Charlie left the goods.

As a new selling day began, the sergeant would take over. It was his job to move supplies from the stash house to the street sellers, or pitchers. The organization had a half-dozen pitchers on 110th Street, all assigned to a specific area. Assisting the pitchers were steerers, who recruited customers, and look-outs, who watched for the police. Around eight o'clock, the sergeant would collect the day's earnings and put them in a bag, which Charlie would then pick up for delivery back to the South Bronx. Normally, the organization took in between $35,000 and $50,000 a week from heroin sales on 110th Street and another $60,000 to $70,000 from nearby crack spots.

The Sunshine Project was putting a dent in those sums. "There's been a lot of heat from the police," Charlie said one morning while chain-smoking Kools in a coffee shop near Columbia University. Overall, he noted, earnings were down about 20 percent. He was not too concerned, though, for the organization was still taking in about $100,000 a week. As for arrests, the damage had thus far been limited to pitchers and steerers. "No higher-ups have been taken," Charlie said matter-of-factly. "Not even any sergeants."

Savvy and cautious, the ranking officers of the organization worked hard to minimize their visibility. "I'm rarely seen," Charlie noted. He worked only at night, a time when police manpower was at its thinnest. And, whenever possible, he traveled in the company of a well-dressed woman, meeting her in a restaurant before making the trip to the mill house. It was she who actually carried the drugs; if the police stopped them, she was far less likely to be searched. Aware that flashy cars could attract attention, Charlie always drove beat-up ones. "You can't be flamboyant," he observed. A sharp but understated dresser, he favored conservative pin-striped pants and nicely tailored sports shirts, and his jewelry—a gold bracelet and a gold ring inlaid with small diamonds—seemed more stylish than flashy.

Not that Charlie was a puritan. Each week he earned between $500 and $1,500, and he spent it squiring an ever-changing roster of young women to discos and after-hours spots. It was a world of abundant booze, easy sex, and reflexive cruelty. Once, Charlie recalled, he was relaxing at a night spot in the Bronx when a crackhead he knew sought him out, begging for a hit. The woman, a one-time beauty, had turned scuzzy and scrawny, and Charlie, eager to be rid of her, agreed to supply her, on the condition that she first perform oral sex on his pet pit bull. Desperate, the woman agreed, but, as she was performing the act, the dog became frenzied and, despite being muzzled, mauled her. "She hasn't been back," Charlie laconically observed.

Such was Charlie's private world. In public, however, he worked hard to appear an upstanding citizen. For five years, for instance, he worked for General Motors at its plant in Tarrytown, New York. He regularly attended a Baptist church and in the summer helped coach a Little League team—even as he was continuing his work in Spanish Harlem. As for his own drug use, Charlie limited himself to beer and pot. In the end, all of his precautions had paid off: it had been more than twelve years since his last arrest.

The pitchers were less fortunate. Working the streets for hours at a time, selling to scores of strangers, they were easy prey for the cops. When buy-and-busts occurred, it was mostly pitchers who got collared.

To the residents of Spanish Harlem, these pitchers embodied the drug trade at its most sinister; they were the dealers and pushers who were destroying their neighborhood. In the drug world itself, the pitchers were figures of contempt. Unlike sergeants and lieutenants, who were salaried, pitchers usually worked on commission, earning $10 to $30 per bundle. And they received none of the fringe benefits officers received. If Charlie was arrested, for example, the organization would hire him a lawyer; pitchers, by contrast, were on their own.

The most striking thing about street sellers was how easily they were replaced. On 110th Street, the process rarely took more than a day. This was not simply a matter of people passing through the revolving door of the criminal justice system. "Very few times do we lock up the same individual over and over," observed Sergeant Ronald Mejia of Manhattan North Narcotics. "The people wanting to sell," he said, shaking his head in wonder, "seem to come out of nowhere."

To UNDERSTAND where those sellers come from, it's necessary to understand where the buyers come from. The huge sums of money exchanged in inner-city drug markets like 110th Street have fed the perception that white middle-class users make up most of the customers. The news media have reinforced this. For instance, the *48 Hours* program on the resurgence of heroin cut immediately from the dealing on 110th Street to a roundtable discussion between Dan Rather and three heroin users—all young, white, and photogenic. Chris, an eighteen-year-old with stylishly tousled hair, was said to have "discovered heroin on the New York nightclub scene." Jason, a clean-cut twenty-two-year-old, predicted that more kids would try it. "It's the hot drug now?" Rather eagerly prompted him. "I don't know if it's hot yet," Jason replied, "but it's definitely on the rise."

Watching the show, one could only conclude that 110th Street was swarming with white well-to-do Americans. And, in fact, it was not hard to find such users there. On a bright autumn afternoon in the fall of 1992, the flow of whites into the area was typically brisk. A sharply dressed couple (he in designer sports shirt, she in tight jeans and black boots) strode down Lexington to 109th Street, where the man found the pitcher he was looking for and quickly made a buy; once it was completed, the woman hailed a livery cab, and the two hopped in and were off. A tall pale man with a flowing brown ponytail and checked flannel shirt lingered on the corner, chatting with steerers, while three motor-cycle toughs with puffed-up chests pushed their way through the crowd— eager, it seemed, to show off their manhood. Through it all, a tall, fleshy young man wearing baggy jeans, work boots, and a Notre Dame cap turned backward on his head leaned against a car, reading a book (Primo Levi's *Survival in Auschwitz*). Overall, in the course of an hour, perhaps fifteen or twenty whites passed through the area.

They were not in the majority, however. A quick glance around the area sufficed to show that the black and Hispanic customers were far more numer-ous. Most were in bad physical shape, with gaunt faces and withered frames. Some walked with canes or were confined to wheelchairs, a sign of circulatory problems brought on by repeated injections; others had grotesquely swollen hands, the result of constant mainlining there. Their clothes, which seemed patched together from thrift shops and trash cans, bore the telltale smudges and tears of life in the street.

Police officers and drug dealers offer strikingly similar estimates as to the breakdown of users on 110th Street. "Maybe a quarter of the customers come from outside Spanish Harlem," said Sergeant Mejia. "Three out of ten at most." Charlie, the drug lieutenant, said that "seventy percent of all our sales go to people who live in East Harlem." Addicts, he added, "don't like to travel much out of the area they live in."

Those who do come from outside the neighborhood generally do so be-cause drugs aren't available where they live, or they cost too much, or are of poor quality. And they resemble not Chris or Jason but Dave, an unemployed twenty-year-old from Paramus, New Jersey. Every morning, Dave would board a bus for the half-hour ride to the Port Authority in Manhattan. There, he would hop on a subway and head for 110th and Lex, where he would seek out a seller he'd done business with in the past and buy a few bags of dope. Merchandise in hand, he would walk toward Central Park, stopping to inject along the way or in the park itself. After that, it was back to the Port Authority and, from there, to Paramus, where he lived with his father (a mechanic) and his mother (a clerk).

Slender and dark-eyed, with abundant brown hair curling out from under a baseball cap and a small gold crucifix hanging from a chain around his neck, Dave had been heavily into drugs since his early teens. His five-bag-a-day habit so consumed him that he was unable to keep a job. Dave did not relish coming into Spanish Harlem; the trip took an hour and a half each way, and he worried constantly about being robbed. But his habit would not let him rest, and dope was all but unavailable in Paramus. "I've got to do this every day," he said one day after copping on 110th Street, his slurred words indicating he had gotten a good bag. "It sucks. It leaves me no money for food or anything else. I don't even have money for a pack of cigarettes."

Fitfully employed, with turbulent personal lives and long histories of drug use—this was the typical profile of the whites visiting 110th Street. In this regard, they did not much differ from the local users. Whether white or black, East Harlem resident or suburban interloper, the buyers on 110th Street all tended to have one thing in common: they were hard-core users, with a compulsive need for drugs.

For such users, the police represented just one more hurdle in the daily struggle to get high. Consider, for example, Luisa, a thirty-seven-year-old Brooklyn resident with large kohl-lined eyes, curly brown hair, and inch-long bright-red fingernails. "The police scare me," Luisa admitted one afternoon, standing in the shadow of Clinton Building Number One. "If they come towards me, I feel my heart beating real fast." Nonetheless, she had been coming to 110th Street almost daily for the last two years. "If the cops are here, I go a block away," she said, adding that it rarely took her more than five or ten minutes to score. If she did not get several bags a day, she would begin to get cramps, headaches, and the other symptoms of withdrawal. "If you're sick, you're sick—you'll do anything to get more dope," she explained. "If it's good, it hits you right away. All your worries are on hold."

For most of the addicts on 110th Street, the main concern is not finding drugs, but paying for them. A committed heroin user might go through five or more bags a day, which, at $10 apiece, requires a steady income. While some addicts hold jobs and finance their habits from their paychecks, most resort to less legitimate means. Among the most common is welfare fraud. In areas like Spanish Harlem, so many people use welfare checks to support their habits that dealers make sure they have extra stocks on hand around the first of the month, when the checks arrive. "Mother's day," they call it.

When the checks run out, many resort to shoplifting; department stores, with their size and bustle, make the fattest targets. For less courageous addicts, there's always panhandling; with crack costing just a few dollars a vial, a half-hour of begging is usually enough to finance a rush. Women, of course, have access to their own special revenue source; in the early 1990s, every major drug market in New York had its own "ho stro"—whore stroll—where rail-thin women stood ready to give blow jobs for a few bucks or a couple of vials of crack.

Ultimately, though, the most ready means of raising money for drugs is to sell them. While some users go into business for themselves, buying a small quantity of drugs wholesale and then selling them on the street, many sign on with an established organization. Drug gangs are always on the lookout for new pitchers, and, given the high risk of arrest, addicts are often the only candidates around. "We know a lot of users willing to work," said Dino, the manager of a spot at 109th and Lexington. "They're constantly hanging around the area, waiting to make a fast buck. Many are sick and looking to get straight. So, if a pitcher is busted, we'll go up to one and ask, 'You got any money in your pocket? You sick? I'll get you straight, and pay you to work.' So they're getting a free high, plus money in the pocket. Naturally, a junkie will jump at a chance like that."

"Just about everybody you see selling on 110th Street is a drug user," said Captain Robert Curley, who succeeded John Stoker as the commanding officer of the 23rd Precinct. "They're all addicted, all selling just to get by. A high percentage of them are HIV-positive. They're in very, very bad shape. And they're easily replaced." Tom Rachko, a Housing Police detective who had worked in East Harlem for nearly a decade, agreed: "Ninety percent of the sellers on 110th Street are users. They're the ones who get picked up the most." In effect, then, the police raids on 110th Street were nothing more than roundups of addicts. And, given the huge number of addicts in the area, the pool of potential pitchers seemed bottomless.

IN LIGHT of this, many law-enforcement officers have concluded that the best place to hit the drug chain is not at the bottom but at the top. But this approach, too, has its limitations, as was apparent from the work of the Manhattan Narcotics Enforcement Unit, a division of the Housing Police that participated in the Sunshine Project. The unit's twenty agents operated out of a cramped office on the ground floor of a housing project at 112th and Fifth. Its mandate was to fight drug dealing in housing projects throughout Manhattan, but, with so small a force, it inevitably spent most of its time in drug-ridden East Harlem. And, within East Harlem, it concentrated on 110th Street.

The unit did have some successes. In late 1992, for instance, it learned from a confidential informant that Hot Stuff heroin, a popular brand on 109th Street, was being stashed in the Clinton Houses. Every morning, the police learned, a packet was dropped off at the project by a courier traveling from the Bronx in a livery cab. One morning, undercover agents staked out the project and, as the shipment arrived, jumped out and seized the sergeant waiting to receive it. Desperate to avoid going to jail, the sergeant agreed to become an informant himself. Loose-lipped, he told the police not only the names of the organization's top members but also their addresses. In short order, the police were able to locate both the head of the organization—a thirty-two-year-old Dominican nicknamed Flaco—and the source of his drugs —a housing complex in the Bronx.

Building a case against the group proved more difficult, for Flaco and his top associates rarely got close to their product. When it became clear that the police were watching, the dealers grew more cautious still. Every time the police learned that a shipment was about to leave for 110th Street, they would post several officers along the expected route, only to find that it had changed. More and more housing agents were assigned to the job, until eventually ten —half the squad—were watching for one vehicle. When undercover buys had to be made, specially trained agents were brought in from the U.S. Bureau of Alcohol, Tobacco, and Firearms (ATF). At one point, the police learned that a rotund dealer named Heavy was driving up from North Carolina to buy Hot Stuff for sale back home, and so they began consulting a DEA task force there. Finally, after months of stakeouts, undercover buys, and car tailings, the Housing Police felt it had a case strong enough to stand up in court. In a series of raids, the unit seized fourteen members of the ring, Flaco among them. Federal conspiracy charges were brought against the lot, and at least half were expected to be put away for life.

"This was a very big case," noted Captain Ronald Welsh, the head of the housing narcotics unit. Based on financial documents seized during the Hot Stuff investigation, Welsh, a laid-back man with a mat of shiny dark hair, estimated that the dealers took in $6 million a year from this one intersection. All in all, he said, the investigation was the most successful his unit had ever conducted.

Unfortunately, its impact was very modest. "There's still heroin on that corner," Welsh glumly noted. No sooner had Flaco's organization been taken out, he went on, than "other guys moved right in, picking up the slack." In all, he said, five or six organizations were battling for control of the spot. Welsh was eager to go after them—indeed, he had already begun investigating one of the groups. His capacity was limited, though. The investigation into Flaco's group had absorbed the energies of six housing officers—three of them full-time—plus one full-time and several part-time agents from the ATF, all toiling over a six-month period.

Even then, the investigation did not get close to the top of the trafficking hierarchy on 110th Street. It did not get close, in short, to Macho, who had undisputed control of the area. Macho derived his power from both his ruthless use of enforcers and his excellent connections to drug wholesalers. Most of the groups active on 110th Street bought their product from Macho, adding their own cuts and brand names. When a gang like Flaco's was taken out, Macho simply sold more heroin to the other groups in the area, or helped a sergeant or lieutenant start a new one.

Of course, the police could go after Macho himself, but the chances of getting him were slim. For he never got near the merchandise. The product he bought was kept in "drop houses" in Queens and Long Island, then delivered directly to his mill house in the Bronx. Macho rarely showed up at the mill house, and he never appeared on the street. Most of the people in his organization did not know where he lived, or even his real name. It was unlikely, then, that a lower-level officer would be able to finger Macho, as Flaco's sergeant had done him.

Even if Macho were somehow nabbed, the flow of drugs to 110th Street would not likely diminish. For there were many other traffickers in the city ready to take his place. New York's drug trade is highly decentralized, with a multitude of organizations jockeying for position. The number of such organizations is anybody's guess, but an informed estimate comes from Walter Arsenault, the head of the Homicide Investigations Unit of the Manhattan D.A.'s Office. An intense man with thick glasses, Arsenault worked on the fifteenth floor of the Manhattan Criminal Courts Building in an office whose walls were covered with grisly photos of executed gang members. In the course of investigating homicides in Manhattan (many of them drug-related), his unit had necessarily become experts on the makeup of the borough's drug gangs. And, as of 1993, the unit had identified more than 140 such groups in Manhattan north of 96th Street alone, with a new one being added every week.

In all, Arsenault said, there were probably 200 such groups in upper Manhattan, with memberships ranging from 5 to 200. Bringing down just one of these organizations could take up to two years, involving as many as twenty-five investigators and prosecutors. Whenever a gang was smashed, the D.A.'s office would call a press conference, and articles reporting the triumph would appear in the next day's papers. By then, however, other groups were already filling the gap.

As long as people kept buying drugs on 110th Street, it seemed, there would be people to supply them. Finding a long-term solution to the drug problem there, then, would require doing something about the hard-core users who sustained it.

6

Explosion

"PLEASE, WE RUN a drug treatment program here," Raphael Flores admonished the scruffy young man sitting on the stoop next to Hot Line Cares. "We can't have people selling drugs here. I'm asking you, with respect—please, don't sell here." Glaring at Raphael, the youth stood up and, without a word, walked off. "He'll be back," Raphael muttered as he watched him disappear down Third Avenue.

Never before had Hot Line had to worry about dealers camping out on its doorstep, but that had changed as a result of the Sunshine Project and the displacement it was causing. And that was not the only problem associated with the operation. In principle, Raphael did not oppose street-level drug enforcement. In many cases, he knew, police pressure was an important factor in driving addicts to seek help. In his experience, however, intensive crackdowns like Sunshine caused addicts to scatter and hide, making them all the harder to reach. "If you arrest them," he observed, "they're not going to come seek help. You make them the enemy."

Even so, Hot Line's workload was continuing to grow, thanks to one of those unpredictable events that so often seemed to sweep the place. In the summer of 1992, a former volunteer who'd been arrested and sent to Rikers Island on a drug charge told some fellow inmates about Hot Line's ability to find treatment beds, and, as word spread, the center was overwhelmed with calls. For Raphael, drug offenders represented a whole new population to work with, and, with characteristic enthusiasm, he began making weekly visits to the detention center, located an hour-long subway-and-bus ride away on a barren island off LaGuardia Airport. After passing through the main gate, Raphael would board the shuttle bus for Cellblock C-73. WELCOME TO THE LARGEST MALE DETENTION FACILITY IN THE FREE WORLD, a sign cheerily greeted visitors as they entered.

Inside, a counselor would escort Raphael down a drearily antiseptic corridor full of inmates in orange uniforms, then through a locked door and into the C-73 drug counseling unit, a bland locker-room-like space. Eventually, a handful of inmates would be brought in to see him, and Raphael would talk with each about his case. It was slow going, however, for many of the clients had complicated criminal histories, and, to Raphael's great frustration, his actual time with them was very limited. On each visit, Raphael would have to wait a half hour or so to be cleared in at the front gate. Then, after arriving at C-73, he would have to wait another twenty minutes for the inmates to arrive. Trying to speed things up, Raphael pressed the head of the counseling unit to give him a permanent pass so that he could come and go as he pleased, but the man kept putting him off. More generally, the counselors seemed actively indifferent to his work.

Raphael could not understand why, until one afternoon when he was eating lunch in the C-73 staff cafeteria. A counselor from another unit who had heard of Raphael's work approached him about visiting some of his clients. After getting grudging permission from the counselors in C-73, Raphael accompanied the man to the Sprungs, a sprawling bubble-enclosed area with endless rows of bunk beds. "Ninety percent of the people here are in for using or selling drugs," said the counselor, whose name was Peter and who ran group sessions in the Sprungs. "And most are nonviolent." In short, these were the low-level drug offenders who were crowding New York's jails and prisons.

Peter led Raphael to a twenty-two-year-old Hispanic man with sharp features, short hair, and a sleepy manner. A user of crack and cocaine, the man had been picked up for selling drugs to an undercover cop. Raphael explained that he was working to get drug offenders into treatment. "If your felony record is serious," he warned, "we might not be able to get you into a program."

"This is my first time in prison," the man said lethargically.

"Would you have any problem going to Albany for a program?" Raphael asked.

"Where's Albany?"

"Three hours north of the city," Raphael said, adding that the program he had in mind lasted a year, with seven months spent in a residence and five in an apartment. "You'll hear of a lot of job openings up there," he said.

"I never heard of a program like that before," the young man said. "It sounds almost too good."

Unfortunately, Raphael had little time to pursue the matter, for he was due back at C-73. On the way over, Peter, referring to the counselors there, observed, "We're not their favorite people." When Raphael looked at him quizzically, Peter explained: "If you rehabilitate people, what happens? You lose bodies." In other words, the counselors at C-73, like many corrections officers, had a vested interest in keeping the inmate population high, and so they saw people like Raphael as a threat. Not surprisingly, he never did get a permanent pass.

Back at Hot Line, too, the staff was encountering numerous obstacles. New to the legal area, Hot Line had little standing with prosecutors and judges and so had limited ability to advocate for inmates. With no legal adviser to consult, the staff frequently got bogged down in technicalities like predicate felonies and plea bargains. Most taxing of all was the trouble the staff was having in distinguishing offenders who really needed help from those who simply wanted out. Raphael tended to be more lenient than his staff, and their disagreements—added to Hot Line's continuing financial woes—were fanning tensions in the office.

One afternoon, for instance, a routine discussion about whether Hot Line should help an inmate charged with burglary flared into a heated argument. "I don't see any reason why this guy should not get into a program," Raphael said loudly. "They call burglary a violent crime. But what *they* call violent and what *we* call violent are two different things."

"A lot of people have a rap sheet that long," countered Alain Bigot, holding his hands wide apart. "They aren't the ones to be helped. Those who are the victims —selling drugs to support their habit—are the ones who should be helped."

"One guy frightened me," said the normally unflappable Marvin. Addressing Raphael, who had come in despite a bad cold, he said heatedly: "You put all your energy into this, to the point that you get sick, and we're not getting a penny for it—not even a cough drop! These people on the phone think we have to do all this for them."

"These guys are totally isolated," Raphael replied, trying to calm everyone down. "They think we've got a big office. But we're only a few volunteers with three phones." Growing reflective, he added, "We're in over our heads. We could do it, if we had the money." Rikers, he observed, "has more heat than we do, more toilet paper than we do—"

"—and three meals guaranteed," Alain put in. "I don't have that."

"We want money!" Marvin declared. "I want a salary. I want to get off welfare."

As things currently stood, however, Raphael barely had enough money for subway tokens. Desperate, he sent out a letter to Hot Line's friends stating that, if new funds weren't soon forthcoming, Hot Line would have to close its doors in December.

In the meantime, the cases kept flooding in. In September 1992, Marvin got a call from Nancy Hamilton. It was five months since Yvonne had entered New Hope, and while neither Nancy nor Marvin had been able to get anything out of the nuns there, they agreed that no news was good news. Now, however, Nancy was calling about her granddaughter. Having recently resurfaced after a six-month absence, Shondelle was completely out of control, getting high, sleeping around, talking back to her elders. With her mother Anne still out hustling, Nancy's daughter Joyce had become Shondelle's legal guardian, but she, too, was at a loss. "You've got to do something about this girl," Nancy pleaded with Marvin, who said to send her over.

Joyce brought her by a few days later. Wearing baggy jeans, gold hoop earrings, and an oversized T-shirt, Shondelle slumped into a chair in front of Marvin's desk, her narrow face steely with indifference. "She's put my mother and me through some *changes*," Joyce sputtered. Shondelle had agreed to go into a program, she said, but when Marvin asked about her drug taking, the girl admitted only to drinking beer and smoking an occasional joint.

Raphael, who had just gotten off the phone, cut in. "If you really want to go into a program, you've got to tell me what you're using and how long you've been using it," he said sternly from behind his desk.

"I already *said* it," Shondelle hissed.

Raphael told her that he wanted her to return the next day at ten to talk more about treatment. "We need to prepare you a little bit," he said.

"She's a good example of teenagers today," Marvin said after they'd left. "Smoking grass, drinking beer, hanging out late at night, dropping out of school. She's at the point where we have to save her." The next day, Marvin took Shondelle into the back room for a tough talking-to. By the end, he had gotten her to confess to smoking "woolas," a marijuana joint laced with crack. Shondelle agreed to go away after her thirteenth birthday, which was a few days off.

Now Marvin had to find her a bed. It would not be easy. So many young people in the city were getting into trouble with drugs, yet the number of facilities in the state catering to their needs could be counted on two hands. In the past, Hot Line had had some luck with Redirections, a private rehab in Liberty, New York, where a trained staff assessed teenagers over a six-week period. Unfortunately, Redirections accepted only clients with private insurance, and Shondelle had only Medicaid. Reluctantly, Marvin settled on Hill House, a more rudimentary facility outside Albany.

On Monday, Shondelle reappeared at Hot Line, ready to go. Given that she could barely read, Marvin decided to accompany her all the way to Albany. After depositing her at the facility and helping her through the intake process, Marvin returned to Hot Line. When he got there, he received a call from Hill House informing him that Shondelle's urine showed adult levels of cocaine. Like her mother Anne, Shondelle was, by the age of thirteen, a chronic drug user. Now, at least, she was in a place that might help.

MARVIN'S ABILITY to get Shondelle into treatment illustrated a key tenet of the Hot Line approach—the importance of working with families. By keeping in close touch with Nancy Hamilton, Marvin had been able to get both her daughter and granddaughter into treatment. "Forget the block, the community, the country," Raphael once observed. "You've got to work with the family."

Yet, for all of his talk about family, Raphael did not have much of one himself. For the last twenty years, he had lived by himself in his sixth-floor walk-up. Despite his many contacts and acquaintances, he had few close friends. In El Barrio, he was widely seen as an anachronism, a relic of an earlier era of social activism. "The Last of the Mohicans," one detox worker said on seeing him after a long absence. Even his staff, watching him labor late into the night with Harlem's outcasts, had little idea of what drove him.

One of seven children, Raphael grew up in a cold-water flat around the corner from his current apartment. When he was eleven, his father, a merchant marine, walked out on the family. Raphael's mother had to go on welfare and an older brother had to drop out of school to take a job. When he was fourteen, Raphael joined a street gang but soon realized he wasn't cut out for it, and he went on to complete high school. After graduating, he enlisted in the Army. While in basic training, he married a young woman from Queens, and for the next three years she would follow him to bases in Alaska and Colorado. The couple returned to New York in 1969 and soon after had a daughter named Monique.

Seeking work, Raphael stopped by Union Settlement House, a social-service agency in Spanish Harlem where he had played as a child, and got a job as a youth counselor. It was 1970, a time of political ferment in El Barrio, and the teens under Raphael's charge talked of joining radical groups like the Young Lords. Raphael instead urged them to come up with practical solutions to the neighborhood's problems, like the heroin epidemic then sweeping it.

One evening, a Puerto Rican teenager strung out on dope stopped by the center, asking for help. After closing the place for the night, Raphael and several of the teens accompanied the boy, whose name was Hector, to Metropolitan Hospital. Because he had no insurance, the hospital would not accept him. Raphael spent the next several hours at a pay phone, trying to find one that would, without success. The teenagers were ready to occupy the hospital, but Raphael convinced them to return with Hector to the community center and continue the search from there. The next day, after dozens of calls, Raphael finally found a hospital in Brooklyn willing to accept him. On arriving, however, they found it was "ladies' day"—only women could be admitted. By then, Hector had had enough and split. Two days later, he was found in the 103rd Street subway station, dead from an overdose.

Devastated, the teens held an emergency meeting to decide what to do. If only there had been a crisis center to which they could have taken him, they told one another. By the end of the evening, they had decided to create one. The community center agreed to donate space, and in July 1970, Hot Line opened its doors. ("Cares" would be added several years later.) The center immediately became a magnet for youths in El Barrio, and Raphael became a big brother to many of them.

His own family life was going less well. Upset by the long hours Raphael was putting in at Hot Line, his wife enrolled in college and volunteered for a political campaign. This did not sit well with Raphael, who had very traditional notions about a woman's proper place, and, their differences growing irreconcilable, they decided to separate. Raphael was given visiting rights with his daughter, but one afternoon, as he went to pick her up, he discovered that his wife had absconded with her. Hiring an investigator, he tracked them down to Norwalk, Connecticut. A nasty custody battle followed, and Raphael lost.

He was crushed. Ever since his own father had walked out on him, Raphael had been determined to be a good one. Now, his daughter had been snatched from him. Seeking an escape, he threw himself into Hot Line even more. It became, in effect, his new family, with plenty of young volunteers to look up to him. Their enthusiasm helped him through numerous crises, as in the mid-1970s, when Hot Line was forced to find new quarters. Raphael eventually located an unoccupied floor in a tenement at 112th and Third. In return for doing maintenance work in the building, Hot Line was allowed to use the space rent-free.

In 1979, Raphael learned of a new Justice Department program to fund grassroots groups working with juvenile delinquents. Applying, Hot Line was one of two dozen groups selected, and over the next three years it would receive several hundred thousand dollars from the federal government. For the first time, Raphael was able to hire a full staff, including an administrator, a youth coordinator—even a part-time psychotherapist. Teen volunteers were paid stipends of $15 a week, with the opportunity to become full-time employees if they excelled.

This expansion came just as East Harlem was being swept by PCP, a powerful hallucinogen that caused users to become aggressive and disoriented. Angel dust, as it was called, was especially popular among teenagers. To fight it, Hot Line sent out squads of youths to talk in schools and put up ANGEL DUST KILLS posters. Outreach teams fanned out onto the street looking for young users and encouraging them to come by Hot Line. At one point, as many as fifteen teenagers were working in the office, answering phones, conducting rap sessions, planning street campaigns.

With the election of Ronald Reagan, however, Hot Line's main funding source dried up, and Raphael found himself with a large staff and few means of supporting it. One by one, staff members drifted away. Urgently seeking new funds, Raphael was eventually able to line up grants from the city's Office of Juvenile Justice and the state's Division of Substance Abuse Services, and Hot Line's budget was nearly back to where it had been.

The center needed every penny, for the neighborhood was being hit by a new plague: crack. Suddenly, a new generation of users was knocking on Hot Line's doors, bringing with them a host of intractable problems like homelessness, AIDS, and illiteracy. Hot Line, which since its founding had been mainly a meeting place for teens, became a full-time drug-referral center, and at home Raphael would get up to thirty calls a night seeking help. Absorbed with clients, he paid little attention to administrative matters, such as vouchering expenses and keeping its books. When staff members warned him about this, Raphael would airily dismiss them. Hurriedly dashing in and out of the office, disappearing for hours at a time without notice, Raphael often seemed as manic as his clients.

In 1988, the state sent a fiscal officer to conduct a routine audit. Looking through Hot Line's books, the officer found that not only was basic documentation missing, but also the program was in complete disarray. After a team of investigators confirmed the findings, the state revoked Hot Line's license, making it ineligible for funds. The Internal Revenue Service, undertaking its own investigation, found that Hot Line had failed to pay thousands of dollars in withholding taxes; it slapped a lien on the center's assets. The city had no choice but to cut off its funds as well. By 1990, Hot Line was virtually bankrupt.

And Raphael was near the breaking point. For twenty years, Hot Line had been the focus of his life, and now it was falling apart. Many of the youths he had trained over the years had moved on to better-paying jobs. His own daughter, now in college, had become something of a stranger to him. Feeling abandoned, Raphael began lashing out at volunteers and alienating potential funders.

He also began drinking. Ever since his days in the Army, Raphael had had a problem with alcohol, and now, as he fought off depression and exhaustion, his drinking began to escalate. Some long-time supporters, fearing he was on the verge of a breakdown, arranged to send him to Sierra Tucson, a blue-chip rehab in Arizona. For thirty days, Raphael got to see the type of treatment real money could buy. In workshops and counseling sessions, he discussed his sense of isolation, his workaholism, his sadness at all the funerals he was attending.

On his return to New York, however, his despair only deepened. From his client work, Raphael knew of a hospital in Poughkeepsie that had an excellent psychiatric ward, and he checked himself in. Over the next three weeks, he attended group sessions during the day and talked with a psychiatric nurse at night. Unburdening himself for the first time, he felt he could finally see the source of his troubles: he was addicted to Hot Line. To get well, he had to break his habit. Returning to the city, he formally resigned from the center, relinquishing control to Marvin. Intent on staying in El Barrio, however, Raphael stopped by Union Settlement, where he'd begun his career, and convinced the staff to provide some office space so that he could continue his work with addicts. But the arrangement quickly soured—among other things, his clients were boosting fixtures from the bathroom—and after four months he was out. Days later, he was back at Hot Line, taking back control from Marvin. Hot Line's situation remained bleak, but Raphael, launching a typically fitful fundraising campaign, managed to obtain $25,000 from the state's AIDS Institute and $30,000 from the city's Department of Youth Services—just enough to keep Hot Line's doors open and himself fed.

Raphael's main sustenance, however, came from religion. In the course of his travails, he had been born again, and, returning to his small, austere apartment at night, Raphael would sit with his Concordance and look up words in the Bible like "sacrifice," "anger," and "fear." Nightly, he would tune in to Family Radio, a religious network based in Oakland. The network featured a call-in show hosted by Harold Camping, a fundamentalist Bible scholar whose ability to quote Scripture on any subject amazed Raphael. Raphael had bought Camping's book *1994?*, which prophesied an end to the world in that year, and, fully subscribing to it, he had come to see his own work as preparation for the final judgment. From his Bible readings, Raphael had concluded that God disapproved of second marriages, and so he had resigned himself to a monastic existence. And it was just as well. "God wants me to be a people worker," he observed one night in the gloom of his living room, "and people who are single have more time for Him."

THE MORE TIME he gave to the Lord, however, the less he had for his own situation, and it was rapidly deteriorating. For months, Raphael had failed to pay his rent, and—thousands of dollars in arrears—he was receiving urgent eviction notices. Every month, he was barely able to scrape together enough money to keep Con Edison from turning out the lights. By November 1992, things had gotten so bad that he decided to take an outside job. An uncle who worked for a company that dubbed video commercials told him of an opening —for a janitor. Shortly after Thanksgiving, he began working at the company's blandly modern office in midtown Manhattan. Now, rather than spend his day counseling addicts, Raphael was cleaning toilets and sinks. Fortunately, the receptionist agreed to take messages for him, and Marvin would call periodically with updates. For several weeks, Raphael managed to juggle it all, but, unhappy with the way he was being treated, he began talking with fellow employees about unionizing. His employers were predictably displeased, and in mid-January 1993, Raphael—certain he was about to be fired—quit. The next day, he was back at Hot Line.

Nothing had changed there, however, and Raphael—setting a new fundraising deadline for April 1993—was growing ever more moody and irritable. Even more indifferent to his appearance than usual, he was showing up at work with rumpled clothes and uncombed hair. If Marvin or Ethel failed to get him a phone number quickly enough, Raphael would angrily rebuke them. Stewing over past injustices, he would bitterly condemn former employees who had deserted him. He was even upset with Monique, who had begun a serious relationship with a young man he disapproved of. Was she, too, going to abandon him?

The explosion, when it came, took place at an antidrug rally called by Angelo and William Del Toro in late March 1993. By this point, the Sunshine Project was in its seventh month, and the Del Toros wanted to take credit for the crackdown. The meeting was scheduled for seven o'clock in the auditorium of an elementary school at 106th and First. Arriving early, Raphael fell into conversation with a middle-aged woman who had a relative with a drinking problem. Saying he could get the man into detox the next day, Raphael handed her a slip of paper with Hot Line's number on it.

As he did, he saw William Del Toro enter the auditorium and, taking a seat, begin talking with constituents. With Hot Line's grant still pending in Albany, Raphael decided to engage in some last-minute lobbying. A rumpled, streetwise man with a nervous smile and a potbelly, Del Toro fidgeted while Raphael made his pitch. When he had finished, Del Toro said that there was little he could do, since the state had not even passed a budget yet. "Yes, but you know they will," Raphael insisted, hovering over him. "If Hot Line doesn't get money, it's going to go out of business after twenty-three years." Del Toro, noting that the meeting was about to begin, suddenly excused himself. Still steaming, Raphael took a seat toward the back of the auditorium, which was packed for the event.

The police were out in force. On the stage with Del Toro were a half-dozen senior officers, including Captain Robert Curley of the 23rd Precinct and Captain Ronald Welsh of the Housing Police Narcotics Enforcement Unit. Sergeant Steve Ringe stood in back, part of an impressive blue phalanx. Bill Del Toro strode to the mike. "We've become prisoners in our own community," he boomed. Saying that he and his brother had received hundreds of calls about the drug problem, Del Toro explained that they had approached the police and demanded action. As a result, he said, the precinct had been rounding up dealers. "We have been cleaning up 110th Street," he proudly exclaimed. "You can walk on 110th and Lexington today, and, at least during daylight hours, it's clean."

"No, no!" people shouted from the audience.

Taken aback, Del Toro immediately sought to pass the buck. "OK, we'll let Captain Curley take the heat on that," he said nervously.

Raphael, who had been shifting impatiently in his chair, suddenly jumped to his feet. "What is the purpose of this meeting?" he bellowed. "Is this public relations?"

"I ask you for some respect," Del Toro shouted back.

"I'm frustrated!" Raphael yelled.

"Everyone in this room is frustrated," Del Toro replied. The crowd applauded.

"Why are there so many police here?" Raphael went on. At this, a woman in the crowd shouted, "Let's not start with the politics!" Raphael reluctantly sat down.

Captain Curley, a large tree trunk of a man with big glasses and dark eyebrows, got up to announce that, in the past month alone, the police had made 379 narcotics arrests in the precinct. He quickly cautioned, however, that "making arrests is not the only approach. We're dealing with a social problem, one that has existed for twenty years. If you think arresting people is going to solve the problem, it's not. Other issues must be addressed. We need more rehabilitation, and education for youngsters." He closed by urging people to join the Drugbusters program.

A slim, fidgety woman stood up. "People are afraid of being rats," she said. Noting that she had recently moved from Brooklyn to Spanish Harlem, she went on: "Our kids are being killed. So I think it's hard for Bill Del Toro and Charlie Rangel to say, 'Help us clean up the area.' There are dealers, dealers everywhere, and we're full of fear. You want me to make a report? I don't want to die."

Raphael could no longer contain himself. Again jumping up, he angrily declared: "Recently, the police broke down the door of a sixty-seven-year-old woman in my building. They thought her place was being used for guns and drugs. They were wrong. The damage hasn't been repaired yet. She met with you, and all you could do, *sir,* was give her an apology. We were hoping you would give her more."

"Those were exceptional circumstances," Captain Curley replied. "It was a mistake. I apologized to her." As a result of the incident, he added, "We've changed our policy on search warrants. The circumstances that led to the existence of that warrant will not recur."

"It's not enough!" Raphael cried. "Her entrance was totally destroyed."

People were now shouting at him to sit down, and he reluctantly did. After a few more questions from the audience, it was time for the evening's main event. From the back of the hall, a police officer rushed down the center aisle, pulled by a ferocious-looking German shepherd on a leash. An officer on stage explained that the dog was part of a special K-9 unit trained to sniff out controlled substances. A packet containing such a substance had been planted near the stage, and the dog nervously sniffed around from one end to the other. Finally, snout to the ground, it began yelping and wagging its tail. Feeling behind a wooden slat, the officer triumphantly held aloft a small plastic pouch. The crowd went wild.

As the meeting broke up, Raphael was still seething. "What are twenty-seven cops doing at a community meeting?" he fumed. To see money being squandered on drug-sniffing dogs while his own staff couldn't afford lunch was too much for him to bear. At this point, he felt, the only hope for change was in Washington. Two months earlier, Bill Clinton had become president, and Raphael hoped the federal government would at last direct its resources at the hard-core users who were at the heart of the nation's drug problem.

Once, in fact, the federal government had done exactly that. It had a drug czar who had, in effect, applied to the nation as a whole the principles Raphael had developed in Spanish Harlem. And the results would prove stunning.

PART TWO

WASHINGTON

7

Apprenticeship

IN 1965, OTTO KERNER, the governor of Illinois, set up a Narcotic Advisory Council to study the state's growing heroin problem. A constant but tolerable condition since the end of World War II, heroin use in Illinois had begun increasing in the early 1960s, and by mid-decade the state was facing the possibility of a full-blown epidemic. The problem was especially acute on Chicago's South Side, a bleak, sprawling district of deprivation and despair. Thousands of residents—mostly black men in their twenties and thirties—had become addicted to heroin, and, like narcotics users everywhere, they were robbing and stealing to support their habit. The city had responded with tough police action, and an estimated 25 percent of all inmates in the state's prisons were drug addicts.

As for drug treatment, it was virtually unavailable. The one public facility offering any type of service was a twelve-bed detox ward at Bridewell, the Chicago House of Correction. Otherwise, the nearest treatment unit was more than three hundred miles away, at the federal narcotics hospital in Lexington, Kentucky. More prison than hospital, the narcotics "farm," as it was called, treated both drug offenders sent by the courts (who lived in locked cells) and addicts voluntarily seeking help. East of the Mississippi River, the narcotics farm was virtually the only institution offering any form of treatment. (A similar facility in Fort Worth, Texas, served all addicts west of the Mississippi.) After receiving counseling, exercise, and vocational training, the addicts would be sent back home. With little follow-up care, however, more than 90 percent of them eventually relapsed.

From this, some public-health officials had concluded that it would be far better to treat addicts in their home communities than in some distant facility. Yet the moral stigma attached to addiction made this impossible. Ever since passage of the Harrison Narcotics Act in 1914—the legal foundation of drug prohibition in the United States—Americans had come to view addicts as dangerous deviants who had to be isolated from society. Drug policy was the preserve of the Federal Bureau of Narcotics and its despotic commissioner, Harry Anslinger. A barrel-chested, bald-headed propagandist, Anslinger was the moving force behind the "Reefer Madness" scares of the 1930s and 1940s, which cast marijuana users as psychotic killers. In 1951, Anslinger's agitation helped persuade Congress to adopt the Boggs Act, which mandated a minimum sentence of two years for first-time narcotics possession. Five years later, Congress made the sale of heroin to minors punishable by death—a stark indication of the depth of public intolerance on the issue.

After the election of John Kennedy, however, the national mood began to change. With the new administration urging greater compassion for the mentally impaired, drug addiction came to be seen as less a criminal condition than a psychological one. In 1962, the Supreme Court ruled that drug addiction was a disease, not a crime. That same year, Harry Anslinger retired from the Federal Bureau of Narcotics, and the seat of decision-making on the issue shifted to the National Institute of Mental Health (NIMH), a division of the Department of Health, Education, and Welfare (HEW). In 1963, a presidential advisory commission on drug abuse issued a report recommending that the federal government reduce the penalties for narcotics offenses and increase funding for drug treatment. On the eve of the fiftieth anniversary of the Harrison Act, then, the era of hostility toward drug addicts was drawing to a close, and local officials across the country were considering what should come next.

In Illinois, the Narcotic Advisory Council held its first meeting on December 21, 1965. Made up of leading judges, doctors, clergymen, legislators, and police officials, the council gathered data on the extent of Illinois's drug problem and on how other states were coping with their own. As they proceeded, however, the council members recognized the need for an experienced adviser. For names, they turned to Dr. Daniel X. Freedman, the chairman of the psychiatry department at the University of Chicago. Recently arrived from Yale, where he had made a name for himself studying the effects of LSD on college students, Freedman knew virtually everyone in the small but growing fraternity of drug-treatment specialists. And, when asked by the advisory council to recommend someone, he did not hesitate. No one in the field struck him as more knowledgeable or insightful than Dr. Jerome H. Jaffe, a psychiatrist on the staff of the Albert Einstein College of Medicine, a division of Yeshiva University, in the Bronx, New York.

THIRTY-TWO YEARS OLD, Jerry Jaffe was a specialist in psychopharmacology, the study of the effects of drugs on the central nervous system. Five feet eight and slightly built, with thinning hair, gold-rimmed glasses, and a wardrobe of white shirts and Sta-Prest pants, Jaffe had the pallor of someone who spent too much time in the lab, which he did. To test the effects of psychotropic substances, he was administering barbiturates and other drugs to a stable of cats, rats, and mice and monitoring their responses. Outside the lab, Jaffe was no less rigorous. Relentlessly logical and analytical, he was reluctant to accept any assertion unsupported by evidence, and he would jump on even the most commonplace assumptions, probing for weaknesses and inconsistencies. He did not except his own statements, appending Talmud-like qualifiers and caveats as he went along. For some, the experience was maddening. Even friends, exposed to his mordant wit and blunt candor, found Jaffe prickly. No one, however, could deny his honesty, his sense of fair play, and, especially, his incisive intellect.

A modest man, Jaffe lived near campus on the ground floor of a two-story house with his wife Faith, an alumna of Bryn Mawr, and their two young daughters. Jaffe's salary, at $6,000 a year, was modest, too, and to supplement it he made house calls in the South Bronx for the HIP health maintenance organization.

His upbringing was no less humble. Jaffe was born in 1933 into a lower-middle-class household in the Germantown section of Philadelphia. His father, a Jewish immigrant from Lithuania, ran a grocery store on the ground floor of the family house. After graduating from high school, Jaffe entered Temple University. Finishing first in his class, he remained at Temple for medical school, paying his way in part by working nights as a bass player in a wedding band. In his final year of medical school, Jaffe read Abraham Wikler's *The Relation of Psychiatry to Pharmacology*, a pioneering work that described how new drugs like Thorazine were being used to treat mental patients. The great pharmacological revolution was on, and Jaffe decided to join it. After graduating from Temple, in 1958, Jaffe, along with his new bride, Faith, moved to Staten Island to begin a year-long internship at a U.S. Public Health Service hospital. As it was coming to an end, Jaffe, facing the physicians' draft, decided to apply for a position at the facility where Abraham Wikler worked, the Addiction Research Center at the federal narcotics hospital in Lexington.

Jaffe was accepted at the hospital, but to his regret he was assigned not to its research center but to its clinical division. It was not a total loss, however, for Lexington had a diverse array of drug users, ranging from street hustlers to jazz musicians, and Jaffe, in counseling them, got a firsthand look at the nature of addiction. In his second year, he was assigned to Lexington's detox unit, where newly arrived addicts were withdrawn from heroin with a synthetic narcotic that had been developed by German scientists during World War II. Methadone, as it was called, helped alleviate the discomfort addicts felt as they were weaned from heroin, and Jaffe, counseling them, became fascinated with phenomena like tolerance, withdrawal, and dependence.

Arriving at Einstein in 1961, Jaffe explored these concepts in his animal experiments. Before long, however, he was dealing with human subjects as well, for addicts he had met in Lexington were seeking him out at his office in the Bronx. As elsewhere, treatment was largely unavailable in New York, and Jaffe did his best to counsel them. From his time at Lexington, however, he knew that psychotherapy alone was rarely effective in curtailing addiction. Seeking a pharmacological agent that might help, Jaffe obtained supplies of a semisynthetic opioid called oxymorphone, which he gave to his patients to inject. (When the Federal Bureau of Narcotics learned of his activities, it sent an agent to protest, but, when Jaffe patiently explained that only a few patients were involved, it left him alone.)

Then, in early 1965, he learned of a fascinating experiment taking place at Rockefeller University, the august research institute on Manhattan's Upper East Side. There, Dr. Vincent Dole, a specialist in metabolic diseases, had teamed with a young psychiatrist named Marie Nyswander to explore new ways of controlling narcotic addiction. Nyswander ran a storefront psychiatric practice in a run-down tenement on 103rd Street in Spanish Harlem, with many heroin addicts among her clients. Several of them agreed to come to Rockefeller to participate in an experiment Dole was conducting. Hoping to find a level at which addicts could be stabilized, Dole was having them injected with heroin. No matter how much they received, however, the addicts would eventually grow tolerant, and Dole would have to keep increasing the doses to keep them from getting sick. Dole then switched to morphine, an opium-derived analgesic, but the same pattern developed, with patients needing a new hit every hour or two. Seeking to withdraw them, Dole used the standard agent, methadone. Because the addicts were so doped up, however, he had to use more than twice the normal amount. After they received several such doses, Dole found to his amazement that the patients were behaving in a more or less normal fashion, with no signs of withdrawal. Experimenting further, he found that methadone, administered in one large dose of 50 to 150 milligrams a day, enabled the addicts to go about their business, free of their hunger for drugs.

Convinced that addiction was a more or less permanent condition, Dole held that addicts had to be maintained on methadone indefinitely, hence the name of the new technique—methadone maintenance. To test its effectiveness, he and Nyswander gained access to a fifty-bed ward at a hospital that would eventually become part of the Beth Israel Medical Center. During a six-week stay there, volunteers were stabilized on methadone, then assigned to an outpatient clinic to receive daily doses of the drug, together with counseling and other rehabilitative services.

Dole began giving some lectures in which he described his findings, and Jaffe, attending them, was impressed. As he knew, methadone was no panacea. Not only was it highly addictive, but people maintained on it often continued to drink and use other drugs. Nonetheless, the discovery that the same agent used to withdraw patients at Lexington could be used to stabilize heroin addicts represented a real breakthrough. Unfortunately, the Dole-Nyswander experiment was proceeding very slowly, and in the meantime addicts were begging Jaffe for help. From his own clinical work, Jaffe did not think it necessary to confine people to a hospital while they were being stabilized. Deciding to conduct his own experiment, he wrote prescriptions for methadone for his patients and sent them to a pharmacy around the corner to be filled. Back at his office, Jaffe would counsel his patients and monitor their progress through regular urine tests. Most, he found, did well even without being hospitalized. (Eventually, the Dole-Nyswander program would move in this direction, offering methadone strictly on an outpatient basis.)

Methadone was not the only new therapy being developed in this period. On Staten Island, two dozen male addicts on probation were living full-time on the grounds of a former convent. Daytop Village, as the program was called, was modeled on Synanon, a live-in community of alcoholics and drug addicts founded in Santa Monica, California, by a recovering alcoholic named Charles Dederich. Like Synanon, Daytop blended the confessional techniques of Alcoholics Anonymous with the confrontational practices of encounter groups, all served up in a boot-camp-like setting. Most of the counselors were recovering addicts, which, it was thought, made them uniquely qualified to help break other addicts of their habits. Good behavior was rewarded with privileges; transgressors were subject to penalties like head shaving and sign wearing. The idea was to break down an addict's personality and rebuild it along more healthful lines. To many psychiatrists, these "therapeutic communities" (TCs) seemed excessively punitive, but Jaffe, knowing how resistant addicts could be to ordinary counseling, felt they had great potential.

By the mid-1960s, then, New York was giving rise to two new techniques for treating drug addicts—methadone maintenance and therapeutic communities. And, from their humble origins at Rockefeller University and on Staten Island, the two therapies would rapidly expand. As they did, however, they became intensely competitive with each other. Therapeutic communities, seeing total abstinence as the only acceptable course, scorned methadone as a "crutch" that was highly addictive in its own right. Methadone advocates, in turn, viewed TCs as little more than penal colonies in which addicts were treated like ex-cons. The factionalism that would become a hallmark of the New York treatment world had begun.

Watching all this unfold, Jaffe was appalled. The two movements seemed almost messianic in nature, with each proclaiming itself the one true way. In reality, both approaches seemed promising. Nor did therapeutic communities and methadone maintenance seem the last word in drug therapy. With his pharmacological background, Jaffe had become interested in a group of drugs, called narcotics antagonists, that blocked the desire for heroin without being addictive themselves. Eager to test them, he obtained supplies of one such substance, cyclazocine, and found some volunteers willing to take it. "The eagerness with which heroin addicts sought such treatment contradicted the belief that they were unmotivated to stop using drugs," Jaffe would later write of the experiment. "It was obvious then that it would be useful to compare treatment with antagonists to treatment with methadone. I had gotten hooked on what works for whom."

It was around this time that Jaffe got his first big break. At Einstein, Jaffe gave the school's basic course on drug addiction. Among those sitting in on it was Dr. Alfred Gilman, the head of Einstein's pharmacology department. Along with Dr. Louis Goodman, Gilman was the author of *The Pharmacological Basis of Therapeutics,* a standard text at medical schools across the country. Originally published in 1940, Goodman and Gilman, as it was known, was due for a revision, and, given the burgeoning literature in the field, the authors decided to include outside contributors for the first time. Impressed with Jaffe's lectures, Gilman asked if he would be interested in contributing chapters on drug addiction and narcotics analgesics. Jaffe, who just a few years before had used Goodman and Gilman at Temple, was flattered and, despite his heavy workload, accepted. When the new volume appeared, in 1965, Jaffe's presence in it marked him as someone to watch in the fledgling field of addiction medicine.

Despite his newfound stature, Jaffe was not completely content at Einstein, for, despite his pleas, its psychiatry department would not provide him the space he needed to conduct clinical tests of a long-lasting maintenance drug called LAAM. And so, in December 1965, when Daniel Freedman approached him about joining the psychiatry department at the University of Chicago, Jaffe was immediately interested. He was further intrigued when Freedman raised the possibility of his serving as an adviser to the Illinois Narcotic Advisory Council—a position that would allow him to test his ideas in the real world. And so, after getting the go-ahead from Faith, who had already had to move three times in the previous eight years, Jaffe accepted Freedman's offer, and in late 1966 he and his family took up residence on the shores of Lake Michigan.

WITH ITS SPACIOUS quadrangles and ivy-covered neo-Gothic buildings, the University of Chicago seemed like a slice of Oxford plopped down amid the decaying flatlands of the city's South Side. The Hyde Park location, while no aid to recruitment, had fostered a strong tradition of service to the local community, and the university's association with the Illinois Narcotic Advisory Council would reflect that. Even as he was setting up his lab at the medical school's Billings Hospital, Jaffe was encouraged to take whatever time he needed to advise the council. Meeting with its members, he shared some of the insights into addiction that he had gained while in New York. Contrary to popular belief, he said, many addicts do want help. To be effective, however, that help had to be responsive to their needs. Addicts were a diverse lot, and so any treatment system had to offer a variety of therapies, expanding those that worked and eliminating those that didn't.

Eventually, the council decided to set up a program along the lines Jaffe had recommended, on one condition—that he agree to run it. With the university's permission, he did. The council's final report, issued in May 1967, closely reflected Jaffe's views. Noting that the state had "done almost nothing other than fill its prisons with addicts," the document asserted that "it is time, long past time, that treatment be an equal partner in the State's response to addiction." It went on:

> There is no such thing as a typical addict. . . . any program which attempts to deal with narcotic addicts as a homogeneous group reachable by a particular program is self-defeating. A variety of fore-care and after-care programs tailored to the needs of the particular addicts and potential addicts they are designed to treat is the key to a successful state program.

Deciding to proceed slowly, the advisory council recommended setting up a pilot program under the aegis of the Illinois Department of Mental Health. To fund it, the state legislature agreed to allocate $1 million, with the University of Chicago picking up part of Jaffe's salary.

It was a unique opportunity: Jaffe was going to get the chance to build a treatment system from scratch, without all the distracting rivalries of the New York scene. Approaching the task as he would a lab experiment, he planned to set up a variety of programs and assign clients randomly to each, then measure the results. In the summer of 1967, he began working full-time on the project, investigating sites and recruiting staff.

In the meantime, word of the success New York was having with methadone had reached Chicago, and Jaffe was constantly being asked for some by the addicts he was counseling. He kept resisting, until January 1, 1968, when one of his patients, a jazz clarinetist suffering from Hodgkin's disease, was refused help at Billings Hospital after the staff discovered he had a heroin habit. Exasperated, Jaffe grabbed a prescription pad in his office. "Today, we start," he declared, then wrote a script for methadone—the first in the state. His staff—worried that he had begun before all the necessary protocols were in place—accused him of jeopardizing the whole project. Jaffe, however, explained that his responsibilities as a doctor took precedence, and in subsequent weeks he would prescribe methadone for a dozen more patients. The Illinois Drug Abuse Program had begun.

Finally, in February 1968, IDAP opened its first formal unit—a methadone clinic located on the ground floor of a three-story building on the western edge of campus. Each of the center's seventy-five clients received liquid methadone mixed with an orange drink, which they consumed on the premises. Each was expected to attend weekly therapy sessions and give three urines a week. Although the opening was not publicly announced, word quickly spread on the street, and within weeks several hundred people had applied for admission. "The problem in Chicago was said to be modest, but when we opened, people came out of the woodwork," Jaffe recalled. Immediately, the search was on for another methadone site.

Meanwhile, IDAP was preparing to open its second unit—a detox ward at Billings. Few such units existed in the country, and all sorts of details had to be worked out, siting among them. The fear of addicts was so strong that hospital workers worried about having them on the grounds; to reassure them, the ward was situated above the hospital's emergency entrance, where security guards were always on duty. The facility would be run by a psychiatrist and a team of nurses, with a parallel group of ex-addicts to oversee the therapy. Patients were expected to stay about two weeks, and a dozen beds were set aside to serve them. Finally, in April, the unit opened, and addicts in Chicago no longer had to be arrested to be detoxed.

All the while, Jaffe was laying the groundwork for Chicago's first therapeutic community. Hoping to find a large house at an affordable price, he canvassed his own neighborhood of Jackson Park Highlands. Located about a mile and a half south of campus, this once-thriving neighborhood had fallen on hard times, and faculty members willing to put up with its high crime rate could live well above their means. The Jaffes lived in an old Tudor mansion with a living room two-and-a-half stories high; nearby were the economist Arthur Laffer, Ramsey Lewis, and Chicago Bears running back Gale Sayers. A few blocks from his own house, Jaffe found a grand six-bedroom mansion that had once belonged to Bo Diddley but was now a vacant eyesore. Because IDAP lacked the funds to buy the house outright, Jaffe signed for it himself, offering his own house as security. Gateway House, as it was called, was modeled on Daytop, with a similarly strict regimen and a required stay of eighteen months. Its forty beds were quickly filled.

By the summer of 1968, then, IDAP had a therapeutic community, a methadone clinic, and a detox unit followed by outpatient aftercare. In line with Jaffe's original plan, addicts were randomly assigned to one of the three programs with the aim of finding which worked best. The addicts themselves kept frustrating the plan, however, for each had his own strong preferences. Quickly adapting, Jaffe scrapped his planned experiment and allowed clients to select their own form of therapy (subject to a counselor's approval). Instead of trying to find the one program that worked best, IDAP would maintain an array of programs to serve clients' various needs. A "multimodality" system, Jaffe called it, and few operations like it existed anywhere else in the country.

With demand continuing to mount, IDAP in the fall of 1968 opened a second methadone clinic, on the second floor of a small bank building at East 79th Street and Stony Island Avenue, in a high-crime, gang-infested section of the South Side. It, too, quickly filled, and again IDAP was hunting for another site. By the end of the year, the program had seven units serving 500 people, and any remaining pretense that it was a pilot vanished. From the city's South Side, the program would expand to the more affluent North Side, and from there to Rockford, Peoria, and East St. Louis.

Along the way, there were inevitable growing pains. The person hired to run Gateway turned out to be a manipulative autocrat with a taste for young girls, and Jaffe had to work behind the scenes to ease him out. Some local black militants objected to having the white-run university operate drug programs in the inner city. Generally, though, the community was supportive, in part because Jaffe had gotten the state to change its civil service laws to make it possible for recovering addicts to work for IDAP, and many had gotten jobs with it. One, a former steelworker and Korean War sergeant named Matthew Wright, became not only a clinical director but also a close friend of Jaffe's, and the two men were a common sight on the South Side as they traveled together to inspect sites and meet with community groups.

Throughout, Jaffe continued to innovate. With hundreds of people on IDAP's waiting list, he set up a pretreatment unit at the 79th Street clinic to provide clients with methadone and limited therapeutic services while they waited for an opening—a way of keeping them from hanging out on the street. For clients who got arrested, became violent, or otherwise had to drop out of a program, he created a reentry unit to provide them skeletal services until they were ready to return. "The main point was to be open and to learn from what you were doing in the field," Jaffe said. "Things are not cast in stone. You have to decide which pieces are good, and which aren't."

One piece that clearly was not good was the detox unit at Billings. Therapeutically, the hospital was performing poorly, with the patients feuding with the staff, and the staff itself divided between ex-addicts and professionals. And the cost—$100 a day per bed—was exorbitant. Unless a patient had special medical problems, Jaffe believed, he could be detoxed just as effectively, and far more cheaply, in a nonhospital setting. As he prepared to close the unit, Jaffe took over a vacant building on the grounds of the Tinley Park Mental Health Center. Located twenty-five miles southwest of downtown Chicago, it had been emptied as part of the movement to deinstitutionalize the mentally ill. From now on, addicts seeking detox would be transported to the center—anchored by a bright, cheery three-story building—and withdrawn over a two-week period, at a cost of just $12 a day.

Experimenting further, Jaffe brought in a team headed by a former Daytop official to create a more flexible type of therapeutic community at Tinley Park. The maximum stay was reduced from eighteen to six months, with the actual length adjusted to each individual's needs. And, while clients still had to earn privileges and could have them revoked for misbehaving, confrontation and ridicule were kept to a minimum. In an even more radical change, Tinley

Park took in not only people committed to abstinence but also methadone clients needing more structure than was available in IDAP's outpatient programs. Eventually, Tinley Park came to serve as a crisis center for clients elsewhere in the system who needed a temporary refuge while trying to stabilize their lives; some stayed for weeks, others for months.

By 1970, the Illinois Drug Abuse Program had fifteen facilities serving more than nine hundred people. And, as new needs arose, Jaffe kept improvising. For clients for whom Tinley Park was too structured, he created Safari House, a short-term residential center located atop a Salvation Army thrift shop; outpatients undergoing a crisis could come here to crash and get emergency help. On the Near North Side, a hippie district full of acid trippers and pill poppers, IDAP took over an abandoned tire factory and converted it into a drop-in center for young people. PFLASH TYRE—BLOWN-OUT MINDS RETREADED, a sign outside declared in psychedelic letters. With so many IDAP clients struggling with problems apart from their addictions, Jaffe set up a special treatment unit that had a psychiatrist to deal with mental problems, a doctor to treat medical problems, and a pregnancy section to help deliver babies.

With the program needing more office space, Daniel Freedman arranged for Jaffe and his staff to move into the Museum of Science and Industry, a majestic Greek temple–like edifice in Jackson Park, between the university and the lake. To help manage IDAP's client base, Jaffe installed a computer system that allowed him at the push of a button to determine an individual's case history. It also allowed him to compile data on the progress of his clients. And many of them seemed to be doing well. The number of clients with jobs increased by about 70 percent over the course of treatment, with most going to work in steel mills or as butchers or cabdrivers. And, according to clients' self-reports, arrest rates for those in the program dropped by about 40 percent.

To make it easier for addicts to apply for admission, Jaffe set up a central intake unit west of the downtown Loop. Here, each new client would fill out a medical history, be examined by a physician, and speak with a counselor. The patient would be informed of the various treatment options available and asked to indicate a preference. If a slot was available, he would be referred immediately; if not, he'd be put on the waiting list. If a client did not thrive in one program, he could be transferred to another. Overall, central intake allowed counselors to keep track of an addict's progress and make sure he didn't fall through the cracks.

Equally pioneering was IDAP's work on the epidemiology of drug use— i.e., how heroin addiction spreads. Under the direction of a young psychiatrist named Patrick Hughes, IDAP sent out field teams into South Side copping zones to interview addicts and gather information about their habits. To establish their credibility, the teams employed recovering addicts, and, to ensure cooperation, offered subjects immediate access to treatment. From the data collected, Hughes was able to track miniepidemics as they struck individual neighborhoods. In some communities, the spread of heroin use resembled outbreaks of infectious disease, with a steep rise in incidence in a very short period. Once he was able to identify such outbreaks, Hughes moved to contain them, converting his research units into outreach teams whose mission was to recruit addicts who might spread the epidemic and place them in programs.

The response was overwhelming. "The community outreach teams showed us that people who don't seek treatment spontaneously may do so if they are asked, and that they do well if they are made to feel welcome," Jaffe observed. Eager to target other neighborhoods, Hughes asked Jaffe to allocate more slots to his outreach teams. With nearly 1,000 people already waiting for treatment, however, Jaffe was reluctant to take slots away from addicts seeking help on their own. Frustrated, Hughes frequently clashed with Jaffe at IDAP staff meetings.

He was not the only one. "Our meetings were so heated," recalled Dr. Edward Senay, a University of Chicago psychiatrist who was one of Jaffe's top aides. "Sometimes I was more afraid in those meetings than on the street." As in New York, sharp divisions arose between devotees of methadone maintenance and adherents of therapeutic communities. There were also racial tensions—most of IDAP's top administrators were white, and most of its clients black—and clashes in lifestyles. As an ambitious social program, IDAP attracted many young activists, and their Aquarian Age ways often clashed with the more staid manners of the physicians and psychiatrists who ran the program.

The problems were exacerbated by Jaffe's woeful management style. Brusque and demanding, he was forever pushing for results, and those who failed to deliver would often feel his scorn. Even those who did well would often not know it, for Jaffe tended to be grudging with praise. In addition, Jaffe disliked confrontation, and so, rather than intervene in conflicts at an early stage, he would allow them to fester. At one point, things got so bad that he had to call in a psychologist to lead the staff in group sessions. In the end, Jaffe managed to keep the lid on by constantly reminding the staff that they were there to serve the needs of clients, rather than the other way around. "Jerry always said that if anything went wrong, it was our fault, not the client's," said Claude Rhodes, an early client of the program who eventually went on to become a clinical director. "It's like the saying 'The customer's always right.' Jerry believed that the client was always right."

And, despite the chaos, most IDAP staff members relished the chance to work with Jaffe. "He was an absolutely brilliant, hardworking guy," Patrick Hughes recalled. "And often he expected everybody else to be as brilliant and hardworking as he was. So he got impatient with us. But those were exciting times. Jaffe's mind was not encumbered by the usual structures. As with the rats in his lab, he'd see the program in experimental terms. He'd say, 'Let's buy that building, set up a clinic, structure it this way, and if it doesn't work, we'll change it, and if it still doesn't work, we'll close it.' "

As word of IDAP's success spread, Jaffe began receiving a stream of visitors, among them government officials, professors, doctors, and foreign dignitaries. One day in June 1970, he got a call from the White House. A domestic policy adviser named Jeffrey Donfeld had heard about IDAP and wanted to see it. Twenty-seven years old, Donfeld was tall, blond, and cocky. Jaffe escorted him to various IDAP installations and showed him the computer system he had set up to keep track of clients. Donfeld took copious notes and, at the end of the day, thanked his host and left for Washington. Jaffe, who was due to give a paper at an upcoming health conference in Geneva, returned to his work. Donfeld's visit, however, was to have profound consequences, both for Jaffe and for the nation's drug policy.

8

To the White House

IF THERE WAS one word to describe Jeff Donfeld, it was contrarian. At a time
when his entire generation was tuning in, turning on, and dropping out, Donfeld liked to boast that he had never been intoxicated, even on alcohol. He
was raised in an affluent Jewish household in Los Angeles not unlike Dustin
Hoffman's in *The Graduate*, but he was not the sort to laugh at the idea of
going into plastics. A brash conservative who despised long hair and psychedelic music, Donfeld attended UCLA, where he became president of the
student body, then went to Berkeley law, where he opposed the Free Speech
Movement. In the summer of 1967, while many of his peers were getting
stoned at rock concerts, Donfeld was interning at Richard Nixon's law firm,
impressing Nixon with pointed questions about Vietnam. Donfeld also began
dating Nixon's daughter Tricia. That did not hurt his chances when, after Nixon
was elected president in 1968, he applied for a job at the White House. Hired
to serve on the domestic policy staff, Donfeld chose drugs as his portfolio—a
ready vehicle for attacking the counterculture he so loathed.

Such an attitude was close to the president's own. A product of the Anslinger era, Richard Nixon felt a reflexive disgust for illegal drugs and the
people who used them. Marijuana, hashish, and LSD were, in his view, turning
a generation of Americans into long-haired, love-beaded, guru-worshipping
peaceniks. During the 1968 campaign, Nixon, in a speech in Anaheim, California, had called narcotics the "modern curse of the youth." "Just like the plagues
and epidemics of former years," he said, drugs "are decimating a generation of
Americans." If elected, Nixon promised, he would triple the number of customs agents and work with friendly nations "to move against the source of
those drugs."

After the election, Nixon entrusted the drug issue to Bud Wilkinson, the former University of Oklahoma football coach. While completely unschooled in the field, Wilkinson was a gridiron legend and symbol of bedrock American values—just the sort to publicize the evils of drugs. In the White House, Wilkinson would launch a variety of PR initiatives, such as meeting with media executives, speaking to community groups, and training youth coordinators. Jeff Donfeld, one of his assistants, specialized in organizing high-profile events in Washington. TV producers were brought to the White House and encouraged to work antidrug messages into their programs. Disc jockeys were urged not to play music with prodrug lyrics. And, in the grandest event of all, the nation's governors were convened in the State Department's auditorium to hear presentations about the menace of drugs, including an emotional address by Art Linkletter describing his daughter's suicide in the wake of an LSD trip.

Gradually, however, Donfeld's contrarian nature began to surface. For all the zest he brought to these events, he could not help recognizing them for what they were—elaborate dog-and-pony shows. And, however much they might help deter kids from using pot, they seemed useless in dealing with more serious problems, like heroin use in the ghetto. With his hard-line views, Donfeld felt little sympathy for addicts, but, as he began reading in the field, he found himself getting caught up in the exciting developments in the treatment world. By the fall of 1969, about 2,000 heroin addicts were receiving methadone in New York, and researchers studying them were finding marked reductions in heroin use, unemployment, and criminal activity.

This last point in particular caught Donfeld's eye. If it was true that heroin addicts committed many robberies and burglaries, as was widely believed, then methadone's seeming ability to reduce recidivism endowed it with great political potential. The risks were high, too, of course. Methadone was so addictive that many users found it harder to kick than heroin. And, while normally dispensed in clinics, the drug could be easily diverted onto the street, giving rise to a black market. The idea that the federal government itself might fund methadone programs seemed far-fetched, especially for a Republican administration extolling God, country, and football.

At the time, the government's efforts in the treatment area were very modest. In 1969, the federal drug budget came to just $81 million. About $43 million of that sum went for treatment, most of it for a dozen or so programs overseen by the National Institute of Mental Health. The remaining funds went for enforcement—mainly to the Customs Bureau, which patrolled the nation's borders, and the Bureau of Narcotics and Dangerous Drugs (BNDD), which targeted trafficking organizations. Acting on his campaign promise, President Nixon nearly doubled the size of Customs and increased the number of BNDD offices abroad from twenty-five to forty-six.

Nixon was particularly intent on stopping heroin at its source. At the time, most of the heroin entering the United States originated in the poppy fields of Turkey's western Anatolia plains. Opium paste extracted from poppy flowers was sold to middlemen, who had it processed into morphine base in the Middle East, which was then shipped to southern France. There, in makeshift labs located in and around Marseilles, chemists employed by the Corsican mafia processed the morphine base into high-grade heroin. The powder was then smuggled into the United States, with New York the most common destination.

This was the famous French Connection, and Nixon was determined to break it. "I feel very strongly that we have to tackle the heroin problem regardless of the foreign policy consequences," he wrote to Henry Kissinger and several other top aides in a September 22, 1969, memo. "I understand that the major problem is with Turkey and to a lesser extent with France and with Italy. In any event, I want the group included in this memorandum to give me a recommendation as to what we can do." Plugging the heroin pipeline thus became a top priority for the White House.

In this climate, Jeff Donfeld remained virtually alone in his interest in drug treatment. That would soon change, however, as the White House became increasingly preoccupied with crime. During the presidential campaign, Nixon had frequently raised the issue, pointing out how, during eight years of Democratic rule, the nation's crime rate had doubled. After the election, Nixon named as his attorney general John Mitchell, whose steely demeanor contrasted with the bleeding hearts who had run the Department of Justice under Lyndon Johnson. At an early meeting of Justice officials and White House aides, Nixon had stressed his desire to bring down the nation's crime rate. Justice officials, however, noted that, in the federal system, law enforcement was mainly the preserve of state and local government, leaving little for the administration to do.

Except in the District of Columbia. Home rule had yet to come to Washington, and both the mayor and city council served at the president's behest, giving him great leverage. In addition, the federal government had abundant enforcement resources in the District. During the campaign, Nixon himself had singled out Washington, where the crime rate had risen even faster than in the nation as a whole. "D.C. should not stand for disorder and crime," Nixon had declared. "Washington should be a model of stability and law and justice in America—and that is what we must pledge ourselves to in a new administration."

In case the White House needed any convincing, the city was hit by a crime wave just as Nixon was taking office; in one incident, a presidential secretary had her purse snatched just outside the White House grounds. On January 31, 1969, Nixon announced a package of emergency measures, including a drastic reorganization of the city's courts, the appointment of new judges and prosecutors, and the hiring of 1,000 new cops. The president also welcomed the appointment of an aggressive new police chief, Jerry Wilson, who, on frequent visits to the White House, joined Nixon in thrashing out ways to improve the local force. The crime rate continued to soar, however, and every

month, when the latest numbers came out, Nixon would call up his adviser
John Ehrlichman to complain.

To the outside world, the balding, impassive Ehrlichman seemed indistin-
guishable from H. R. Haldeman, the dour, unswervingly loyal chief of staff. In
private, however, Ehrlichman was wry, personable, and pragmatic. After serving briefly as White House counsel, Ehrlichman became Nixon's domestic
policy adviser, and he assembled about him a band of like-minded aides. And,
faced with the crime problem in the District, he turned to the most trusted of
them, Egil Krogh, Jr.

Thirty years old, Krogh was the White House's Mr. Fix-it, the man called
on to solve its most intractable problems. "Bud," as he was known, would arrive
every morning at seven-fifteen at his office in the ornate, French Empire–style
Old Executive Office Building (OEOB) next to the White House, and he would
rarely leave before eight or nine at night. Ruggedly handsome, with a square
jaw, dark eyes, and a receding hairline, Krogh had ten aides of his own, and he
needed every one, so broad were his responsibilities. They included corrections, legal services, transportation, the Justice Department, and "internal security," which consisted mainly of keeping order during the large antiwar
demonstrations that periodically rocked the capital. (When Nixon made his
famous predawn visit to the Lincoln Memorial in May 1970 to talk with antiwar
protesters, Krogh was by his side.) Paralleling his grueling work pace, Krogh
jogged five miles a day, a lone figure in a gray sweatsuit circling the Ellipse
behind the White House.

For all his drive, though, Krogh projected a sense of decency and earnestness that was rare in the Nixon White House. He got it from his father. A
self-made Norwegian immigrant, Egil Krogh, Sr., rose to become a vice president at the Marshall Field department store in Chicago before moving the
family to Seattle. When Bud was fourteen, his father, a heavy drinker and
smoker who was interested in Christian Science, said he would forgo alcohol
and tobacco if his son promised to do the same; Bud did so with a handshake,
and in later years he would never waver. In Seattle, the Krogh family became
friendly with a local zoning lawyer and fellow Christian Scientist named John
Ehrlichman, and young Bud grew close to him. After graduating from Principia
College in Illinois, Krogh spent three-and-a-half years in the Navy, then enrolled in the University of Washington Law School. After getting his degree in
the summer of 1968, he went to work for Ehrlichman's law firm. After Nixon
was elected, Ehrlichman asked Krogh to come to work for him in Washington.
Just months out of law school, Krogh was on his way to the White House.

Like many Nixon aides, Krogh was young and inexperienced, but he had
an aptitude for grasping the nub of a problem, then finding the right people to
solve it. The objective was to get results, not pursue an agenda. When, for
instance, the United States was hit by a rash of airplane hijackings, Krogh was
given the job of stopping them. While some politicians favored calling out the

military, Krogh put together a more measured series of steps, including the installation of metal detectors in airports, and the problem was soon brought under control.

In addition to all his other responsibilities, Krogh served as the White House's liaison to the District of Columbia. And so, when John Ehrlichman was ordered by Nixon to bring down the city's crime rate, it was natural for him to look to his young aide. Krogh knew nothing about crime, but he characteristically embarked on a crash course. "I rode around town in squad cars to see with my own eyes the kinds of things we could support the police with," he recalled. Working closely with Jerry Wilson, he helped step up recruiting efforts for the department, procured a helicopter for its use, and had sodium-vapor lights installed on the city's streets.

The more Krogh looked into the District's crime problem, however, the more he realized he would have to tackle its drug problem. Like most other large cities, D.C. was being overrun by heroin addicts. Under orders from Wilson, the police were making more drug arrests, but Krogh worried that such actions, by driving up the price of heroin, would cause addicts to commit even more crimes. And so he began investigating what might be done about them.

To that point, Krogh's involvement with the drug issue had been limited to the international side. With the White House seeking to break the French Connection, Krogh had been placed in charge of the effort. In late 1969, he had gone to Paris to see what the French were doing about the Marseilles heroin labs. Not much, he was told by the U.S. ambassador, Arthur Watson. The French, Watson said, regarded drugs as an American problem and so felt little need to act. Meeting with French officials, Krogh stressed that relations between the two nations would suffer if stronger measures were not taken. Even more troubling to Krogh were the internecine battles taking place between Customs and BNDD. In France, as in the rest of the world, the two agencies were so busy fighting one another that they had little energy left for the traffickers, and Krogh, back in Washington, had to work endlessly to patch up their differences. All the while, he was consulting with U.S. officials in Ankara, exploring ways of convincing the Turks to curtail local opium production.

Now, in addition to fighting the drug trade abroad, Krogh was having to confront it at home, too. Gradually nudging aside Bud Wilkinson (who eventually left the White House in frustration), Krogh began asking Jeff Donfeld about his research, and the young lawyer eagerly shared his findings on methadone and its seemingly miraculous ability to reduce drug-related crime.

Krogh also sought out a local treatment expert named Robert DuPont. Few people in the District knew more about heroin addicts than the tall, gangly, sandy-haired psychiatrist. A graduate of the Harvard Medical School, DuPont had come to Washington in 1966 to work at the National Institutes of

Health, then had gone on to counsel inmates at the D.C. Department of Corrections. From his sessions with those inmates, DuPont became convinced of the close connection between drugs and crime, and, seeking corroboration, he hired a team of researchers to interview inmates. Of the two hundred interviewed, fully 45 percent were found to be heroin users—strong evidence of the drug-crime link. Interested in how other cities were dealing with their heroin problems, DuPont went to Chicago to meet with Jerome Jaffe and see his multimodality system in action. Back in D.C., he convinced Mayor Walter Washington to let him set up a pilot version of that system, and in the fall of 1969 methadone for the first time became available in the nation's capital.

In early 1970, DuPont met with Krogh at his grand, high-ceilinged office at the OEOB. A man of missionary-like exuberance, DuPont (no relation to the Delaware family) gushingly described the success he was having with methadone, especially in reducing crime. When Krogh asked if he would like to expand his program, DuPont immediately said yes, and Krogh quickly found the necessary funds. On February 19, 1970, the Narcotics Treatment Administration (NTA) opened its doors. Like the Illinois Drug Abuse Program, it offered not only methadone but a variety of treatments. And, like IDAP, it was immediately swamped with applicants. With the White House's backing, the NTA soon had more than 2,000 slots.

Krogh closely monitored the results. "The District of Columbia became a laboratory in my mind," he recalled, "a place where we could put more funding into treatment and see what happened." If crime went down in the District, then a case might be made for expanding treatment nationally. "The administration's emphasis had been so overwhelmingly on the law-enforcement side," Krogh said, "that I concluded that if we could get a substantial portion of the addict population into some kind of treatment program, where they would have a chance to function and not be driven to commit street crimes, that would be a very important contribution to the law-enforcement side." For the first time, a U.S. official was thinking of the drug problem in terms of both supply and demand.

To get a sense of what a national treatment system might look like, Krogh sent Jeff Donfeld on a tour of programs. On June 9 and 10, Donfeld visited a half-dozen facilities in New York, including Daytop Village, Phoenix House, and a methadone clinic. From there, he went to Chicago—a trip he had long anticipated. "I had been traveling around the country," he recalled, "talking with program directors and experts in the field, and all roads seemed to lead to Jerry Jaffe as the brightest, most respected guy in the field." Jaffe spent the better part of a day showing Donfeld his handiwork.

Brimming with impressions, Donfeld summarized them in a tart sixteen-page memo to Krogh. Noting at the outset that "drug rehabilitation is a virgin, yet fertile area for social and political gain," Donfeld was nonetheless dismissive of most of the programs he'd seen. "With one exception," he wrote, "personnel of each program had something disparaging to say of another program, ostensibly because they are all competing for the same dollar but probably because each is a very parochial zealot believing that his program is the true panacea."

The one exception was IDAP. "Jaffe was the most impressive man I met on the trip because he was not a dogmátist, he thinks in broad management terms, is politically sensitive and recognizes that modalities must be meticulously evaluated in order to empirically determine success," Donfeld observed. He wrote enthusiastically of IDAP's numerous innovations, including Tinley Park ("it is not the intense, moralistic, rigid approach of Daytop"), the use of computers to collect data, and the reliance on epidemiological data to locate new treatment sites. Donfeld also praised Jaffe's personal style, noting that he "maintained a low profile from day one. He always made sure he could deliver more than he promised."

As for IDAP's core feature—the multimodality approach—Donfeld was more cynical. "Different strokes for different folks," he flippantly called it. Narrowly focused on the need to reduce crime, Donfeld was interested in just one modality. "Methadone," he wrote, "is a benign addiction for it allows the addict to function normally, be employed, pay taxes and stay out of jail. The choice is between methadone addiction and death for some addicts, imprisonment for many more and a crime infected society."

Donfeld's memo was reinforced by the reports Krogh was getting from Bob DuPont. In one four-month period, only 2.6 percent of those enrolled in his program had been arrested, compared with 26 percent of those who had tried to become abstinent and 50 percent of those who had dropped out. Summing up these results in a memo to Ehrlichman, Krogh wrote that DuPont's progress "gives us some assurance" that the idea "to go forward with development of a nation-wide addict treatment policy is correct."

Krogh's enthusiasm for methadone was certainly ironic. As a student of Christian Science who abstained from alcohol and tobacco, he could have been expected to shun a highly addictive substance like methadone. From a pragmatic standpoint, however, the narcotic seemed to offer a way out of the administration's crime predicament, and, with the 1972 election looming, Krogh stepped up his campaign to win White House approval for a national treatment system with methadone at its core.

To do that, he had to win over John Ehrlichman. A practicing Christian Scientist, Ehrlichman felt far more constrained by his beliefs than Krogh. Because of them, he recalled, "I kind of recused myself from health issues." In the case of methadone, he added, "I felt incompetent to make a judgment on physiological questions of that kind."

As a step toward winning Ehrlichman over, Krogh convinced him to set up a task force to study the feasibility of a national treatment program. The group would consist of representatives from eight federal agencies and be chaired by Dr. Bertram Brown, the director of the National Institute of Mental Health. A thirty-nine-year-old Brooklyn-born psychiatrist, Brown was a natural to head such a group. NIMH was the government's lead agency in providing drug treatment, and Brown—a one-time aide to President Kennedy—was well regarded in the largely liberal mental-health field.

Krogh was dubious, however. For NIMH had shown little interest in the plight of drug addicts. The hundreds of community mental health centers it ran across the country seemed more interested in helping middle-class neurotics than inner-city junkies. Moreover, NIMH, with its psychiatric orientation, could be expected to shun a pharmacological agent like methadone.

In light of this, Krogh persuaded Ehrlichman to set up a parallel panel of experts from outside the government. And, to head it, he wanted Jerome Jaffe. Donfeld was sent to recruit him, and the two met in New York in late October. The White House, Donfeld told Jaffe, wanted him to assemble a group of experts to suggest what the government should be doing in the area of drug treatment. The report could not exceed one hundred pages, had to be completed in four weeks, and had to be kept strictly confidential.

As a registered Democrat, Jaffe felt in a quandary. "I was far more conservative than the average psychiatrist, but not enough to think that I should be a Republican, God forbid," he recalled. But, presented with an opportunity to affect national drug policy, he felt obligated to accept Donfeld's offer. Concerned that four weeks was not enough time to produce a quality report, however, he coaxed an additional two weeks out of Donfeld, and the deal was done.

Back in Chicago, Jaffe began calling around to some of his colleagues to ask them to join the project. It was a tough sell. Opposition to the war in Vietnam was at its peak, and few people in the public-health field wanted to be associated with Richard Nixon. Appealing to their sense of history, however, Jaffe managed to put together a stellar eleven-person team, including Dr. Jonathan Cole, the superintendent of Boston State Hospital, and Edward Brecher, a noted science writer who was in the process of completing his landmark book *Licit and Illicit Drugs*. Over the next month, the group would gather on three weekends to discuss what should go into the report. When it was time to write it, Jaffe tethered himself to the dining room table in his house, and, with editing and typing help from Faith, rushed to complete it. Finishing two days before Christmas, he sent off the 134-page manuscript to Donfeld by special courier.

Meanwhile, the government task force was completing its own report. Ignoring the White House's request for a broad interagency study, Bert Brown —a canny, stiff-necked man—had assigned a handful of NIMH aides to draft it, and the finished product faithfully reflected the NIMH view of the world. Praising traditional psychotherapy, the report said that creating systems "for delivering psychiatric care to drug abusers should have high priority" in any national treatment program. As Krogh had feared, the report expressed strong doubts about methadone, chiding public officials for their "pell-mell rush to get thousands of addicts on the drug without due consideration of the possible long-term consequences." Full of hip sixties-style sociologizing, the 119-page report called the extent of the drug problem in America "relatively small" and said the response to it "should probably be titrated to the need rather than the outcry." Accordingly, the report stated, any growth in spending should be "moderate" and any programs undertaken "experimental" in nature.

The Jaffe report, by contrast, termed heroin addiction a serious national problem that required bold government action. Questioning the effectiveness of psychiatry, the document stated that "for half a century, attempts have been made to treat narcotics addiction (as well as alcoholism) through various forms of psychotherapy, and even therapists themselves are almost unanimously agreed that the addictive states are peculiarly resistive to this approach." Methadone, it went on, showed far more promise. While duly noting the drug's drawbacks, the report asserted that studies of it had "uniformly indicated that significant numbers of hard-core heroin users can be changed to law-abiding, job-holding, non-heroin using citizens." The report called for spending $15 million over two years to create 15,000 new methadone slots, as well as for setting up IDAP-type systems in cities without existing programs.

After the many exhausting weeks of work, Jaffe eagerly awaited the White House's response. It came on January 6, 1971, in the form of a two-paragraph note from Richard Nixon thanking him for his "diligent leadership" in preparing the report. Other than that, Jaffe heard little, and, concluding that his handiwork had been consigned to some storage bin, he turned his attention back to his work in Chicago.

Bud Krogh was in fact distracted in this period. On the morning of December 21, 1970, Elvis Presley had suddenly appeared at the northwest gate of the White House with a handwritten note requesting a meeting with the president to offer his help in fighting drugs. Since this was Krogh's area, he was asked to handle the matter. Having grown up listening to Elvis, Krogh was thrilled at the possibility of meeting him, and, calling the president's office, he quickly arranged a meeting between the two men for twelve-thirty that afternoon. Presley showed up wearing tight dark-velvet pants, a matching cape, a flouncy white shirt open to below the chest, and a gold medallion hanging from his neck. Krogh ushered him into the Oval Office, then stood to one side and took notes as Presley showed Nixon photos of his wife and daughter, denounced the Beatles for being "anti-American," and described how he had been studying "Communist brainwashing" and the "drug culture." Then, getting at what seemed the real purpose of his visit, he asked the president if he could help him get a badge from the narcotics bureau to add to his collection. "Bud, can we get him a badge?" Nixon asked his young aide. Krogh said he thought he could, and, escorting the singer back to his office, procured for him the coveted credential. To Krogh's disappointment, Elvis never did follow up on his offer to help the administration fight drugs.

In terms of dazzle, the Jaffe report could not quite compare, but when Krogh finally got around to it, he found it exciting in its own right. A "seminal document," he would later call it. The report took on added significance when the FBI released its crime stats for 1970. While the nation's crime rate had increased by 11 percent, Washington's had fallen by 5.2 percent—the first decline in the capital in years. In interviews, Chief Jerry Wilson and other city officials cited a host of factors, among them the increased size of the police force, the use of more aggressive tactics—and the growing availability of drug treatment. By the end of 1970, the Narcotics Treatment Administration was treating more than 2,500 people, and, as the FBI figures showed, most of the reduction in crime occurred after the NTA had become fully operational.

The results from Krogh's D.C. lab removed any remaining doubts he had about the need for a national treatment system. Hoping to prod the White House, he asked Donfeld to draft an options paper for the president's top domestic advisers. Sitting down with both the Jaffe and Brown reports, Donfeld extracted the key recommendations of each and summarized them side by side, accompanied by pithy commentaries of his own. On methadone, he noted that, while many important philosophical and political issues remained to be worked out, "in 1972, citizens will be looking at crime statistics across the nation in order to see whether expectations raised in 1968 have been met. The federal government has only one economical and effective technique for reducing crime in the streets—methadone maintenance."

Interestingly, John Mitchell, the attorney general, was open to the idea of expanding methadone. Elliot Richardson, the secretary of health, education, and welfare, was not. A large-scale methadone program, he wrote in reply to Donfeld's memo, "may court potential disaster. We would be forced into a posture of pushing this program without the support of a generally accepted consensus of scientific knowledge and in the face of the judgments of our professional advisers." Richardson expressed support for a $60 million increase in funding for treatment and prevention, with a small portion earmarked for a scientific evaluation of methadone's effectiveness.

The $60 million figure struck Krogh as reasonable, but, unless a generous share of it went for methadone, he believed, the desired payoff in crime reduction would not occur. To resolve the issue, Krogh arranged for a showdown on April 28, 1971, in John Ehrlichman's office. Attending were John Mitchell, Elliot Richardson, Bert Brown, Krogh, and Donfeld. It pitted the young but self-confident Donfeld against the regal Richardson and the bulldog Brown. "It was exhilarating, being up against those renowned people," Donfeld recalled. "They were advocating the psychotherapy-TC modality. I was advocating this substitute addiction that I felt would help address what was perceived to be a major problem in the United States. And Ehrlichman listened."

By the end of the meeting, all had agreed that the administration should be doing more on drug treatment, but the methadone issue remained unresolved, and Ehrlichman, engrossed in other issues, put off a final decision.

THERE MATTERS would probably have rested had it not been for the actions of two members of the House Foreign Affairs Committee—Robert Steele, a Republican from Connecticut, and Morgan Murphy, a Democrat from Illinois. In April 1971, the two congressmen went to South Vietnam to investigate reports of growing heroin addiction among U.S. troops there. According to the press, Vietnam had been flooded with cheap, 95-percent-pure heroin from the Golden Triangle region of Laos, Thailand, and Burma. "Drugs," *Time* stated, "are rapidly becoming as great a threat to American forces as the enemy."

On April 29, Steele, back from his trip, visited the White House to brief Bud Krogh and General Alexander Haig, deputy director of the National Security Council. Based on his interviews, the congressman said, he believed that 10 to 15 percent of all GIs in Vietnam were addicted to heroin, with as many as 25 percent in some units. And it was not just the war effort that was at stake. With the United States withdrawing 1,000 troops a day from Vietnam, many addicts were already on their way home, bringing with them their craving for drugs and experience with guns.

Krogh was not surprised by Steele's figures. He had visited Vietnam the year before and seen how widely drugs were used there. After a long period of having denied the problem, the Pentagon was now cracking down on it, stepping up interdiction efforts and importing dope-sniffing dogs. Soldiers caught using drugs were subject to arrest and court-martial. The main effect, however, had been to clog the military justice system without doing much to reduce consumption.

Clearly, something had to be done, and for advice Krogh turned to the man who seemed most knowledgeable about drugs. After months of hearing nothing from the White House, Jerome Jaffe in early May 1971 was summoned to Washington to discuss the GI drug problem. Jaffe had been nowhere near Vietnam, but, hearing Krogh's description, he made some inferences based on his own experiences in Chicago. While Steele and others were talking about tens of thousands of *addicts* in Vietnam, Jaffe assumed that the heroin-using population there was more diverse, including also new users as well as people in the process of becoming dependent. The key was to find a way to prevent the dabblers from becoming addicts, and to break the addicts of their habits. From Krogh's remarks, it seemed clear that the military's harsh approach was not working. The pace of military justice was too slow, and the penalties too remote. "It seemed self-evident that a small but certain consequence would change behavior more than a catastrophic but highly unlikely one," Jaffe observed. "And what might such a consequence be? You can't get on the plane." GIs were so desperate to leave Vietnam, Jaffe reasoned, that the idea of delaying their departure by even a few days could provide a powerful deterrent.

Earlier in the year, Jaffe, attending a conference in Toronto, had learned of a new process, called FRAT (Free Radical Assay Technique), that allowed for assembly-line-like urine testing, and he had ordered one of the machines for use in Chicago. If such a device was used in Vietnam, Jaffe said, soldiers could be tested as they prepared to board the plane to return home. Those who tested positive would be subject not to imprisonment or court-martial but to a mandatory stay in Vietnam of two weeks or so to be detoxed. As word of the testing spread, Jaffe said, many of those not yet addicted would probably stop on their own so as not to delay their departure. If the White House wanted, Jaffe said, he would be happy to sign over use of his machine.

Listening to his proposal, Krogh could see some immediate problems. For one thing, it would require the Pentagon to *reduce* the penalties for drug use—something it was loath to do. Civil libertarians, meanwhile, would surely object to the procedure on privacy grounds. But the idea had one undeniable merit—it might actually work. Sending Jaffe back to Chicago to await further word, Krogh sent a seven-page memo to Ehrlichman urging him to proceed on the drug issue. Referring to the "Vietnam and DoD Powderkeg," Krogh wrote that "addicted veterans must get treatment but Defense and the V.A. cannot agree on who has responsibility for these people. As a consequence, over-burdened treatment programs in the U.S. are sinking with additional veteran junkies." He added:

> The President, on many occasions, has declared that solutions to problems of drug abuse have no higher priority in his Administration. But the reality is that much more needs to be done to bring about substantively effective programs in rehabilitation, prevention and research. Law enforcement and diplomatic overtures to other countries —Turkey, France, and Mexico—have been effective, but more here needs to be done. Bluntly, Mitchell has taken his job a lot more seriously than Richardson and Bertram Brown have taken theirs.

Krogh went on to urge creation of a new agency within HEW to be headed by Jaffe, "the undisputed leader in America in narcotic addict treatment programs."

Ehrlichman continued to stall. But the Vietnam issue would not go away. G.I. HEROIN ADDICTION EPIDEMIC IN VIETNAM, the *New York Times* declared on its front page on May 16. Shortly thereafter, Congressman Steele scheduled a press conference to release his report on Vietnam. The White House's nervousness was apparent in a memo to Krogh from White House aide Donald Rumsfeld:

I called Congressman Steele Monday before his Tuesday press conference with the thought that it might moderate anything he might
say against the Administration. He was friendly and indicated that he
would be interested in cooperating with the Administration on any
legislative initiatives, if he agrees with them, obviously. One specific
thing he mentioned was the possibility of some legislation to deal
with returning veterans who are drug addicts.

Steele's report was blunt. If drug use continued to spread among the troops in
Vietnam, it stated, "the only solution" would be "to withdraw American servicemen from Southeast Asia."

With the drug problem threatening to undermine the administration's
Vietnam policy, Ehrlichman finally decided to act. On May 26, he and Krogh
asked H. R. Haldeman for a meeting with the president, and two days later
they were brought in to brief him on the drug proposal. Krogh was well aware
of what he was up against. While Nixon had spoken only sporadically about
the drug issue, his comments were invariably fierce. Heroin traffickers, he
believed, deserved the heaviest possible penalties, including death. Marijuana,
meanwhile, stood for everything that was wrong with the country. For Nixon,
"marijuana was part of a larger tapestry," John Ehrlichman recalled. "The
people who were demonstrating against what he was doing in Vietnam, the
wearing of long hair, and the smoking of dope were all part of a picture. These
were people he had no use for."

Yet, as with China and the environment, Nixon's ideological convictions
on drugs were tempered by a strong dose of pragmatism. While helping to
build up the Bureau of Narcotics and Dangerous Drugs, for instance, Nixon
had few illusions about its effectiveness. Krogh recalled a White House meeting at which John Ingersoll, the bureau's director, briefed the president on its
achievements: "Ingersoll told Nixon that seizures of heroin were up, arrests
were up, more investigations were under way. He just laid out a whole list of
operational indices of success. The president then said, 'Let me ask you this,
are we taking one step forward and two steps back? Is there any less narcotics
coming into the United States? Are we solving the problem?' And there was
just silence."

Such silences left Nixon open to a new approach. And, at the May 28
meeting, Krogh briefed him on the heroin situation and the threat it posed to
the administration, both in Vietnam and urban America. Already overwhelmed
with junkies, the nation's treatment facilities faced the prospect of dealing with
thousands of returning vets, he said. Krogh went on to describe his meetings
with Jerome Jaffe and his imaginative scheme for dealing with the GI drug
problem. Krogh also mentioned his idea of creating a new federal agency to
set up treatment programs nationwide, an initiative that, he said, might help
reduce crime.

Listening intently, Nixon immediately saw the appeal of Krogh's proposal. By setting up a new agency to deal with the drug problem as a whole, he could divert some of the attention being paid to the situation in Vietnam. In the process, he could be seen as acting dramatically to confront a serious social problem threatening the nation's young. Ehrlichman's shorthand notes of the meeting captured the president's thinking:

> Handle so we get Jaffe for Narc generally,
> not vets or the war— . . .
> Use by younger people
> Then, subsidiary, hit vets . . .
> Highest level—
> Π [Ehrlichman's symbol for the president] setting up new org—not
>   just vets . . .
> $120 MM
> Get it out of NIMH

This last notation showed that even Nixon was aware of the NIMH situation. The president wanted a dynamic new agency, headed by the outsider Jaffe. And, in agreeing to set up such an agency, Nixon was implicitly approving a government role in dispensing methadone.

Without telling him what was afoot, Krogh called Jaffe back to Washington on May 30 for further consultation on Vietnam. As expected, the Defense Department was balking at the drug-testing scheme. A briefing had been scheduled at the Pentagon, and Donfeld and Jaffe—already an hour late— hurried over. Expecting to meet with a few researchers, Jaffe instead found himself in a room full of generals and admirals irritated at having been kept waiting. Introduced as a consultant to the president, Jaffe described his idea for reducing drug use through urine testing. The generals sourly responded that, given the complex logistics of bringing the troops home, ordering them to provide urine specimens was out of the question. "I cannot believe," Jaffe bluntly replied, "that the mightiest army on earth can't get its troops to piss in a bottle." Perhaps something could be in place by September, the generals said. Losing patience, Jaffe snapped, "Gentlemen, the White House wants something done about the problem a little sooner than that, and I feel certain that I can find a few civilians who will be willing to aid me in getting this effort under way. If you will help me make transportation arrangements and will bring me a phone I will make a few calls." Taken aback, the officers took a brief recess, then reluctantly pledged their cooperation.

Krogh, who had dealt with the military on countless occasions, was startled when told of Jaffe's performance. Only someone unschooled in the ways of Washington could have acted so nervily in the face of so much brass. The meeting reinforced Krogh's notion that a nonbureaucrat like Jaffe should head the new treatment agency he had in mind, and that he should be able to invoke the authority of the president.

Jaffe was told none of this, however, and a week later he was called back to Washington. Only after arriving was he told that he was to see the president. "If I'd known I was going to meet him, I would have dressed better," Jaffe recalled with a laugh. "I was wearing a shleppy wash-and-wear suit and a psychedelic tie that one of my daughters had given me. And I would have gotten a haircut. I had sideburns almost down to my jaw." Arriving at the Oval Office with Krogh and Donfeld, he found waiting for him Ehrlichman, Haldeman, and, of course, the president. Awestruck at being in the White House, Jaffe collected himself enough to describe his plan for dealing with drug use in Vietnam. Nixon was more interested in the domestic aspects of the problem. According to Donfeld's notes of the meeting, Nixon raised the subject of methadone, asking if it "was worse than heroin." Jaffe described the success he was having with the substance in Illinois, with a 40 percent reduction in crime observed among those using it. For a national program, Jaffe went on, the goal should be "to make treatment available to all heroin addicts so that no one had to commit a crime to support a habit because they cannot get treatment."

Giving vent to his dour opinion of the bureaucracy, Nixon stressed the need to bring in people "from outside of the government to help run the program" and to inject "a sense of urgency." "The President," Donfeld wrote, "said that no one's feelings should be spared and that he wants this agency to have terrific clout. The President wants the Department of Health, Education and Welfare to be shaken up, he wants budgets cut and government hacks fired. . . ."

As the session was drawing to a close, Jaffe casually mentioned some research being done on an insect that ate poppy plants. Perking up, Nixon got on the phone to Secretary of Agriculture Clifford Hardin and asked him about a drug-eating insect he had heard of that was bred in such a way as to ensure its own destruction. Hardin had no idea what he was talking about. Putting the phone down, Nixon noted that the insect "died after intercourse," which led one member of the group to crack that it should be called the "screw-worm." And on that surreal note the meeting broke up.

Still in the dark, Jaffe returned to Chicago. Meanwhile, Krogh was putting the finishing touches on the new treatment office. He was also stepping up the campaign against the French Connection. As a result of his prodding, the French government had agreed to add dozens of agents to its antinarcotics squad, and they were pursuing the Corsican traffickers with new vigor. In Turkey, a new government had been installed by the military earlier in the year, and, fearful of losing U.S. military aid, it seemed receptive to the idea of curtailing local poppy cultivation. To increase the pressure, Krogh arranged for the U.S. ambassadors to Turkey, France, and other heroin-producing nations to come to Washington and meet with the president. At the meeting, Nixon stressed his determination to secure the Turks' cooperation and said that, to get it, he was willing to pay them up to $50 million in compensation.

On June 17, Krogh called Jaffe back to Washington. Showing up at his office, Jaffe was immediately led into the Cabinet Room in the White House, where Nixon was meeting with a bipartisan group of congressmen. While Jaffe watched, Nixon announced that he was mounting a major new offensive against drug use and, to lead it, was creating a new Special Action Office for Drug Abuse Prevention, with Jaffe in charge. As Jaffe later recalled, the statement "left me too shocked to say to the president that no one had asked me."

At the end of the two-hour session, Nixon escorted Jaffe to the press room in the West Wing of the White House, where he announced that he was declaring drug abuse "public enemy number one in the United States." "In order to fight and defeat this enemy," he stated, "it is necessary to wage a new, all-out offensive." To underwrite the effort, Nixon went on, he was requesting $155 million in new funds, of which $105 million would go for treating and rehabilitating addicts. Nixon added:

> I very much hesitate always to bring some new responsibility into the White House, because there are so many here, and I believe in delegating those responsibilities to the departments. But I consider this problem so urgent—I also found that it was scattered so much throughout the government, with so much conflict, without coordination—that it had to be brought into the White House. Consequently, I have brought Dr. Jaffe into the White House, directly reporting to me.

And so, for the first time in U.S. history, a president had declared war on drugs. And Richard Nixon, the apostle of law and order, was going to make treatment his principal weapon. As his general, he was enlisting a young Jewish Democratic psychiatrist with no experience in national politics. And so, at the age of thirty-seven, Jerome Jaffe was going to get a chance to apply to the nation as a whole the lessons he had learned during his long apprenticeship in Lexington, New York, and Chicago.

9

The Great Experiment

To HOUSE the new Special Action Office for Drug Abuse Prevention (SAODAP), Bud Krogh had obtained one of the colonial townhouses that lined Jackson Place, on the west side of Lafayette Square, just across from the White House. Elegant brick structures with electrified gas lamps out front, the Jackson Place townhouses were reserved for high-priority projects, and the White House's decision to locate the new drug office in one of them showed the importance it was attaching to the new drug offensive. As Jaffe recalled, "This was the first time in fifty years that people had said, 'Let's really try to make a commitment to reducing demand, rather than suppressing supply.' I believed that an opportunity like this would come once in a lifetime."

He had little time to savor the moment, however. According to a June 1971 Gallup poll, Americans considered drugs the nation's third-most-serious problem, behind Vietnam and the economy. In New York City, nearly a hundred people were dying of drug-related causes every month, while in Detroit seven people were gunned down in a gangland-style war the same week SAODAP was created. And now thousands of heroin addicts from Vietnam were on their way home. "Each returned planeload of G.I.s adds to the drug malaise at home," *Time* declared.

From the start, Jaffe was clear about his priorities. In terms of sheer numbers, marijuana was the most widely used illegal drug in the country, and public officials from the president on down were loudly denouncing it. Jaffe was not among them. From his clinical work, he knew that most people who used marijuana did not become dependent on it, nor did they suffer serious health problems. Heroin, by contrast, was highly addictive, generated much crime, and caused frequent overdoses. No one knew how many heroin addicts there were in the country—estimates ranged from 250,000 to 600,000—but

Jaffe believed they constituted the heart of the nation's drug problem, and that treatment was the best way to deal with them. At the time, virtually every large city had long waiting lists, and getting rid of them became Jaffe's top goal.

The obstacles he faced were tremendous. With so few people in the government experienced in drug treatment, he would have to build SAODAP (pronounced SAY-oh-dap) from scratch. Even as work crews were carting in furniture and secretaries were appearing out of the woodwork, Jaffe was calling around to friends and colleagues, trying to persuade them to come to work for Richard Nixon. That task was made all the more difficult by the rumors swirling around the mental-health field. "It is plain that the shots will be called, not by Dr. Jaffe, but by Nixon and Atty. Gen. John Mitchell," one newsletter stated, adding that some observers "are accusing Jaffe of selling his scientific credentials to the highest bidder."

Within the government itself, meanwhile, responsibility for the drug issue was divided among fourteen different agencies. In the past, each was accustomed to setting its own agenda; now all were expected to take orders from an unknown physician heading an untested office. And, legally, that office didn't even exist yet. On June 17, the White House had sent an authorization bill to Congress, and both houses—controlled by Democrats with their own ideas about drug policy—were spoiling for a fight.

All of these concerns, however, were overshadowed by Vietnam. SAODAP had been created largely because of the GI drug crisis, and if Jaffe failed to resolve it, nothing else would matter. While in Chicago, he had arranged for the FRAT urinalysis machines to be flown in cargo planes to Vietnam and installed at the military bases at Long Binh and Cam Ranh Bay, the two main points for soldiers departing the country, or "DEROSing" ("date of expected return from overseas"). At midnight on June 17, the military announced that all returning servicemen would be tested for drugs immediately prior to their departure for the United States. Those who tested positive were to be kept in-country for seven days to detox; once free of drugs, they were to be transported to the United States and referred to a VA or DoD treatment center. To facilitate the program, Secretary of Defense Melvin Laird issued a memo stating that anyone testing positive for drugs would not be subject to disciplinary action under the Uniform Code of Military Justice. With a stroke of the pen, the Nixon Administration had effectively decriminalized drug use within the military.

With many questions remaining in the program, however, the White House wanted Jaffe to take a firsthand look. And so, on July 6—his thirty-eighth birthday—he left for Vietnam. He was accompanied by a handful of aides, including Jeff Donfeld and Dr. Beny Primm, the director of a methadone program in Brooklyn. In Saigon, the group was to be met by Bud Krogh, who had left Washington two weeks earlier on an around-the-world tour of narcotics-producing nations.

Krogh's trip went well. In Paris, he found French officials in a newly receptive mood, owing to reports in the French press about the growing heroin problem at home, and he was taken to see heroin labs that had been seized in southern France. In Turkey, Krogh, working with Ambassador Arthur Hadley, helped put the finishing touches on a deal in which the Turks agreed to ban all poppy production beginning in the summer of 1972, in return for $35 million in U.S. aid. After stopping in Lebanon and India for briefings with the U.S. ambassadors there, Krogh went on to Thailand and Burma, where, working with CIA agents, he organized a clandestine campaign to attack opium caravans as they descended from the highlands of the Golden Triangle.

Arriving in Vietnam, the ever-energetic Krogh set off on a one-man fact-finding tour. From the DMZ in the north to Bac Lieu province in the south, he hopscotched the country in a Huey helicopter, interviewing officers and enlisted men about the prevalence of drug use among the troops. Heroin, he recalled, "was not a problem—it was a *condition*. It was not everywhere, but it was sufficiently available so that to think that the military was going to stop it by interdiction was crazy."

When Jaffe and his party arrived, Krogh went to the airport to greet them. Jaffe, who had gotten sick on the plane ride over and would battle a fever throughout his four-day stay, nonetheless managed to attend scheduled briefings with Ambassador Ellsworth Bunker and General Creighton Abrams and to visit the two DEROSing sites. They were real eye-openers. Soldiers preparing to leave for the United States were being led into cramped tents and told to pee into a bottle. The bottles were then transported in giant wooden trays to the FRAT machine, a long metal contraption that resembled a desk with control panels. Within thirty seconds of receiving a specimen, the machine would spit out a reading as to whether the provider had used opiates within the previous seventy-two hours. Those testing positive were escorted to the detox area, a barbed-wire enclosure in which they were forced to go cold turkey in 110-degree heat. In all his years in the drug field, Jaffe had never seen anything quite so primitive. He was further troubled by reports that soldiers were paying supervisors hundreds of dollars for clean urines. The FRATs themselves seemed to be producing numerous false positives. Obviously, many kinks remained to be worked out.

As the delegation prepared to leave, however, it got some good news. Of the 22,000 servicemen tested to that point, about 4.5 percent had been confirmed positive for opiates, a rate well below the 10 to 15 percent cited by Steele and Murphy. On their return journey, Jaffe, Krogh, and Primm on July 17 stopped by the western White House in San Clemente to brief the president. Joined by John Ehrlichman, the group sat around a white patio table in the estate's sunlit garden. Uncharacteristically upbeat, Jaffe told Nixon that the progress in Vietnam had been "remarkable" and that a key factor was the president's "very clear message that no punitive action is going to be taken against men who seek treatment for a drug problem or who accept treatment after we've detected it on the basis of these tests." Visibly pleased, Nixon said that it was "quite clear" that "the problem's been blown up far greater than it actually is."

After the briefing was over, Ehrlichman asked Krogh back to his office for a private chat. The previous month, the *New York Times* had published excerpts from the Pentagon Papers, and Nixon and Kissinger—still furious—wanted to know more about Daniel Ellsberg, the man responsible for leaking them. Krogh, Ehrlichman said, seemed just the person for the job. Handing him a file on the case, Ehrlichman recommended that he read Nixon's book *Six Crises,* especially the chapter on Alger Hiss. Krogh, ever loyal, duly accepted the assignment.

On the car ride from San Clemente to the airport in San Diego, Jaffe recalled, Krogh "seemed very serious. He said, 'I have a very important assignment.'" Jaffe gave the matter little thought, however, for, back in Washington, he had a thousand details to attend to in connection with Operation Golden Flow, as the military had nicknamed the Vietnam program. Among other things, he wanted to institute better safeguards against cheating and to upgrade the detox centers. Contacting his colleague Matt Wright in Chicago, Jaffe arranged for him to assemble a team of IDAP graduates and fly to Vietnam to train detox counselors. At home, meanwhile, Jaffe was pushing the VA to create a network of facilities to treat returning addicts. At every point, however, he was meeting resistance, and to overcome it he would seek Krogh's support.

Krogh was leading a strangely bifurcated life that summer. On the one hand, he was energetically carrying out the assignment he had been given in San Clemente. Summoning Krogh to the White House, Nixon fumed that the administration was drowning in leaks, and that he wanted Krogh to plug them. In response, Krogh commandeered Room 16 in the Old Executive Office Building and set up a special investigations unit. To help run it, he brought over a gung-ho aide from the Treasury Department named G. Gordon Liddy. Krogh had worked with Liddy on both narcotics and gun-control matters, and while many found him overly zealous, Krogh admired his verve and self-confidence. Joining Liddy were a former CIA agent named E. Howard Hunt and a Kissinger aide named David Young.

The Plumbers Unit was born. Coming under its influence, the normally straight-arrow Krogh found himself contemplating all sorts of extralegal schemes, including one to obtain the psychiatric files of Daniel Ellsberg. In August, Krogh would give Liddy and Hunt permission to break into the Beverly Hills office of Ellsberg's psychiatrist, Dr. Lewis Fielding. The job was carried out by Cuban operatives over the Labor Day weekend. They found nothing on Ellsberg, but they did leave behind a huge mess. Trying to make the operation look like the work of a drug addict, the Cubans littered the floor with pills they had found in the office. Shown photos of the scene, Krogh was horrified by the damage and immediately ruled out any more such jobs.

While engrossed in these clandestine matters, Krogh was also tending to Jaffe's pleas for help with the drug offensive. "I was the logjam breaker of last resort," Krogh said. "If Jaffe and his guys couldn't get something done, they would call me up, and my job would be to go to the Cabinet secretary and say, 'This is something the president would probably want.' If that didn't work, I'd go to the president himself and say, 'Here's what we want to do.' And he gave us support almost every time."

By September 1971, Operation Golden Flow was more or less in place, and there was little more Jaffe could do about it other than await the results of the monthly urine screens. Finally, he was able to devote himself to establishing his office. Despite SAODAP's status as an arm of the White House, Jaffe was free to hire whomever he wanted. "I didn't ask people's political affiliation," he observed. "I was concerned only about competence." His deputy director, a former prosecutor named Paul Perito, had helped out on the Kennedy campaign in 1960 and served as chief counsel to Representative Claude Pepper's Select Committee on Crime. Profane and pugilistic, the bantam-sized Perito had risen from Boston's North End to attend Harvard Law School on a scholarship, an accomplishment he was not shy in sharing with others. "On the day I was confirmed," he recalled, "Haldeman came by the office and said, 'You represent the smallest minority group at the White House—an Italian Catholic Democrat who went to Harvard and worked for JFK.'" At SAODAP, Perito noted, "the inner circle was made up of mostly Italian and Jewish Democrats."

The one exception was Jeff Donfeld, who was Jewish but not, of course, Democratic. Krogh assigned him to SAODAP both to work as a liaison with the military and to keep an eye on the office. "Commissar," he was called, after his insistence on knowing the political consequences of every SAODAP act. Still, as a cofounder of the office, Donfeld had a vested interest in making it work. "The White House wanted Donfeld to be its eyes and ears," Perito said, "but we converted him, and he became a good soldier."

Even with his newly enlarged staff, however, Jaffe found himself hamstrung, for the legislation to authorize his office remained stalled in Congress. In the Senate, such prominent Democrats as Edmund Muskie and Harold Hughes were pushing the White House to turn SAODAP into a "superoffice" with control over not only treatment and prevention but also law enforcement. The White House resisted. "We regarded treatment and enforcement as separate missions," Krogh recalled. "On the treatment side, we wanted doctors and lawyers who were really dedicated to helping people who were ill. Lawenforcement people had a different mind-set. If the two groups were working together in the same place, they wouldn't be able to function well."

In the House, meanwhile, Paul Rogers of Florida was pressing the White House to make the National Institute of Mental Health the lead agency for the drug offensive. Given NIMH's preoccupation with middle-class whites, Jaffe was opposed. "We wanted to make sure the new money would go for inner-city addicts," he said. The issue would not go away, however, due to the tireless efforts of Bert Brown. Smarting over losing control of the drug issue, Brown was rallying his friends in the psychiatric community against the new office. Among them were some of Jaffe's closest colleagues. For example, Jonathan Cole of Boston State Hospital, who had sat on Jaffe's White House task force, asserted in a statement to Congress that "consolidation of everything within a single director in a potentially restrictive and totalitarian manner does concern me since it might reduce experimentation and lead to everyone following a party line which may or may not be a productive one."

Daniel X. Freedman was even more outspoken. Freedman, of course, had been instrumental in getting Jaffe involved in drug policy in the first place. But, jealous of his protégé's rapid rise, he had begun spreading vicious rumors about him, claiming that he had sold out to the Nixon Administration and left a mess behind in Illinois. Feeding his ire was a curious incident that occurred at a meeting with Krogh in the Old Executive Office Building. Frustrated over the continued resistance to the SAODAP bill, Krogh heatedly remarked, "Anyone who opposes us, we'll destroy. As a matter of fact, anyone who doesn't support us, we'll destroy." Jaffe, who was present, thought that Krogh was referring to people inside the administration, but Freedman took the remark as a personal threat, and he promptly leaked it to the press, helping to polarize the debate further.

On October 22, 1971, Jaffe—feeling his once-in-a-lifetime opportunity slipping away—vented his exasperation in a three-page memo to Krogh. NIMH, he complained, "has taken advantage of our precarious position" by withholding information and intimidating SAODAP consultants. "In addition," Jaffe wrote, "rumors of lobbying of Congress by NIMH (not in support of the bill) are rampant. It is impossible to tell how much of this is normal resistance and how much, if any, is deliberate undercutting of the President."

Luckily for Jaffe, the head of NIMH's Division of Narcotic Addiction and Drug Abuse was an old friend, Karst Besteman. A stolid fireplug of a man with a large bald head and a deliberate speaking manner, Besteman had spent seven years working at the Lexington narcotics farm, two of them overlapping with Jaffe's time there. He now began paying quiet visits to Jaffe's office to discuss ways of getting treatment dollars into the field quickly. Under standard procedure, the government was supposed to send out requests for proposals and wait for the responses to trickle in, then deliberately review them. To expedite the process, Jaffe and Besteman decided to send representatives into the field to solicit proposals, then subject them to quick review. Besteman recalled spending a day in Detroit briefing officials about what they should be doing in the field. "We had the money, but there was a lot of resistance to going into the drug area," he observed. "People would say, 'You want me to take these people in? They're crooks!' " Eventually, though, Besteman found some willing applicants, and, before long, money was heading to the dope-plagued city.

As long as his office remained in limbo, however, there was a limit to what Jaffe could do. And the White House was growing impatient. In December 1971, Donfeld sent Jaffe a memo stating that "while many of SAODAP activities to date will be of significant long term benefit for the federal effort . . . we are doing little to impact immediately either on the problems at the local level or on the political process. In order to achieve both ends—practical and political impact by November 1972—I suggest targetting significant resources on a number of cities in order to achieve short term results, specifically a demonstrable reduction in crime such as has occurred in Washington, D.C., and Atlanta, Georgia." Appending a list of thirty-one target cities, Donfeld asserted that "programs must be serving clients by June 1972 prior to the summer crime peak."

For Jaffe, it was a time of deep frustration. On the one hand, he was becoming a minor celebrity in Washington. At his office, he was receiving a constant flow of congressmen, foreign officials, and reporters eager to hear about the great Nixon drug offensive. Indulging the White House's interest in enlisting famous names in the antidrug cause, he met with Sammy Davis, Jr., James Brown, and Art Linkletter. On January 20, 1972, the night of the State of the Union address, the Jaffes were invited to a dinner at the White House and seated next to the Nixons.

Whenever possible, however, Jaffe avoided such events. "I always tried to get other people to go," he said. "The task was to make a change." PERLE MESTA HE'S NOT, declared the headline of a magazine profile about him. Arriving at night at the roomy house he and Faith rented in the Virginia suburbs, Jaffe would plant himself at the dining-room table and labor away on briefing papers, congressional testimony, and speeches. With the SAODAP bill still bottled up in Congress, however, he felt as if he were moving in place.

Then, suddenly, the logjam broke. For months, the rate of positive urines in Vietnam had been steadily declining, and in February 1972 it dipped under 2 percent. PROGRESS SEEN IN DRIVE TO CURB GI DRUG USE IN VIETNAM, the *Washington Post* declared. "By far the most important innovation appears to have been the urine test which made it vastly more difficult to take heroin without getting caught," correspondent Peter Osnos wrote.

With the GI drug problem coming under control, the opposition in Congress quickly evaporated, and in mid-March 1972 Congress voted unanimously to pass the authorization bill. Under it, SAODAP was to remain in existence for three years, at which time its duties were to be taken over by a new National Institute on Drug Abuse to be housed within HEW. With the new funding in the legislation, federal spending on treatment and prevention in 1973 would come to $420 million—more than eight times the amount when Nixon took office. In all, demand-side programs were absorbing two-thirds of the federal drug budget, compared to one-third for the supply side—the reverse of what might have been expected from the hawkish Nixon. As Donfeld noted, "It took a law-and-order president to go up against the law-and-order establishment and say, 'Let's give this a try.' "

AT LONG LAST, Jaffe would have the resources and authority he needed to tackle the nation's drug problem. His staff, which over the preceding months had inched up to 65, would quickly expand to 140, most of them housed in the New Executive Office Building, located behind the Jackson Place townhouses. With the election fast approaching, he had less than eight months to achieve his goal of getting rid of the nation's waiting lists. As a first step, he needed to know how many people were actually on those lists, and so in early spring he sent out 100 government inspectors to visit programs across the country. Within weeks, the results were in. The numbers ranged from 5 in Poughkeepsie, New York, and 25 in Atlanta to 1,064 in San Francisco-Oakland, 4,168 in Los Angeles, and a whopping 16,713 in New York City. Overall, an estimated 30,000 addicts were waiting for treatment, in most cases methadone.

Seeking a quick solution, Jaffe again began plotting with Karst Besteman. They ultimately came up with a scheme so sensible and straightforward that no one had ever thought of it before: They would buy up the lists. Using a formula worked out by SAODAP, the government would pay programs a set amount for each person treated. "We had a vision—X number of slots had to be created by the end of the year," Besteman recalled. "And we worked our fannies off to bring it about."

The biggest push came in the cities with the greatest need—New York, for example. In response to the city's pressing heroin problem, Mayor John Lindsay had set up an Addiction Services Agency to provide treatment to addicts. By the spring of 1972, the agency—funded by both the city and the state—was operating thirty-seven methadone clinics serving more than 5,500 people. Thousands more were being helped by the Beth Israel Medical Center, now the largest private provider of methadone in the country. Despite this expansion, hundreds of people were applying for methadone every week, and the wait for a slot in some parts of the city exceeded six months. To address the situation, Jaffe made repeated trips to the city, meeting with the mayor and public-health officials, and before long millions of dollars in federal treatment funds were headed New York's way.

In his drive to expand capacity, Jaffe gained the Nixon Administration some strange bedfellows. One day, for instance, two SAODAP representatives showed up at the Haight-Ashbury Free Medical Clinic in San Francisco. The clinic had been set up in 1967 to minister to the Haight's hippies; by 1971, the flower children had given way to heroin addicts and speed freaks, many with serious medical problems. For support, the clinic had relied on rock benefits organized by Fillmore impresario Bill Graham, but after the bloodshed at the

Rolling Stones' Altamont concert, this was no longer feasible. "We were struggling to keep going," recalled Dr. David Smith, the clinic's director. "And suddenly these government officials appeared," offering support.

The staff was suspicious. "We saw ourselves as a civil rights movement for addicts; the government was putting people in jail," said Smith, a down-to-earth, square-jawed man with an air of earnestness accentuated by his thick-lens glasses. But Smith had met Jaffe on a visit to Chicago and could vouch for his credentials, and so the clinic decided to submit an application. Soon it was receiving hundreds of thousands of dollars in federal aid.

The money did not flow without conditions. If a program had a low retention rate, SAODAP would send in a team to investigate. "We didn't mess around," Karst Besteman recalled. "We'd say, 'We're coming in on Tuesday—have your staff ready.' The program would then be given ninety days to take corrective action." If it didn't, SAODAP would send in auditors from an accounting firm. If the program still didn't respond, SAODAP would oust its director and install a new one. The process was "highly authoritarian," Besteman acknowledged, but it did guarantee a minimum level of care.

Jaffe became so engrossed in his work that he sometimes went whole days without seeing his kids. Jim Gregg, SAODAP's associate director for management, said he would sometimes get calls from Jaffe at five o'clock on a Sunday morning. "He had no sense of time," Gregg observed. "If something crossed his mind, he'd feel at liberty to call at any time of the night or day." Gregg compared working at SAODAP to his experience at NASA in the mid-1960s, when it was seeking to put a man on the moon. "There was a real sense of purpose and mission," he said.

As he carried out that mission, however, Jaffe came under increasing attack. Methadone was the main flashpoint. As the number of methadone clinics increased, the black market in the drug flourished. In some cities, more people were overdosing on methadone than on heroin. THE "CURE" THAT CAN BE A KILLER, declared a headline in the New York Times. "Every time someone sold a dose of methadone illegally, it was a front-page headline," Jaffe observed. "We felt under siege all the time." "The methadone king," he was called.

The label was unfair, for methadone was not the only type of program the Special Action Office was funding. In line with Jaffe's multimodality philosophy, in fact, the office created twice as many slots in drug-free programs as in maintenance ones. And, while the diversion of methadone was undeniably a problem, it paled when compared to the many addicts whose lives it helped stabilize. Diversion itself became less of a problem after the government, under Jaffe's direction, issued regulations to control distribution. Still, Jaffe would continue to be pummeled by editorialists, political activists, and some black leaders.

The attacks from within the government, however, were far sharper. Even after the SAODAP authorization bill passed, the office continued to be harassed by NIMH, with Bert Brown as ever in the lead. NIMH personnel were routinely withholding data from SAODAP, delaying the awarding of contracts, letting projects drag on endlessly. Unless such obstacles were removed, Jaffe felt, the whole drug initiative would be imperiled. The White House agreed. Ever since Brown had hijacked the interagency task force, it had regarded him with suspicion, and, with Jaffe complaining about him nonstop, it was agreed that Brown should go.

During a tennis match at the White House, John Ehrlichman informed Elliot Richardson of the plan to oust Brown. Richardson asked to talk with Jaffe first. On May 12, 1972, Jaffe met Richardson for lunch at his dining room at HEW. Everything was in place for Brown's head to roll. Yet, at the critical moment, Jaffe backed down. Perito was outraged. "I told Jerry that, as a small Italian kid, I always had to get the first punch in," he recalled. "He said Bert Brown was a good guy. I said, 'Fuck him.' Brown was kicking the shit out of the White House and should have been fired. But Jerry didn't take his gun out of his holster."

The incident was not an isolated one. As in Chicago, Jaffe shrank from making tough personnel decisions. And he was so focused on his mission that he often behaved insensitively, even abrasively, toward those around him. If he had an urgent project, he would sometimes assign it to two or three different people without telling them—a recipe for strife. In Chicago, staff tensions had remained manageable; in Washington, they were amplified by the high-pressure atmosphere of the White House. Struggling to keep up with the crushing demands on his time, Jaffe began neglecting basic administrative duties. "This would be a very good day for you to catch up on the tremendous backlog of paper on your desk" went a typical comment on his daily schedule.

By the summer of 1972, things in the office had gotten so bad that the White House commissioned a management audit from Peat Marwick. Its findings, presented to Jaffe in memo form, were unsparing. "The staff," it stated, "sees apparent contradictions in decisions, reversals of policies, duplication of assignments, and so forth, which they believe result in the development of many projects without direction, confusion as to priorities, and a lack of responsiveness by the staff." Observing that SAODAP's image "is often a negative one," the memo noted that "professional staff openly speak of Special Action Office problems and personalities to third parties. Our internal problems are well known by our few friends and many detractors around town."

Interestingly, the memo attributed many of SAODAP's problems to its lack of political savvy:

While there is a general understanding that we are responsive to the White House, Congress and OMB, most of the staff believes that they are "apolitical" and above politics. This has created problems in our relations with Congress, OMB and with the rest of the Federal bureaucracy. It is folly to believe that the President would establish an office to handle purely technical problems of drug abuse prevention. . . . While we need not be "political" in our actions, neither should we delude ourselves that the agency is above political considerations.

This went to the heart of SAODAP's dilemma. On the one hand, Jaffe had been selected to run the drug office on the basis of his expertise on drugs. And, drawing on it, he had already managed to defuse the Vietnam drug crisis and was working to do the same with the national heroin epidemic. Yet the political needs of the Nixon Administration kept intruding—especially as the reelection campaign got under way.

An early instance came in January 1972, when the White House set up an Office of Drug Abuse Law Enforcement (ODALE) to create joint federal-local strike forces to fight the street-level drug trade in cities across the country. Given the dispersed nature of that trade, it was unclear how much such an office could accomplish. In an election year, though, that did not much matter. "The street pusher program is good politics and has widespread acceptance wherever it's talked about," John Ehrlichman wrote to Nixon on February 8, 1972.

ODALE's director, Myles Ambrose, an ebullient Republican who had previously served as commissioner of customs, was full of brash schemes for snagging drug dealers, and Nixon sent him around the country to tout the administration's get-tough policy. And, as his stature at the White House rose, Jaffe's fell. "Myles became the point man for the administration," Jaffe recalled. "He was more partisan, more Republican, more in tune with the constituency that Nixon needed to appeal to for the election. I was fairly neutral politically, and too professorial to be of much use in a campaign." By the time of the convention, in August, Jaffe observed, "I got the feeling that we'd had our bite of the apple."

Despite it all, Jaffe was making steady progress in the campaign against the waiting lists. By late 1972, the number of clients in federally funded programs had increased to 60,000—three times the level of October 1971. And the effects were evident in clinics around the country. "All indicators are that waiting time is decreasing substantially," stated a SAODAP internal memo. In New York City, it added, the average wait "has dropped from six months to two to four weeks."

Meanwhile, Egil Krogh's campaign against the world narcotics trade was taking hold. In a single week in July 1972, French agents destroyed three heroin labs, one of them reportedly large enough to supply a fifth of all the addicts in the United States for a year. In three separate raids, the governments of Argentina, Brazil, and Venezuela confiscated 285 pounds of U.S.-bound heroin, while Thai agents seized eleven tons of opium along the Burmese

border. And, after some tough diplomacy, Washington persuaded the government of Paraguay to extradite Auguste Ricord, a major Corsican trafficker who
had taken refuge there.

Suddenly, the French Connection was in disarray. And the impact was
soon apparent on the street. "Our concentrated effort to curtail the heroin
traffic in the United States is having dramatic results," the BNDD stated in an
October 24, 1972, report. "These results have been emphasized by the existence of a heroin shortage in the Eastern half of the United States. This
shortage, which has been developing over the past several months, is most
apparent in those cities which have historically been supplied by European
sources."

The combination of reduced heroin supplies and increased treatment
capacity was beginning to have a tangible effect. TURNAROUND ON DRUGS?
the New York Times asked in a September 5 editorial. "It is clear that a dozen
years of dizzy upward spiral in drug-related deaths here has mercifully slowed,"
it stated. In another encouraging sign, fewer arrestees were being picked up
with drugs in their system. Most remarkably, the city's crime rate dropped by
21.1 percent in the first five months of 1972, compared to a 10.6 percent
increase in the same period the previous year. "I, for one, feel we're really
gaining on the whole heroin problem in New York City," Gordon Chase, the
city's health administrator, was quoted as saying.

Washington, D.C., was reporting similar progress. As 1972 unfolded, the
number of people dying from heroin-related overdoses was declining steadily;
in September the city recorded not a single heroin overdose death (although
three people died from methadone). And the city's crime rate plunged 30
percent in the first quarter of the year.

The District was not alone. Seventy-two of the nation's largest cities,
including Chicago, Detroit, Los Angeles, and San Francisco, experienced a
drop in crime. For the nation as a whole, crime rose just 1 percent in the first
half of the year—the smallest rate of increase since the FBI began issuing
quarterly reports in 1960. And, while the precise reasons for the drop were
difficult to pinpoint, officials in both Washington and New York cited the
increase in treatment availability as a key factor. The heroin drought in these
and other large cities probably played a part as well, though in many of them
crime began to fall well before the shortages in supplies appeared.

From a political standpoint, the matter was even more clear-cut. "Was the
drop in crime a result of the tremendous increases we had made in the drug
program?" Egil Krogh would later ask. "The answer is, I don't know. Was it a
success from a political perspective? The answer is, Heck, yes, it was a slam-
dunk great success."

And the White House moved quickly to capitalize. Although the nation's
crime rate had jumped nearly 30 percent during Nixon's first three years in
office, the 1 percent rise in the first half of 1972 allowed the president to claim
that he had delivered on his promise to reduce crime. And he did just that in

a national radio address delivered three weeks before the election. Having brought the "frightening trend of crime and anarchy to a standstill," Nixon declared, his administration was winning "the battle against the criminal forces in America." In the District of Columbia, he proudly observed, crime had declined by 50 percent since the start of his term. And, through bureaucratic shake-ups and energetic diplomacy, he stated, his administration had stemmed the "raging heroin epidemic" of the last decade.

The strategy that Bud Krogh and Jeff Donfeld had devised to bring the crime rate down had worked more brilliantly than they had ever dreamed. And the key to that strategy had been the priority given to expanding treatment capacity. "We increased the funding for everything," Krogh observed, "but the major increase was on the demand side."

WATCHING THE ELECTION RETURNS, Jaffe felt a small measure of satisfaction. While the outcome had never been in doubt—Nixon defeated George McGovern by 18 million votes—Jaffe had personally helped to contain two potential problems, the GI drug epidemic and the increase in street crime. And, within days, he got his reward: a demand that he submit a letter of resignation.

Jaffe was not being singled out. *All* presidential appointees were required to submit such letters—part of Richard Nixon's plan to avoid complacency in his second term. In a meeting with White House staff shortly after the election, a strangely downbeat Nixon observed that most second terms ended up as failures—an "exhausted volcano" was his term—but his was going to be different. No longer having to worry about getting reelected, Nixon was now free to pursue his true beliefs. Adding to his dark mood was the nagging problem of Watergate. Prior to the election, the White House had managed to keep the scandal under wraps, with few news organizations pursuing it aside from the *Washington Post*. Now, however, every reporter in Washington was on the story, and Nixon wanted to shed those in his administration whose sympathies might be suspect.

Jaffe did not fall into that category, and so his letter of resignation was not accepted. Like many other White House officials, however, he found the whole experience highly deflating. He was further distressed by developments at the Old Executive Office Building. Convinced that his domestic policy staff had become too large and operational, Nixon wanted to transfer some power back to the Cabinet departments. In each, though, he wanted loyalists on whom he could rely. And he wanted Bud Krogh, who had been working to bring a new subway to Washington, to become undersecretary of transportation. It was a heady promotion for the young aide, but, as a result, SAODAP was going to lose its chief protector. From now on, the drug office would come under the mantle of two young aides—Walter Minnick and Geoffrey Shepard—who, while bright and energetic, had neither Krogh's influence nor his emotional attachment to the program.

In mid-December 1972, Jaffe, seeking a break from all this, decided to attend the annual meeting of the American College of Neuropsychopharmacology. It was taking place at the Caribe Hotel in San Juan, Puerto Rico, and three hundred mental-health professionals gathered there to discuss treatment and drink piña coladas. Given SAODAP's exertions on behalf of drug addicts, Jaffe could have expected a rousing reception, but the fact that he had carried out those efforts on behalf of the odious Richard Nixon remained a sore point with many ACNP members. The keynote speaker, Matthew Dumont, the director of drug rehabilitation programs in Massachusetts and a well-known critic of methadone, denounced the administration for its "scapegoating of minority groups" and "conceptual blurring between persecution and treatment." "By and large," Dumont thundered, "we have adopted the values of cops, the sensibilities of liberals, and the technologies of physicians. The result has been a mishmash of interventions which are nothing less than behavioral trade-offs, social controls masquerading as therapies."

Dumont's remarks were greeted with loud applause. Jaffe, who had little taste for public combat, remained silent. But Dr. Roger Meyer, a Harvard psychiatrist and SAODAP consultant, rose to denounce Dumont's speech. A form of "fascism from the left," he called it, rooted in a dangerous "self-hatred" that was undermining respect for medical professionalism. Meyer's remarks, however, got lost in the overall din of criticism of SAODAP, which, Jaffe later observed, marked the "high point" of the "mau-mauing" directed at the office.

IN THE END, however, the main threat to Jaffe's work came not from the left but from the right. And the alarm went off not in Washington but in Albany, New York. There, on January 3, 1973, New York Governor Nelson Rockefeller delivered his annual State of the State address. It was Rockefeller's fifteenth such speech, and the legislators gathered for it expected nothing out of the ordinary. They were thus stunned when he let loose a fierce attack on New York's drug problem. "The crime, the muggings, the robberies, the murders associated with addiction continue to spread a reign of terror," Rockefeller declared.

> Whole neighborhoods have been as effectively destroyed by addicts as by an invading army. We face the risk of undermining our will as a people—and the ultimate destruction of our society as a whole. This has to stop. This . . . is . . . going . . . to . . . stop.

Noting that "all the laws we now have on the books won't work to deter the pusher of drugs," Rockefeller proposed a draconian set of new ones. Anyone convicted of selling heroin, methadone, LSD, amphetamines, and hashish— no matter how small the quantity—was to receive a mandatory sentence of life imprisonment. And, to "close all avenues" of escape, Rockefeller said, the new laws would forbid all plea bargaining and chances of parole. "These are drastic measures," Rockefeller acknowledged, but, he added, "I am thoroughly convinced, after trying everything else, that nothing less will do."

Rockefeller's proposals were indeed tough. Sending a seller of heroin away for life was harsher than the penalty for murder, which at least allowed for the possibility of parole. And the criticism was furious. The *New York Times* editorialized that the governor's "simplistic, lock-'em-up-for-life-for-everyone proposal" was a "gross disservice that made adoption of a responsible program less likely than ever." An analysis conducted by Mayor Lindsay's office warned that if Rockefeller's proposals became law, the state's prison population—then about 13,000—would exceed 80,000 within ten years.

What made the speech all the more surprising was that it came from a man who had long supported drug treatment. The rapid expansion of methadone programs in New York City would have been impossible without Rockefeller's generous backing. What's more, that investment seemed to be paying off. Politically, though, the governor's proposals were more understandable. Rockefeller was contemplating a run for president in 1976, and, having been thwarted by the Republican right on three previous bids, he hoped to make a preemptive strike by attacking drug dealers.

Reading Rockefeller's remarks, Jaffe felt a sense of dread. Since the early 1960s, the nation had been moving steadily away from mandatory drug sentences. In 1970, Congress had passed a law eliminating all such penalties at the federal level, and most states had followed suit. One of the key lessons of the whole Vietnam episode, Jaffe believed, was the value of replacing severe, remote penalties with shorter but more certain ones backed by treatment. Now, Rockefeller was talking about sending away dealers for *life*. And not just major traffickers, but also street-level addict-sellers. "For them, what you want is to create just enough pressure to change what they do," Jaffe observed. "There are ways to do that other than providing longer and longer sentences. Sending a low-level dealer away for years and tying up a scarce resource like a jail cell, then turning the person loose—it just didn't make sense."

Jaffe got a chance to put his objections to Rockefeller in person. The governor—expecting that the new penalties would push many addicts to seek help—had approached the White House about obtaining more treatment funds. To discuss the matter, Jaffe in early February 1973 went to see Rockefeller at his plush townhouse-office in midtown Manhattan. After assuring the governor that SAODAP would provide the desired funds, Jaffe expressed his reservations about the governor's plan. "I tried to be diplomatic," he recalled. "I pointed out that, under his proposals, someone would be better off murdering a policeman than getting sentenced for selling drugs."

Rockefeller listened politely but was unmoved. According to a White House summary of the meeting, the governor wanted "to make his law enforcement effort a model for the nation. He emphasized that the possibility of serving a life sentence would have a considerable deterrent effect on young people's involvement with drug pushing or use." Under the heading "Recommendations," the memo stated: "Determine from John Ehrlichman and Ken Cole [a White House adviser] what steps they are willing to take to make Governor Rockefeller's approach a national model."

The White House needed little encouragement. Polls taken in New York showed two-thirds of the public supporting Rockefeller's stance. Determined not to be outflanked, Nixon asked Ehrlichman to prepare a new package of drug penalties for a major speech on crime and drugs that he was scheduled to give in mid-March. Though less severe than Rockefeller's measures, the proposed package called for a sharp escalation in federal penalties, with anyone convicted of selling up to four ounces of heroin subject to a mandatory minimum sentence of five years.

Until now, Jaffe had managed to accommodate himself to Nixon's hardline views. But imposing lengthy sentences on low-level drug felons violated his most basic principles, and he set out his reservations in a March 9 memo to Ehrlichman. "While such a bill's appearance of toughness may generate an emotionally based favorable reaction initially," he wrote in his professorial manner, "that reaction is not likely to persist in the face of analyses which show the bill to be counterproductive even in strictly law enforcement terms." Jaffe went on to propose a "much more responsive and responsible option"—a "public announcement timed to coincide roughly with the first anniversary of the statutory creation of the Special Action Office detailing the very real progress which has been made both in curtailing narcotic supplies and in providing treatment."

Eventually, some minor changes were made in the proposal, and Jaffe—swallowing his reservations—acquiesced. And, on March 14, Nixon sent his proposed Heroin Trafficking Act to Congress. Two weeks later, he announced his intention to create a new superagency to fight drug traffickers. "The cold-blooded underworld networks that funnel narcotics from suppliers all over the world into the veins of American drug victims are no respecters of the bureaucratic dividing lines that now complicate our anti-drug efforts," Nixon stated. ". . . I therefore propose creation of a single, comprehensive Federal agency within the Department of Justice to lead the war against the illicit drug traffic." Barring congressional action, the Drug Enforcement Administration would come into being in sixty days.

On the same day the DEA was unveiled, the *Los Angeles Times* ran a front-page story on Jaffe's memo to John Ehrlichman. NIXON ANTIDRUG BILL CRITICIZED BY AIDE, read the headline atop the article. The White House was furious. In a memo to Ehrlichman's office, Geoffrey Shepard wrote,

> This will teach Jaffe not to write to JDE [Ehrlichman]!! I am sure that his is the office which leaked it since I still have the original. . . . Jaffe is very worried (rightfully!) since it seems to show his disagree-

ment with our bill. Actually, he was satisfied with it when it finally went and supports it. He wants JDE to know he is very upset about the leak and told the reporter it was only preliminary commentary on a draft. I told him to write me, but never John, in the future.

Jaffe wrote a letter offering to resign, but it was refused. A few days later, however, the White House informed him that it was revoking his White House mess pass.

As it happened, the same day the *Times* story appeared, the FBI released its crime figures for 1972. They were stunning. Of the 154 U.S. cities with a population of 100,000 or more, 94 reported decreases. The crime rate fell 4.1 percent in Chicago, 4.5 percent in Philadelphia, 8.8 percent in Boston, 15.8 percent in Detroit, 18 percent in New York, and 19 percent in San Francisco. For the nation as a whole, the crime rate in 1972 fell 3 percent—the first decline in seventeen years.

There were other encouraging numbers. In the first two months of 1973, the number of narcotics-related deaths in New York City, Cook County (Chicago), Washington, D.C., and San Francisco County declined 48 percent compared with the same period in 1972. And, according to the new Drug Abuse Warning Network (DAWN), the number of drug-related visits to hospital emergency rooms fell by 4 percent. In New York, meanwhile, the number of drug-related hepatitis cases plunged from 386 in the first quarter of 1971 to 318 in the same period in 1972 and just 89 in 1973.

By far the most dramatic changes were taking place in Washington, D.C. —Egil Krogh's laboratory. In the first quarter of 1973, the city recorded just one heroin overdose death—down from a peak of twenty-five in the same period in 1971. (Six people did die from methadone overdoses.) And Washington's crime rate dropped a remarkable 26.9 percent in 1972—the largest decline of any major city in the country. No doubt the expansion of the D.C. police department had played a part in this; by this point, the force had some 5,100 officers, 2,000 more than four years earlier. Interestingly, though, the number of heroin arrests in D.C. actually declined in this period, from 3,144 in 1971 to 2,108 in 1972. Testifying in Congress about the drop in crime in the capital, Chief Jerry Wilson said that his department

has long recognized and repeatedly stated that in order to bring the problem of drug abuse under control in the District of Columbia, a sound program of treatment had to be present as an alternative for the drug addict. . . . I have no question that much of the reduction in crime that has been achieved in this city is a result of the narcotic treatment program, as well as the court reorganization and increased police and other efforts that have been made under President Nixon's program.

In New York, as in Washington, the drop in crime was occurring despite a sharp falloff in the number of drug arrests, from 52,479 in 1970 to 16,403 in 1973 (the result of a decision by the police to deemphasize street-level arrests). It was also occurring without any of the harsh sentences mandated by the Rockefeller Laws, which did not take effect until May 1973. More generally, the decline in overdose deaths and hospital visits was occurring without any rise in incarceration rates. From 1971 to 1972, in fact, the number of federal and state inmates actually *fell*, from 198,061 to 196,183. Clearly, the expansion in drug treatment had played a key part in the progress being made.

FOR EGIL KROGH, these numbers should have been a source of deep satisfaction. He was unable to mull them, however, because of the spreading tentacles of Watergate. A congressional investigation led by Senator Sam Ervin was turning up illegalities almost daily, and the White House's effort to cover up its misdeeds was quickly unraveling. In early April 1973, White House counsel John Dean, fearing that he was being set up for a fall, began cooperating with federal prosecutors. Among his revelations was the part the White House had played in the break-in into Dr. Lewis Fielding's offices. The White House's involvement first became public on April 26, at the espionage trial of Daniel Ellsberg, then under way in Los Angeles. Suddenly, Krogh's role in the incident was front-page news, and two weeks later he was forced to resign. (Both Haldeman and Ehrlichman had stepped down in late April.) It was a sudden, wrenching end to a career that had been so full of promise, and Krogh, who would eventually plead guilty to violating Fielding's civil rights, and who would serve four months in federal prison, would spend the rest of his life regretting that monumental lapse of judgment in the summer of 1971.

Needless to say, with all this going on, the White House staff had little time to talk about drug policy; all they cared about was staying out of jail. Jaffe was so wrapped up in his work, however, that he took his lack of access as a personal affront. His sense of isolation deepened when Paul Perito resigned in April, taking with him the last rampart against total anarchy. Jaffe's desk became lost under the mounting paperwork, and the sniping within SAODAP was turning lethal. Feeling harassed and unappreciated, Jaffe barricaded himself in his office, burying himself in his work.

Sensing that his days in Washington were numbered, he rushed to put in place the remaining elements of his national treatment system. By the spring of 1973, so many slots had been created that some cities had excess capacity, and Jaffe, seeking to take advantage, was setting up mechanisms to coax more addicts off the street. Building on Pat Hughes's work in Chicago, Jaffe was urging cities to create outreach teams to scour copping zones. To make it easier for addicts to gain access to programs, Jaffe was issuing contracts to cities to set up IDAP-like central intake units. And, to help get more drug offenders into treatment, he was expanding SAODAP's Treatment Alternatives to Street

Crime program (TASC), a forerunner of the drug courts that were to become so popular two decades later.

When he agreed to become SAODAP's director, Jaffe had taken a two-year leave of absence from the University of Chicago. It was now coming to an end. In addition to wanting to return to his research, Jaffe hoped to spend more time with his kids, who'd become virtual strangers. The Special Action Office itself was due to be downsized, and Jaffe did not want to wield the ax. Mentally and physically, he was near collapse. "I had made enough enemies, enough compromises," he observed. "Working at a place with someone like Haldeman at the top was pretty stressful. They were very, very tough people. You felt you couldn't make any mistakes. From day one, there was not a day on the job that I enjoyed."

And so, on May 29, 1973, Jaffe sent Richard Nixon a letter of resignation. In it, he recounted what he felt were SAODAP's accomplishments—the expansion of national treatment capacity, the curtailing of the Vietnam heroin epidemic, the drop in overdose deaths, the decrease in crime. "In its first two years," Jaffe noted, "the Special Action Office has moved the country a little closer to your goal of reducing the high cost of drug abuse to the people of America."

Five days later, he got a note back from Richard Nixon. Expressing "deep appreciation and admiration" for Jaffe's "outstanding service" and "forceful and imaginative leadership," the president accepted his resignation. And so on June 17, 1973—the second anniversary of SAODAP's birth—Jerome Jaffe stepped down as the nation's drug czar.

10

The Retreat

THE INDIGNITIES Jerome Jaffe had to endure did not end with his resignation from SAODAP. Through the summer of 1973, he would remain on the Nixon Administration's payroll, working to address a shortage in the supplies of medical morphine that had developed as a result of the Turkish opium ban. In early August, he went on the *Today* show to be interviewed by Barbara Walters about the Nixon drug program. While offering his usual qualifiers, Jaffe managed to be positive, noting that, for "the first time in the history of this country," the government had made help available to all addicts who wanted it. The White House was pleased, and a staff member wrote a memo recommending that Nixon meet with Jaffe to convey his thanks. Geoffrey Shepard of the domestic policy staff vetoed the idea. "I already called Jaffe and thanked him for the TODAY appearance," he peevishly jotted on the memo. "He is still on our payroll at SAODAP and should be expected to do a decent job on appearances. He is a good man and has worked hard for us, but he gets very strange ideas at times. We should not expose him directly to the President in a phone call or individual meeting."

Jaffe's relations with the University of Chicago were no less strained. Originally, he had planned to rejoin its faculty, but Daniel Freedman remained so hostile as to rule out that option. Fortunately, Jaffe had another offer, from Columbia University, and in the fall he and his family relocated to New York, with Jerome becoming a professor of psychiatry and Faith setting up house in nearby Scarsdale. For the first time since 1967, Jaffe was able to return to his true love, psychopharmacology. And, as his focus, he chose a substance that had been off-limits during his time at SAODAP: nicotine. Although smoking caused more than 400,000 deaths annually, the subject was politically taboo, and any time Jaffe tried to mention tobacco (or alcohol) in policy statements, the White House staff would resist. Now, freed of such constraints, he began exploring a phenomenon that had always fascinated him: the behavioral similarities between heavy smokers and opiate abusers. And, just as he had sought to make treatment more available to heroin addicts, he now began testing ways of breaking smokers of their habits. So, two decades before it became a political issue in Washington, Jaffe was studying nicotine addiction at his office at the Columbia-Presbyterian Medical Center in upper Manhattan. Thus engrossed, he attempted to forget the painful denouement to his brief career in Washington.

Yet his legacy there would remain strong. In just two years, Jaffe had helped create a comprehensive public-health system for dealing with drug addiction. Its centerpiece was a national treatment network offering help to all those who wanted it. To run it, Jaffe had trained a cadre of treatment specialists, a small but dedicated fraternity able to carry on his work. All had endured the SAODAP initiation rite, working long days over many months to provide services to addicts. The fraternity had its own look—rumpled clothes, unkempt hair, glasses, pencils in shirt pockets.

Above all, the fraternity had a code, a set of principles that summed up Jaffe's approach to drug abuse. Its core was simple. Chronic drug users are at the heart of the nation's drug problem. Those users are a heterogeneous lot, requiring a diverse array of services. The government has a responsibility to make sure such services are available and effective. Law enforcement has a role to play in curtailing drug abuse, but only as an adjunct to rehabilitation. And those two functions should remain separate at all times. Maintaining the nation's treatment network was simply too complex a task for those entrusted with it to be distracted by meetings with drug agents or visits to foreign lands. At all times, efforts to reduce the demand for drugs had to take precedence over efforts to reduce the supply—the essence of the public-health model Jaffe had championed.

Already, that model had demonstrated its ability to reduce the level of drug abuse in the United States. Given the nation's political culture, however, it was highly vulnerable to attack. And, from the day Jerome Jaffe resigned, there would be a steady retreat from it. Initially, the backsliding was barely perceptible. In fact, the man chosen to succeed Jaffe was one of his leading disciples. As the head of the district's Narcotics Treatment Administration, Robert DuPont had helped convince the Nixon Administration to undertake its treatment initiative in the first place. Under his leadership, the NTA had attracted so many visitors that he had had to hire someone just to show them around. The program had generated hundreds of research papers, and DuPont himself had written more than fifty.

A graduate of Emory College in Atlanta and the Harvard Medical School, DuPont had been inspired by President Kennedy's call to public service, and, while completing his psychiatric residency in Boston, he had found time to counsel inmates at the Norfolk State Prison. To fulfill his obligation under the physicians' draft, he had won a coveted slot at the National Institutes of Health. From there, he went on to the D.C. Department of Corrections, where he did his pathbreaking work on the crime-drug connection, then set up a Jaffe-style treatment system in the District.

While an intellectual disciple of Jaffe's, DuPont presented a strong personal contrast. A lanky six-feet-five, with chiseled features and neatly combed hair, DuPont had none of Jaffe's brooding ambivalence or maddening indecisiveness. A man of great enthusiasm, he threw himself into causes with a zest bordering on the evangelical. And, where Jaffe was ornery and independent-minded, DuPont was personable, relaxed, and reliable—precisely the qualities needed to stabilize the operation Jaffe had created.

It would, however, be a much-reduced operation. For the sense of crisis surrounding the drug problem had faded, and DuPont's main task would be phasing out SAODAP and establishing its successor, the National Institute on Drug Abuse (NIDA). In the end, thirty or so staff members would move with DuPont to NIDA's new office, located in a glass-and-steel box in Rockville, Maryland. Rather than two hundred steps from the White House, the federal drug office was now out in the suburbs, a fourth-tier agency buried deep inside HEW. And, while the federal treatment budget was not cut, few new initiatives were undertaken. "We lost our momentum," Robert DuPont would later observe. "The priority and focus of the issue declined, and so the game became holding on, rather than expanding. We lost our morale—and direction. And that continued into the Ford Administration."

SHORTLY AFTER Gerald Ford became president, DuPont was summoned to the White House to brief him. Ford was about to meet Luis Echeverría, the president of Mexico, and that nation's heroin industry was on the agenda. Heroin was hardly a new phenomenon in Mexico. Since World War II, Mexican traffickers had grown opium poppies in the Western Sierra Madre mountains. The brown heroin produced from those poppies was consumed almost entirely in the United States, where it accounted for about one-third of the market. The dismantling of the French Connection had created new sales opportunities there, however, and Mexican traffickers, rushing to exploit them, had quickly expanded local poppy cultivation. Within months, beat-up Chevrolets and Fords were rolling across the 2,000-mile U.S.-Mexican border, carrying heroin hidden in spare tires and specially built gas tanks. The drought in the United States had proved very short-lived.

DuPont knew next to nothing about Mexican heroin. In line with the Jaffe code, he had focused his energies on dealing with drug use in the United States. With the president asking to be briefed, however, he quickly caught up on developments to the south. And, despite his nervousness, his meeting with Ford went well. But the issue was bound to resurface, and DuPont, wanting to be prepared, decided to visit Culiacán, the violent capital of the Mexican heroin trade. "It was like Dodge City," DuPont recalled. "The streets were full of bodyguards with machine guns. Even the Rotary Club had been taken over by narcotics traffickers."

DuPont was hardly the only U.S. official to take the Mexican opium tour. State Department officers, White House aides, congressmen, and journalists all went tromping about the poppy fields of the Sierra Madre. "Mexico was where the action was," DuPont noted. Yet, in partaking of it, he was ignoring Jaffe's injunction against foreign travel. And, sure enough, while DuPont and his fellow officials were distracted by Mexico, a surge in heroin use in the United States was causing a run on treatment clinics, with waiting lists again appearing.

Belatedly recognizing the urgency of the situation, the White House in April 1975 set up a task force to study it. It was placed under the direction of Richard Parsons, a young aide to Vice President Nelson Rockefeller. A black man of bearlike proportions, Parsons (who would go on to become president of Time Warner) set up a review team to match, with a twenty-person task force backed by working groups involving more than eighty people. The result, a 104-page *White Paper on Drug Abuse,* was one of the most enlightened documents on drugs ever produced by the federal government. Noting that "not all drug use is equally destructive," the paper asserted that "we should give priority in our treatment and enforcement efforts to those drugs which pose the greatest risk." Rating drugs according to their abuse potential, the white paper ranked heroin at the top, followed by amphetamines and barbiturates, with marijuana at the bottom. Whatever the drug, the government was urged to concentrate its efforts on "chronic, intensive users."

After four months of work, then, the White House task force had largely recapitulated the Jaffe code. And, in line with it, it urged the government to intervene quickly in the current crisis. "Nearly everyone from the treatment community contacted in the course of the study named 'limited treatment capacity' as the single most important issue in drug abuse treatment and rehabilitation," the *White Paper* stated. Accordingly, it called on the government to "undertake a high priority analysis of treatment capacity" and submit a recommendation to the president by December 1, 1975.

No such action was taken, however. Instead, the White House continued to focus on stopping heroin at its source. Rather than create more treatment slots at home, the administration sent the Mexican government Bell helicopters and fixed-wing spotter planes to be used in spraying poppy fields. In 1976, federal spending on drug enforcement would for the first time catch up with that on treatment and prevention—a key signpost on the road away from the public-health model.

THE FOCUS on treating heroin addicts was being further eroded by the new attention being paid another drug: marijuana. By the mid-1970s, an estimated

25 to 30 million Americans had tried it, including Jack Ford, the president's son. *High Times* magazine, with its cannabis centerfolds and marijuana growing tips, was available on neighborhood newsstands, while the cast of *Saturday Night Live* could barely make it through a show without at least one drug joke. ("Football's kinda nice," George Carlin cracked on one program. "They moved the hash marks in. . . . The guys found 'em and smoked 'em anyway.")

Once a symbol of protest and rebellion, then, pot was going mainstream. But the nation's marijuana laws had not kept pace. Every year, more than 400,000 people were being arrested on marijuana charges, mostly for possession, and stories abounded of college students being thrown into jail for having a joint on them. In Texas, pot possession was a felony punishable by up to life in prison.

Leading the campaign for change was the National Organization for the Reform of Marijuana Laws. As Washington lobbying groups went, NORML was pretty low-rent—a one-man show run out of a ground-floor apartment. But that one man, Keith Stroup, was endlessly resourceful. Magnetic and mercurial, Stroup (rhymes with "cop") had shed his Southern Baptist roots in small-town Illinois to become a flamboyant presence on the Washington scene. Politically, Stroup emulated Ralph Nader, using the techniques of consumer activism to advance the cause of an illicit drug. Personally, his model was Hugh Hefner. Stroup, in fact, was a frequent visitor to the Playboy Mansion, and the Playboy Foundation was his chief backer. With his long hair, wire-rimmed glasses, and rousing speaking style, Stroup was tirelessly touring the country, inveighing against the madness of the nation's marijuana laws.

Stroup, who smoked pot regularly and openly, believed that marijuana should be fully legalized. After consulting some grayer heads, however, he decided the nation was not quite ready for such a step. Instead, he took his cue from the National Commission on Marihuana and Drug Abuse. Set up in 1970 by Congress and appointed by President Nixon, the commission was a decidedly mainstream group, its members including two U.S. senators, two U.S. representatives, and a Republican governor. But their final report, issued in March 1972, turned out to be quite lenient. The "experimental or intermittent use" of marijuana, it stated, had resulted in "little proven danger of physical or psychological harm." The commission nonetheless rejected outright legalization on the grounds that "it would institutionalize availability of a drug which has uncertain long-term effect." Instead, it recommended that marijuana be *decriminalized.* Anyone smoking pot in public would be subject not to arrest but to a fine, much as one would for speeding. The production and distribution of marijuana, however, would remain fully prohibited.

The report did not sit well with Richard Nixon, who summarily rejected it. For Keith Stroup, though, it offered an establishment seal of approval for marijuana reform, and, following the commission, he took decriminalization as his top goal. And, in an encouraging early sign, Oregon in 1973 became the first state in the nation to decriminalize pot.

Seeking to boost NORML's visibility, Stroup invited Bob DuPont to address its third annual conference, scheduled for November 1974. DuPont was very tempted. Pot was not harmless, he believed, but the idea of sending people to jail for smoking it seemed preposterous, and so he, too, had decided in favor of decriminalization. Under Nixon, he had had to keep such views to himself, but, with Ford now in office, he was free to speak his mind, and he accepted Stroup's invitation. In his talk, DuPont made it clear that he was not endorsing marijuana use, given its possible health consequences. Nonetheless, he said, those consequences should not be allowed to obscure the "well-documented, harmful social effects of the marijuana laws on the public well being." All criminal sanctions for marijuana possession, he declared, should be eliminated.

The nation's drug czar had publicly embraced decriminalization. And, over subsequent months, he would fervently promote it. "I'd always been a person with a lot of enthusiasm," DuPont noted, "and I was feeling enthusiastic for my new mission. I was captured by the idea of decriminalization." In 1975, five more states—Alaska, California, Colorado, Maine, and Ohio—would decriminalize pot, with Minnesota joining them the following year.

Overall, then, the nation seemed well on its way to adopting decriminalization. Yet the debate over pot was having the side effect of diverting attention from the more pressing problem of heroin, and support for the public-health model continued to ebb.

THE ELECTION of Jimmy Carter seemed certain to change that. Few other politicians had shown as much interest in the subject of drug addiction, or compassion for its victims. Unlike Richard Nixon, who had refused to step foot inside a treatment facility, Carter, while governor of Georgia, had spent a full afternoon at Bob DuPont's Narcotics Treatment Administration in Washington. Back in Georgia, Carter had decided to set up a similar program. And the man he chose to run it, Dr. Peter Bourne, had become a close friend. After the election, Carter appointed the British-born psychiatrist to be his drug adviser, with an office in the West Wing of the White House. Bourne, Carter told the press, was "probably the world's foremost expert on heroin, cocaine, and marijuana—even alcohol—all the drugs that are bad."

It was only a slight exaggeration. Urbane, erudite, and charming, the thirty-seven-year-old Bourne was something of a wunderkind in the drug field. A graduate of Emory College at the age of nineteen, he had written dozens of papers on the psychology and treatment of addiction, plus a highly praised book, *Men, Stress, and Viet Nam.* As the head of Georgia's statewide treatment system, he had emerged as a leading figure among methadone providers. He had set up an alcohol program in the Atlanta city jail, dealt with bad acid trips as a volunteer at the Haight-Ashbury Free Medical Clinic, and, from 1972 to 1974, served as SAODAP's assistant director, working closely with Jerome Jaffe. Bourne, in short, was a core member of the treatment fraternity.

Yet Bourne did not relish his fraternity status. In contrast to most members, with their button-down shirts and off-the-rack sports coats, Bourne wore elegant three-piece suits. With his stylishly cut dark hair, sensitive eyes, and shy smile, he had the debonair look of a young Alec Guinness. While at home discussing withdrawal symptoms and opiate receptors, he much preferred topics like the Chinese Cultural Revolution and the poetry of Dylan Thomas. A licensed pilot, Bourne at one time owned a house in Aspen, Colorado, where he ran an art gallery and hung out with local luminaries like Hunter Thompson. With his wife Mary King, who had once worked for SNCC, the radical civil rights group, Bourne considered himself as much a political activist as a caring physician. And these two sides of his personality were constantly at war.

His interest in medicine came from his father, Dr. Geoffrey Bourne, an eminent medical scientist from Australia who had discovered vitamin C in the human body. Bourne was working at Oxford when his son was born, and Peter as a youth gravitated to the Young Conservatives. When he was a teenager, however, his father, accepting a post at Emory, moved the family to Atlanta, and Peter, exposed to the raw racial politics of the South, became radicalized. While attending the Emory Medical School, he invited a group of students from nearby Morehouse College to attend a meeting on campus, causing an uproar. "I was regarded as a subversive," Bourne recalled.

It was not the last time. In 1964, Bourne, drafted into the Army, was assigned to the Walter Reed Army Institute of Research in Washington, where he began studying the body's reactions to stress. The Army found his work promising enough to send him to Vietnam to study soldiers in combat. For several months, Bourne flew around with helicopter ambulance crews, collecting urine samples from medics to be analyzed in Washington. He also spent time with a Green Beret unit near the Ho Chi Minh Trail. On several occasions, Bourne himself saw action, for which he was later awarded a Bronze Star. By the time he returned home, however, he had become thoroughly disillusioned with the war. And, while his work at Walter Reed was attracting national attention, including a laudatory article in *Time* magazine, Bourne was becoming active in the antiwar movement. While completing his psychiatric residency at Stanford, he helped found Vietnam Veterans Against the War.

As exciting as all this was, Bourne feared becoming politically marginalized, and in 1969 he accepted an offer to return to Atlanta to help establish a health center on the city's predominantly black south side. The following year, he was asked to set up Georgia's first community mental health center. Unlike many such centers, Bourne welcomed heroin addicts and, to treat them, he obtained one of the state's first methadone licenses. Among the regular visitors to the center was Rosalynn Carter, and soon Bourne was being invited to meals at the Governor's Mansion, where Jimmy often joined them. At Carter's urging, Bourne agreed to set up a statewide treatment system, and before long it was serving more than 10,000 people. In 1972, after accompanying Carter to the Democratic National Convention in Miami, Bourne sent him an eleven-page handwritten memo describing why he should run for president. A series of strategy sessions followed, and by September the candidacy had become a reality.

Amid all this, Bourne received a visit from Egil Krogh. Krogh had heard a lot about the brilliant young physician in Atlanta and, convinced that SAODAP needed more hands-on expertise, had come to see him. Impressed, he persuaded Jerome Jaffe to invite Bourne to join his staff. Carter opposed the idea, fearing that the state's treatment system would collapse without him, but Bourne convinced him that he could be of more use to him in Washington, and so in the fall of 1972 he became SAODAP's assistant director. Once a month, Bourne would fly to Atlanta to participate in secret strategy sessions for the Carter campaign. In 1974, he left SAODAP to work openly on the campaign, and he and his wife began holding small cocktail gatherings in Washington to spread the word about the Georgia peanut farmer. In a gushing profile of Bourne in the *Washington Post,* Carter was quoted as saying that Bourne was "about the closest friend I have in the world." That did not sit well with Carter's Georgia-based advisers, notably Hamilton Jordan and Jody Powell, who never did like Bourne's British airs, and the psychiatrist-activist quickly found himself on the sidelines.

Having tasted the thrill of power, however, Bourne was eager to regain it. After Carter's election, he recalled, "my goal was to be in the White House and have an office in the West Wing." That he was granted. When told that his portfolio was to be drugs, however, Bourne balked. "I was tired of drugs and didn't want to be typecast as dealing only with them," he observed. Informed that his title was to be special assistant to the president for drug abuse, Bourne complained in a memo that it should be "Special Assistant for Mental Health, Drug Abuse, International Health and the White House Fellows Program, although I realize this is a little long. . . . I have specifically discussed with the President the need to maintain a broad designation if I took on the drug responsibility, and he agreed." In a compromise, Bourne was made special assistant to the president for health issues.

Constantly trying to expand his domain, Bourne began peppering the president with memos recommending grand initiatives to combat world hunger, reduce poverty in the Third World, and wipe out infectious diseases in Africa. Viewing himself as a sort of humanitarian emissary at large, he was always rushing off to meetings with officials from Iraq, Cuba, and other pariah nations, seeking to use health initiatives to build diplomatic bridges. Nothing much came of these projects, however. As far as Carter was concerned, Bourne had always been his drug adviser, and he was stuck with the job.

In one concession, Bourne was given control over the supply side as well as the demand side of drug policy. "I was the first person who had authority over all aspects of the drug issue," he observed. This, however, represented a clear violation of the church-state provision in the Jaffe code. In a further transgression, Bourne decided to emphasize the supply side. As he later explained, "We were still under the shadow of the Turkey agreement and of the breaking of the French Connection, and we had a feeling that you really could have some dramatic impact in stopping the flow of heroin into the country."

Focusing on the international side also allowed Bourne to indulge his taste for adventure, and in the spring of 1977 he and Mathea Falco, the State Department's narcotics adviser, went to Mexico to examine the opium eradication program launched by the Ford Administration. In Mexico City, the two had amicable conversations with Mexico's attorney general and defense minister. Using the aircraft Washington had provided, Mexican security forces were pelting the opium fields of the Sierra Madre with the herbicide 2,4-D. In addition, the Mexicans explained, they were spraying the local marijuana crop. The Mexicans feared that the revenues from this trade were being used to finance local insurgent groups. The herbicide being used in this case was paraquat, a highly toxic weed killer made in Europe. To gauge its effect, Bourne and Falco went to Oaxaca, where they boarded a helicopter for a ride to a nearby marijuana field. Back in Washington, Bourne sent Carter a glowing report, noting that "everyone I spoke to both in the Mexican government and in the U.S. mission felt the opium eradication program had been almost 100% successful this growing season."

Bourne would return to Mexico several times, each visit leaving him more optimistic than the last. He also went to Colombia, a major source of marijuana and cocaine, and the Golden Triangle region of Southeast Asia, whose opium industry was thriving. On these trips, Bourne came to rely on the DEA. "If you went to Thailand or Burma," he observed, "there was a permanent DEA guy there in the embassy, and having him be helpful to you was important." When Jimmy Carter moved to eliminate a proposed budget increase for the DEA, the agency's director, Peter Bensinger, implored Bourne to intercede. "He came to me wringing his hands, saying, 'You've got to go to the mat with Carter on this,' " Bourne said. "And I did. I got the money reinstated. I did it knowingly to invoke gratitude—to keep Bensinger on my team."

The federal treatment budget, meanwhile, was entering a period of steady erosion. During the Carter years, government spending on drug treatment would remain flat, which, given the period's high inflation rates, meant a steady reduction in real terms. This occurred as many cities, facing fiscal crises of their own, were slashing their treatment budgets. In New York, where waiting lists had reappeared, the city abruptly shut down its Addiction Services Agency, taking itself out of the treatment business. In Washington, D.C., budget cuts forced the Narcotics Treatment Administration to close its doors to new patients for three months, even as the demand for slots was growing. And, in Chicago, Jaffe's beloved Illinois Drug Abuse Program was being dismantled as the state withdrew from the project, thus depriving it of the centralized control that had been so critical to its success. Absorbed as he was in his foreign ventures, Peter Bourne paid these ominous developments little heed.

To THE EXTENT that Bourne did concentrate on domestic issues, it was marijuana, not heroin, that engaged him. This was not by choice. In the overall scheme of things, pot seemed to Bourne a trivial matter. Yet it would not go away, due in part to Keith Stroup. With the Democrats in the White House, Stroup was determined to press his cause. Soon after the inauguration, the New Mexico state legislature was scheduled to take up the decriminalization issue, and Stroup, hoping to score a coup, wanted Chip Carter, the president's son (and a confessed pot smoker) to testify. He asked Bourne to help, and, to his surprise, Bourne agreed. On February 2, 1977, he sent Hamilton Jordan a memo titled "The Need for Chip Carter to Lobby for the Marijuana Decriminalization Proposal Currently Pending in New Mexico." "It would be very helpful," Bourne wrote, "and would very likely assure passage of the bill if Chip Carter would spend a day in New Mexico meeting with legislative leaders and perhaps testifying on the President's position before the appropriate committee."

Politically, of course, having the president's son testify in favor of decriminalization would be suicidal, and the idea was quickly dropped. When informed of the decision, Stroup, irate, called up reporters to tell them that Hamilton Jordan had kept Chip from testifying. When the story hit the press, the White House was furious, and Bourne, himself flabbergasted at Stroup's behavior, cut off contact with him.

The NORML lobbyist would not be denied, however. In the spring of 1977, President Carter sent Bourne a handwritten note asking him to "prepare an overall message" on drugs. Bourne immediately went to work. His draft was unremarkable, save for a section calling for decriminalizing marijuana, which Carter was on record as supporting. Feeling the draft needed more work, Stuart Eizenstat, Carter's top domestic adviser, sent it to a speechwriter named Griffin Smith. A lawyer in his early thirties, Smith had met Keith Stroup while working as a legislative aide in Texas in the early 1970s, and he now solicited his advice on the marijuana section of the speech. Jumping at the opportunity, Stroup began sending Smith memos suggesting possible language, and Smith incorporated whole chunks intact. "Marijuana has become an established fact throughout our society, and the sky has not fallen," went one passage.

When Eizenstat saw the draft, he erupted. "I am very concerned about the marijuana section of this message," he wrote Carter on July 7, 1977, warning that it would "certainly be the headline story in the message." The speech was sent back for further revision, and the most offensive passages were deleted. Nonetheless, the final version, sent to Congress in August, retained much of Stroup's language. "We can, and should, continue to discourage the use of marijuana, but this can be done without defining the smoker as a criminal," the message stated in a passage lifted almost verbatim from Stroup. Noting that states that had already removed criminal penalties for marijuana "have not noted any significant increase in marijuana smoking," the message supported legislation to "eliminate all Federal criminal penalties for the possession of up to one ounce of marijuana"—the same level supported by Stroup.

As Eizenstat had predicted, the president's support for decriminalization was big news. CARTER SEEKS TO END MARIJUANA PENALTY FOR SMALL AMOUNTS, the *New York Times* declared on its front page. It was a great victory for Stroup and NORML. With the president of the United States now on board, the decriminalization juggernaut seemed unstoppable.

Far from boosting the promarijuana movement, however, Carter's speech would mark its high point. For, unknown to Peter Bourne, Keith Stroup, and everyone else in Washington, a fierce backlash against pot was brewing—one that would not only halt the march toward decriminalization but also inflict lasting damage on the public-health model Jerome Jaffe had established.

11

The Counterrevolution

THE COUNTERREVOLUTION began, coincidentally enough, in Atlanta, the political home of Jimmy Carter and Peter Bourne. The spark came on a hot, muggy night in August 1976, in the suburban backyard of Ron and Marsha Keith Schuchard (pronounced SHOE-hard). The Schuchards lived in Druid Hills, an enclave of stately homes, rolling lawns, and flowing wisteria across the city line from Atlanta. Ron was an assistant professor of English literature at Emory, which was just down the street; Keith (as her friends called her) had a Ph.D. in English literature and taught at a nearby community college. The only sour note in their otherwise idyllic lives was the personality changes they saw coming over their daughter. About to turn thirteen, she had gone from being a playful burst of sunshine to a moody and lethargic squall. Once an avid tennis player, she now wanted only to hang out with her friends. When she asked to have a birthday party, her parents, taking it as a positive sign, fired up the barbecue.

The hamburgers went uneaten, however. The kids—many of whom were strangers to the Schuchards—retreated to the far corners of the backyard, away from the festive lanterns that had been strung up. Inside, one red-eyed girl tried to use the phone but had trouble dialing; an older boy barged through the kitchen without introducing himself. Cars filled with teenagers cruised out front amid shouts of "Where's the party?" Retiring upstairs, the Schuchards, peering out the window, could see lights flickering at the edge of the yard. Around 1 A.M., after the last of the kids had gone, the couple went outside in their pajamas and, crawling around with flashlights in the wet grass, found crushed cans of malt liquor, empty bottles of wine, and—most disturbing of all—marijuana butts and roach clips.

At last, the Schuchards felt, they had found the cause of their daughter's dourness. It was not adolescent rebellion, nor emotional growing pains, but pot. Like many members of their generation, the Schuchards had had little experience with the drug. During their undergraduate days in Texas, in the early 1960s, beer was by far the drug of choice. Returning to Texas for graduate school after a three-year teaching stint in East Africa, however, they found pot everywhere. The Schuchards had no interest in trying it, but one day some friends served them marijuana-laced brownies without telling them, and they remained stoned for days—an experience that left them full of dread about the drug. Moving to Atlanta in 1969, the couple felt they had left all that behind, but now, at their daughter's birthday party, pot was literally in their own backyard. "We had a sense of something invading our families, of being taken over by a culture that was very dangerous, very menacing," Keith Schuchard observed.

A tall, large-boned woman in her mid-thirties, with a Gatling-gun speaking style, boundless energy, and an unshakable faith in her own opinions, Keith Schuchard demanded from her daughter a list of all the youths who had attended the party, then spent a day calling around to their parents and explaining what had happened. Many were defensive and hostile, but Schuchard eventually persuaded thirty of them to meet with her. After sharing what they knew, the parents decided to get tough. For two weeks, their children would be grounded. That would be followed by a strict curfew, with parental chaperoning to all events—even school dances. The "Nosy Parents Association," the kids called them, but the parents would not relent.

Many others remained aloof, however, and Schuchard, intent on winning them over, began reading up on the risks of marijuana. Using the research tools she'd developed while writing her eight-hundred-page dissertation ("Freemasonry, Secret Societies, and the Continuity of the Occult Traditions in English Literature"), she pored through medical journals and pediatric reviews. In the end, she found only one item that seemed to take the dangers of marijuana seriously: an interview in *Science* magazine with Dr. Robert DuPont. While reaffirming his opposition to sending pot users to jail, the NIDA director noted his concern over the rapid spread in marijuana use, especially among young people. Impressed, Schuchard sat down at her manual typewriter and banged out an emotional letter explaining that she belonged to a group of parents who were concerned about growing marijuana use among their children but frustrated at not being able to find any material on the "serious behavioral changes" and "deterioration of values" that pot caused. Could DuPont help?

Reading her letter, DuPont was leery. He knew Druid Hills well from his days at Emory and found it hard to believe that marijuana had so thoroughly penetrated it. He was not reassured by Schuchard's writing style, with its overripe prose. To make sure she wasn't crazy, he had an assistant talk to her by phone. Assured she wasn't, DuPont arranged to see her during a scheduled visit to Atlanta in early June 1977. DuPont met first with a group of students, who told of how pervasive pot use had become in their school, then with their parents, who expressed their concern over the drug's corrosive effects on the community.

DuPont came away feeling troubled. For more than two years he had been speaking out forcefully in favor of decriminalization. Now, in Atlanta, he had come face-to-face with the consequences: soaring pot use among kids, and panic on the part of their parents. Those parents were so different from the public-health officials he had worked with over the years in the fight against heroin. For the first time, DuPont recalled, he had encountered "real people" who "cared about drugs in a direct, personal way." The heart of the drug problem, he felt, was not heroin addiction, which affected a small, marginalized population, but pot smoking, which touched so many families. This ran directly counter to the Jaffe code, with its emphasis on hard-core users, but DuPont felt strongly that the future of the issue lay with the parents, and overnight he became a convert to their cause. Never again would he speak out in favor of decriminalization. Seeking further to atone for his past views, DuPont asked Schuchard if she would be interested in writing a handbook for parents on how to prevent drug abuse.

Schuchard was so taken with the idea that she quit her teaching job to pursue it full-time. For help, DuPont directed her to Tom Adams, a San Francisco-based prevention specialist who worked frequently with NIDA. Adams, in turn, put Schuchard in touch with drug-abuse professionals around the country. To her dismay, none shared her concern about marijuana. "These people are the enemy," Schuchard recalled thinking.

Schuchard was rescued from her isolation by a neighbor, Sue Rusche. One day in the fall of 1977, Rusche stopped by a local record store with her two young boys and several of their friends to buy a *Star Wars* record. In the store, Rusche was shocked to find a display case full of bongs resembling space guns, pot pipes shaped like Frisbees, and other paraphernalia clearly aimed at kids. Hurrying the boys out of the store, she returned with Schuchard to buy some of the items. Driving around Atlanta, the two women found several other stores selling rolling paper, roach clips, and coke spoons.

If anyone needed proof that the drug culture was out to recruit young people, this was it. "The head shops and the paraphernalia were a gift," said Rusche, a vibrant dark-haired woman who, while more amiable and accommodating than Schuchard, felt no less strongly about the issue. "They helped parents struggling with children with drugs to come out of the closet." Rusche and Schuchard began giving talks at PTA meetings, using a bag full of bongs to illustrate their concern. They also circulated petitions demanding that store owners remove the offending items; most immediately complied.

Hoping to mobilize other parents, Rusche, with Schuchard's help, formed Families in Action—the first organization of parents in the nation dedicated to fighting teenage drug use. In an early test, the group organized a campaign to get the Georgia state legislature to pass a law banning the sale of drug paraphernalia. (It would easily carry.) Meanwhile, Rusche and Schuchard, seeking to learn more about the drug scene, began reading *High Times, Head,* and other drug magazines. To their dismay, they found them filled with blatant come-ons to kids, with ads featuring bongs for "Tots Who Toke" and articles advising teens how to order LSD through the mail. They also learned that paraphernalia manufacturers were helping to fund NORML and were preparing to cash in on the anticipated changes in the law. "Carter Proposes Decrim!" an ad in *High Times* proclaimed. "Paraphernalia Industry Boom Expected."

"We were feeling undermined daily by things the government was doing," Schuchard observed. "Peter Bourne was going strong."

Ever since meeting Bob DuPont, Schuchard had been complaining to him about the president's drug adviser and his liberal views on marijuana. Defending his old friend, DuPont sent Schuchard some copies of his speeches. When she remained unpersuaded, DuPont, learning that Bourne was scheduled to visit Atlanta to give a speech in early December 1977, arranged for Schuchard to meet him. Attending his talk, Schuchard was disappointed by Bourne's cavalier remarks on marijuana. Meeting with him afterward, she began pouring forth her concerns about teenage drug use. Bourne countered by asking Schuchard how she would feel if her child were forced to spend two years in prison for using pot. Back and forth they went, until Schuchard, exasperated, pulled out her "secret weapon," a shopping bag full of head magazines and manuals. Glancing at the ads and articles extolling drug use, Bourne seemed genuinely dismayed, but after a short interval he excused himself and rushed off.

Seething, Schuchard fired off a scorching letter to DuPont. "I know this sounds harsh," she wrote, "but, for all his urbane charm and intelligence, Dr. Bourne seemed more difficult to communicate with about this problem than our image-conscious P.T.A. matriarchs and ex-basketball coach school-principals—and communicating with them is like talking into the tailfeathers as the ostrich blithely buries his head in the sand!" She sent another letter to President Carter, warning him that, by tolerating Bourne and his work on behalf of decriminalization, he was "sitting on a political powder keg." "We seem to be so preoccupied with heroin addicts (1% of the population)," she complained, "that we have formulated no clear national policy towards beginning, youthful users of non-addictive but still hazardous drugs." The letter was ignored. As long as Bourne remained drug czar, Schuchard and her fellow parents had little chance of penetrating the White House.

AND PETER BOURNE'S position certainly seemed secure. The centerpiece of his drug program—the eradication campaign in Mexico—was coming along splendidly. Throughout the Sierra Madre, poppy plants were shriveling, and the flow of Mexican heroin into the United States was dwindling. Once again, shortages were showing up in the nation's cities, and the number of overdose deaths went from 1,800 to 800 in just two years. "The overall success which we have achieved in the drug area during the last ten months continues to be sustained," Bourne stated in a report to the president in late November 1977.

Feeling expansive, he decided to drop by the bash that NORML was throwing in early December to mark the end of its annual conference. If nothing else, Keith Stroup knew how to throw a good party, and the event, held in a posh Dupont Circle townhouse, drew several hundred lawyers, congressional aides, politicians, bureaucrats, and lobbyists, plus assorted marijuana growers and paraphernalia merchants. Waiters carried silver trays bearing caviar and thick joints rolled from the finest grass. Around ten o'clock, a charge went through the crowd: Peter Bourne had arrived. Mobbed by well-wishers, he was quickly escorted upstairs to a private room where the inner circle was gathered. Among those present were Hunter Thompson, David Kennedy (Robert's son), and Keith Stroup. A small, bulletlike container of coke was being passed among the people in the room. Bourne stayed for a short while, then headed back downstairs and left. Rumors quickly spread that the drug czar himself had indulged in the drug-taking. When questioned by journalists, Stroup refused to comment.

As 1978 began, the ties between NORML and the Carter Administration seemed unshakable. Several NORML staff members were given a tour of the White House, and the staffs of NORML and the White House squared off in a softball game.

The good feelings would soon evaporate, however, and Peter Bourne's Mexico program would be the cause. Paralleling the campaign against poppies, the Mexicans had kept up their offensive against marijuana. The Mexicans claimed that all plants sprayed with paraquat died on contact, but there were reports that traffickers were harvesting contaminated leaves and shipping them to the United States. When the U.S. government tested some shipments seized along the border, it found that some were indeed poisoned. Washington refused to intervene, however, and Keith Stroup, sensing a potent organizing tool, began accusing the administration of "cultural genocide." The administration's main defender was Peter Bourne, who argued that, because marijuana was illegal, the Mexicans had every right to destroy it.

Ironically, even as Stroup and his backers were attacking Bourne, the parents in Atlanta were gathering to do the same. In her ongoing search for allies, Keith Schuchard had been introduced to Thomas "Buddy" Gleaton, an associate professor of health at Georgia State University. A former junior-college football coach with a doughy face and easy smile, Gleaton, every spring, held a conference for drug-prevention specialists from throughout the Southeast. By Gleaton's own admission, the conferences had become rather dull affairs, and he was resigned to more of the same for the upcoming session in

May 1978. Then Schuchard came by. For five hours he listened to her describe
her research on marijuana and her organizing activities in Atlanta. Finding her
to be a breath of fresh air, or, more accurately, a gale-force wind, Gleaton,
hoping to liven up his conference, invited her to deliver the keynote.

She did not disappoint. Giving voice to all the rage that had built up in
her over the last two years, Schuchard declared that "many parents, myself
included, have called drug abuse agencies or counselors to ask for information
and advice when they learn that their child or his friends are using marijuana.
Often they are told, in mocking tones, 'Don't over-react; it's just pot; all the
kids do it.'" Denouncing the "youth culture" and its slick come-ons to kids,
Schuchard said that the main reason for the conference was to tell parents to
"trust your gut instincts as parents: you have every right to worry about the use
of any psychoactive drugs, especially illegal drugs, by your child."

After the AP sent out a story about the conference, the phone in Buddy
Gleaton's office would not stop ringing. "I was barraged with requests for
information from parents," he said. To serve them, he and Schuchard decided
to set up a new organization, called Parents' Resource Institute for Drug
Education, or PRIDE.

By mid-1978, then, the marijuana issue had spawned two bitterly opposed
but equally determined middle-class movements, each seeking to wrest control
of the nation's drug policy. In a strange exchange of roles, the guerrilla-like
NORML had become the political insiders while the suburban moms were the
insurgents. "We were the real counterculture," Schuchard would say years
later, sitting in the kitchen of her home in Druid Hills. From time to time, the
conflict between the two groups would flare into the open, with parents showing up at Keith Stroup's speeches to heckle him, and High Times calling Sue
Rusche the "dragon lady."

In the end, though, there was one thing on which the two groups could
agree, and that was their antipathy to Peter Bourne. One false move and they
were ready to pounce. And he soon made it. One day in early July 1978, an
assistant named Ellen Metsky approached Bourne complaining of anxiety and
depression. In his capacity as a psychiatrist, Bourne wrote her a prescription
for fifteen Quaaludes, a popular tranquilizer. To protect Metsky's privacy,
Bourne made out the script to a fictitious "Sarah Brown." Metsky gave the slip
to a friend, who took it to a People's Drug Store in suburban Virginia. A state
pharmacy-board inspector happened to be present, and, asking the woman for
identification, arrested her when she couldn't produce it. Because of Bourne's
position, the U.S. attorney general's office was notified, and within days the
story was on the front page of the Washington Post. CARTER AIDE SIGNED
FAKE QUAALUDE PRESCRIPTION, the headline read. Bourne was put on paid
leave pending further investigation.

The same day the Post story appeared, Keith Stroup was approached by a
reporter for Jack Anderson and asked to confirm reports that Bourne had used

cocaine at the NORML party the previous December. Still steaming over the paraquat issue, Stroup told the reporter that he would no longer deny the charge. The next day, Anderson, appearing on *Good Morning America,* announced that Bourne had used cocaine at the NORML party. At the White House, Bourne gave his version of the story—that while the people around him at the party had used cocaine, he personally had not. By that point, it did not matter. The simple fact that the president's drug adviser had been present while cocaine was being used was sufficient, in the current circumstances, to seal his fate. In an emotional letter of resignation, Bourne wrote the president that, if he had made any mistakes, "they are of the heart and not of the mind." With a flourish, he added, "I fear for the future of the nation far more than for the future of, Your friend, Peter G. Bourne."

THE DEPARTURE of Peter Bourne would mark a watershed in U.S. drug policy. For all his personality quirks and lapses in judgment, his globe-trotting and love of technology, Bourne had remained an adherent of the Jaffe code, with its belief in the primacy of hard-core drug use and the government's responsibility to treat it. Though battered, the public-health model had remained largely intact on his watch.

On the surface, his successor, Lee I. Dogoloff, seemed likely to carry on that tradition. A longtime member of the treatment fraternity, Dogoloff in 1969 had worked for Robert DuPont at the D.C. Department of Corrections, then served as his deputy at the Narcotics Treatment Administration. In 1972, Dogoloff went to work for SAODAP, supervising its relations with state and local governments, and two years later he followed DuPont to NIDA. Under President Ford, Dogoloff was brought into the Old Executive Office Building to help write the *White Paper on Drug Abuse.* After Jimmy Carter's election, he had stayed on as Peter Bourne's deputy.

Unlike Jaffe, DuPont, and Bourne, however, Dogoloff was not a physician. A native of Baltimore who had short curly hair and a chunky build, Dogoloff had attended the University of Maryland, then gone on to earn a master's degree in social work at Howard University. And, while active in the treatment world, he had had limited experience with addicts. As Bourne's deputy, in fact, he had been put in charge of drug prevention. Few areas in the drug field were less glamorous or more amorphous. Seeking inspiration, Dogoloff had convened a group of drug-prevention specialists from around the country, but they seemed to have little clue about how to keep people from using drugs. "I came away from the discussions understanding as little as I did going in," Dogoloff recalled. "Then Buddy and Keith came to see me."

With the help of their congressman, Billy Lee Evans, Gleaton and Schuchard had arranged a series of interviews in Washington. Most did not go well. Trudging from meeting to meeting at NIDA and HEW, the two Atlantans would pour out their concerns about the rise in pot use and its effect on young people. Invariably, they were met with condescension and eye rolling. Then they visited Lee Dogoloff. Seeing these two wild-eyed Georgians enter his office, he was initially skeptical, too. But Gleaton, noticing a photo of Dogoloff's three children, said that he wanted to talk to him not as a professional but as a father. And, as he and Schuchard described their alarm at the expanding drug culture, their anger at the scornful attitudes of drug-abuse professionals, and their efforts to prod parents into taking more control of their kids, Dogoloff grew excited. "It all began to make sense to me," he recalled. "What I hadn't realized before was that drug-abuse 'professionals' were supplanting what families should have been doing." Schuchard and Gleaton "gave me the answer," he went on. "If we could support parental involvement at the grassroots level, there was a promise of turning things around. They crystallized my thinking."

That crystallization represented a dramatic turnaround on Dogoloff's part. As a longtime upholder of the Jaffe code, he had accepted certain key principles about drug abuse, including the distinction between hard and soft drugs, and between chronic and casual use. The *White Paper on Drug Abuse,* which he had helped write, had been emphatic on this point, stating that "the largest portion of the drug abuse problem (and the portion where efforts at reduction should be focused) is created by chronic, intensive users of drugs." In siding with the parents, however, Dogoloff was accepting the notion that experimental pot use was the real core of the nation's drug problem.

To a degree, his concern was understandable. In 1975, the University of Michigan, in an annual survey of high school seniors, found that 27.1 percent had used pot in the previous thirty days; by 1978, that number was up to 37.1 percent. The proportion of those using *daily* had gone from 6 percent to 10.7 percent. In other words, one of every nine high school seniors was getting stoned every day. And they were smoking an average of three-and-a-half joints a day. Wasted, they were falling asleep in class, neglecting their homework, botching exams. Something indeed needed to be done.

Yet marijuana was hardly the only problem kids faced. At their daughter's birthday party, for instance, the Schuchards had found empty beer cans as well as marijuana butts. Yet it was only the latter that had vexed them. As Keith Schuchard would later explain: "Marijuana alarmed us because kids were doing it everywhere. They weren't drinking during school, but they were smoking pot during school. Because it was easier to conceal." Marijuana, she added, was a "gateway drug" that led inexorably to the use of harder drugs like heroin and cocaine. Worse, she said, marijuana had a "whole culture around it" preaching that the drug was fun. "We didn't have anybody preaching to kids that alcohol and cigarettes were going to save them. There was not an aggressive culture directed at kids on those." As a result, she said, "kids smoked marijuana much more often than they smoked cigarettes or used alcohol."

The numbers, however, did not back this up. According to the University of Michigan survey, 72.1 percent of all seniors polled in 1978 said they had

had a drink in the past month—nearly double the number that had had a joint. And 40.3 percent said they had engaged in binge drinking, i.e., had five or more drinks in one sitting, over the past two weeks—nearly four times the number who had smoked pot daily. As for marketing, the ad campaigns mounted on behalf of Budweiser and Miller were far more aggressive than anything being done to promote pot. And, by all accounts, young beer drinkers were far more likely than pot smokers to get into fights, smash up their cars, and engage in casual sex. As for the claim that marijuana was a gateway drug, the National Commission on Marihuana and Drug Abuse had firmly rejected it. While marijuana users were somewhat more likely than nonusers to try other drugs, the commission had found, "only a small portion" were "likely to become persistent, frequent users of these other drugs. The majority appear to experiment only."

Of course, even the small number of marijuana smokers who went on to become chronic users of other drugs were a serious concern; over time, they would swell the ranks of those in need of drug treatment. The key, it would seem, was finding a way to keep kids who experimented with drugs from getting into trouble with them. Yet, in their furious intolerance of all forms of illegal drug use, and in their general indifference toward alcohol, the parents seemed to have broader considerations in mind. As Lee Dogoloff would later put it, the parents were pursuing a cultural agenda whose goals included "changing permissive social attitudes, as well as strengthening the family. The authority of the family in the post-Vietnam period had really been eroded, and this was a way of giving parents a sense of competence once again." Rather than approach the drug problem in public-health terms, then, the parents saw it in moral ones. And, accordingly, they regarded full opposition as the only acceptable course. "Zero tolerance," they called it.

BY THE FALL of 1978, parent groups were sprouting in suburban communities across the country. In Naples, Florida, a wealthy businessman named Bill Barton and his wife Pat—concerned about their daughter's relationship with a drug dealer—organized parents to pressure the police to crack down on dealing at a local high school. In Sacramento, California, a schoolteacher named Carla Lowe was leading a campaign to get the state to ban the sale of drug paraphernalia. From her base in Short Hills, New Jersey, a suburban housewife named Geraldine Silverman was touring the state, lecturing PTAs on the hazards of marijuana use. Even Ross Perot was getting in on the act, organizing chapters of Texas mothers into a statewide campaign called Texans' War on Drugs.

Journalists, who had once written so favorably about NORML, saw a fresh story in the new movement. NBC News, for instance, ran an hour-long antimarijuana special called "Reading, Writing, and Reefer." Produced with the help of Robert DuPont and Keith Schuchard, it portrayed a nation of schoolchildren turned into zombies by pot. "That's when we knew we were in trouble," Keith Stroup recalled. "After years of focusing on young college kids locked away for long periods for smoking grass, all of a sudden NBC was looking at kids smoking at ten and eleven. And it was downhill from there." At the end of 1978, Stroup would leave NORML to start his own law practice.

In Washington, meanwhile, Lee Dogoloff was pushing the parents' agenda. In early 1979, the White House launched an Adolescent Drug Abuse Prevention Campaign, which, as he put it in a memo to Stuart Eizenstat, was designed "to discourage drug use among our youth by providing accurate information to parents, teachers and other key community leaders." Dogoloff also moved to remake the National Institute on Drug Abuse. As the bastion of the professionals who had for so long dismissed the marijuana issue, NIDA represented to the parents all that was wrong with national drug policy. In 1978, the parents lost a key ally when Bob DuPont—a Nixon-Ford holdover —was forced to step down as NIDA's director, but they gained a new one in his successor, Dr. William Pollin, a mild-mannered technocrat who was not about to stand up to the militant mothers. Flexing their muscle, the parents convinced Dogoloff and Pollin to convene a panel of outside experts to review NIDA's literature on marijuana and "reach consensus on a clear health statement," as Dogoloff put it in a memo.

The main flashpoint, however, was the handbook Keith Schuchard was writing. Bob DuPont's original idea had been for her to describe her campaign to mobilize parents in Atlanta, but Schuchard had insisted on including medical information about the risks of marijuana. Most of NIDA's staff—upset at lending the agency's imprimatur to this English teacher—refused to cooperate with her. There was, however, a growing legion of antimarijuana researchers on whom Schuchard could draw, and she packed her manuscript with their views. After handing it in, she and her husband left for Greece, where he was beginning a Fulbright. While she was away, the NIDA staff went to work, shearing away what they saw as her more extreme claims. When the new version reached her in Greece, Schuchard was irate at the extensive revisions that had been made, but, eager finally to get the thing out, she gave it her approval.

Even in its watered-down form, *Parents, Peers, and Pot* was vintage Schuchard. Published under her maiden name (Marsha Manatt), it began with a vivid account of her organizing experiences in Atlanta. There followed a scalding critique of the "youth culture" and its tendency to undermine "the traditional adult authorities who could nurture a young person's ability to reject drug use." The core of the ninety-eight-page booklet, though, was its long and dire description of the health risks of marijuana. Among other things, Schuchard asserted that pot caused lung and bronchial damage, induced acute panic reactions, impaired the body's immune system, altered "the relative roles of the right and left hemispheres of the brain," and decreased the level of sex hormones, causing "enlarged breasts" among adolescent boys. And, without qualification, Schuchard asserted that marijuana was the "gateway" into illicit drug use in America.

To the dismay of NIDA's staff, *Parents, Peers, and Pot* became an instant hit. Eventually, more than one million copies of the manual would be distributed, making it the most widely circulated publication in the institute's history.

NIDA WAS NOT the only organ of government to feel the parents' wrath. In late 1979, Joyce Nalepka, a housewife turned antimarijuana activist in Silver Spring, Maryland, learned that the Senate Judiciary Committee was preparing a revision of the federal criminal code that, among other things, would decriminalize the possession of up to thirty grams of marijuana (slightly more than an ounce). Incensed, Nalepka prodded Charles Mathias, a Republican senator from Maryland and a member of the committee, to hold hearings on the health consequences of marijuana. Prior to the start of the hearing, Nalepka convinced a local Safeway to provide her 50 one-ounce jars of dried parsley—each roughly equivalent to the amount of marijuana in question. Along with two other Maryland moms, she distributed the jars in the Senate. The hearings themselves, held in January 1980, were attended by parents from around the country, and they were so insistent on being heard that a full day was set aside for their testimony. In her own statement, Nalepka said, "The most important credential I can give you to substantiate my testimony is that I am a mother, not a doctor, not a scientist. I am here to protect my children. I am also here to protect my neighbor's children and the children of this nation." It was a statement to which no member of Congress had a retort, and by the end of the hearings decriminalization was effectively dead.

For the parents, the hearings were a milestone, showing one another how widely shared were their concerns. Peggy Mann, a New York writer who was turning out furious antipot pieces for publications like *Reader's Digest,* raised the idea of forming a national organization to push the parents' agenda. It was decided to take up the issue at Buddy Gleaton's upcoming conference, to be held in Atlanta in April. Now called the PRIDE conference, the event drew such luminaries as Lee Dogoloff, Robert DuPont, Senator Sam Nunn, and Atlanta Mayor Maynard Jackson. Meeting in Buddy Gleaton's living room, the movement's leaders decided to set up a National Federation of Parents for Drug-Free Youth (NFP), to be based in Washington. Among those named to the board were Keith Schuchard, Buddy Gleaton, Sue Rusche, and four other Atlantans—a tribute to that city's role as the cradle of the new antimarijuana movement.

Interestingly, even as the parents were preparing to push their cause in Washington, the nation was being hit by a new wave of heroin. The source this time was the Golden Crescent region of Afghanistan, Iran, and Pakistan, where opium production was booming. With the Mexican heroin industry in disarray, traffickers from this area were rushing to fill the gap. Even the old French

Connection reemerged as Italian and French traffickers succeeded in reestablishing their networks. Once again, the success of the supply-side effort had proved very fleeting. And this time, with the Soviet army in Afghanistan and the Ayatollah Khomeini ruling Iran, there was little Washington could do about it.

Reflecting the sharp increase in supplies, New York, Philadelphia, Washington, and other East Coast cities experienced a sudden surge in addiction. Unfortunately, the nation's treatment centers—badly neglected over the past four years—were ill-prepared to deal with it, and the wait for treatment lengthened. "We may be at the edge of a precipice with regard to the Middle Eastern/South Asian heroin problem in the U.S.," a worried Dogoloff wrote to Stuart Eizenstat. Scrambling to respond, the administration sent $10 million in emergency treatment funds to the affected cities, and the crisis was narrowly averted. The experience, however, showed what could happen when the government took its eye off the problem of hard-core drug use. With a new administration preparing to take office, though, it was not clear how much the lesson sank in.

12

Dismantlement

IN LATE MAY 1981, Jerome Jaffe received an invitation to a tenth-anniversary celebration of the founding of the Special Action Office for Drug Abuse Prevention, to be held in Washington on June 17. At the time, Jaffe was working as a professor of psychiatry at the University of Connecticut School of Medicine in Farmington, outside Hartford. He had transferred there in 1979 after spending six years at Columbia University. From a professional standpoint, his time in New York had been very satisfying. His research on smoking and nicotine addiction had established him as a leader in that field. Among other things, he had coined the phrase "compulsive smoking syndrome" to describe smokers' dependence on cigarettes and, after strenuous efforts, convinced the American Psychiatric Association to include it in its new edition of the *Diagnostic and Statistical Manual of Mental Disorders.*

But the psychiatry department at Columbia had proved to be highly fractious, and Jaffe had confided his unhappiness to, among others, Dr. Roger Meyer, the chairman of the psychiatry department at the University of Connecticut Medical School. Just as Meyer had come to Jaffe's aid at the 1972 conference in Puerto Rico, so he now invited him to come to work for him in Connecticut. There, Jaffe, in addition to continuing his research on tobacco, began to study alcoholism and its links to depression. Working in Connecticut was pleasant enough, but he could not escape the sense of being on the sidelines, and so he welcomed the opportunity to return to Washington and see old friends.

About fifty SAODAP alumni, plus their wives and friends, showed up for cocktails and dinner at the Ft. McNair Officers Club. Robert DuPont, Peter Bourne, Lee Dogoloff, and Paul Perito were all there. Regrets were sent by Jeff Donfeld, now working as a real estate lawyer in Los Angeles, and Bud

Krogh, who was struggling to resume his legal career in Seattle. Jaffe, who had taken inches off his sideburns but put them on around his waist, gave a speech that was at once wry and wistful. After reading a telegram from Richard Nixon, who sent his "warm regards" to the former SAODAP workers, Jaffe noted that the drug office had established the notion that there are "two sides" to the drug problem, supply and demand. "Americans had always given lip service to the notion of redemption of the sinner," he said, "but the dollars usually went into fire and damnation." As a result of SAODAP's efforts, he added, recovery from drug addiction "is not just a rare, theoretical possibility—it is common and documented."

While conceding that Nixon may have gone overboard by declaring a "war on drugs," Jaffe suggested that such rhetoric may have been necessary to mobilize people. "If the trumpet give an uncertain sound," he said, recalling a quote from Nixon, "who shall prepare himself for the battle?" "For one brief period," Jaffe concluded, "we believed we could make a difference. We gave of ourselves, unselfishly and unstintingly. For a brief period the word bureaucrat was not a reproach, but an accolade. And we made a difference—we left a legacy."

As Jaffe's tone made clear, the SAODAP experience, though only a few years past, already seemed part of some distant era. The sense of mission that had spurred the office seemed a quaint relic at a time when the nation's treatment system was under assault from neglect, inflation, and the changing political climate. Five months earlier, Ronald Reagan had swept into office proclaiming a new political and cultural agenda, and in the drug field all anybody wanted to talk about was marijuana. Alluding to this in his remarks, Jaffe said, "Why is it, that when marijuana kills a neuron in the cortex or the bone marrow, it is so much more fascinating than when alcohol kills a thousand cells or tobacco causes cancer in those who only inhale the smoke others breathe out?"

Most of those in the room were sympathetic, but even here, among the charter members of the treatment fraternity, a rift was opening. Lee Dogoloff, after leaving office, had gone to work for the National Federation of Parents, the antipot organization he had helped found. And Bob DuPont, now working at an outfit called the American Council on Marijuana and Other Psychoactive Drugs, was leading a campaign against marijuana ("the single biggest new health threat in the nation," he called it in a newspaper column). And so, on that June night at Ft. McNair, the joy of reunion was tempered by the melancholy awareness of old colleagues moving apart.

BY CONTRAST, the atmosphere at the annual PRIDE conference, held that same spring in Atlanta, could not have been more electric. About five hundred people from thirty-four states had shown up, and, with a sympathetic president now in the White House, the anger and alienation that had so suffused the movement were giving way to a new sense of excitement and expectation. Keith Schuchard, who in the past had glowered like an Old Testament prophet, now sounded her own call to battle. "The dream we dared to speak of rather timidly three years ago in this auditorium," she declared, "seems well on its way to realization—that is, the growth of the parents' movement for drug-free youth from a handful of scattered individuals and groups to an increasingly cohesive, articulate, and powerful national movement."

Among those listening to Schuchard was Ann Wrobleski, a member of the staff of First Lady Nancy Reagan. Tall, handsome, and strapping, Wrobleski seemed older than her twenty-eight years. That was due in part to her appearance: Wrobleski favored the sculpted hair and matronly dress common in Republican lunch-club circles. Her manner was no less mature. Polite and charming, Wrobleski projected a sense of self-assurance without seeming arrogant about it. Her poise, together with her political experience (she had worked for several House Republicans) and connections (her husband worked at the Heritage Foundation), had landed Wrobleski a position as Nancy Reagan's projects director.

It was not a trivial job. For, like all first ladies, Mrs. Reagan needed a project. Lady Bird Johnson had highway beautification, Betty Ford had women's rights, and Rosalynn Carter had mental health. While Ronald had been governor of California, Nancy had worked with the Foster Grandparents Program, but the prospect of hanging out with senior citizens over the next four years did not excite her. Drugs did. Her interest in them went back to the late 1960s, when she had had to cope with her children's open experimentation. During the 1980 campaign, Mrs. Reagan had taken time out to visit a Daytop facility in New York, and the reception had been rousing.

When word of Mrs. Reagan's interest in drugs appeared in the press, she received calls from several friends offering encouragement, Ross Perot among them. She also heard from Patricia Burch, a board member of the National Federation of Parents. Burch was well connected in the new administration. Her husband Dean had been chairman of the Federal Communications Commission under Nixon and had since held a number of influential positions in the Republican Party. Thin and affable, with an air of suburban elegance that made her seem stylish even in slacks and sandals, Pat Burch belonged to a Christian study group that met every Friday at the home of Joanne Kemp, the wife of Congressman Jack Kemp. In 1979, Joyce Nalepka, the Silver Spring antipot activist, had addressed the group, and Burch, taken with the cause, decided to enlist.

With the election of Ronald Reagan, a social friend, Burch was determined to recruit the White House as well. Among the members of her Bible group was Susan Baker, whose husband James was the new White House chief of staff, and through her Burch arranged a meeting with Nancy Reagan. In early March 1981, she and two other NFP board members spent ninety minutes with the first lady, telling her about the growing use of marijuana among young people and how the parent movement was fighting it. Interested but wanting to know more, Mrs. Reagan had sent Ann Wrobleski to the PRIDE meeting in April.

Like many members of her generation, Wrobleski had always thought of drug abuse as "people shooting up in the ghetto," as she put it, not kids smoking pot. In Atlanta, however, she was "taken aback by the fervor of the parents. There was a lot of pain and suffering and anger—at the government, and at so-called drug-abuse professionals. You could taste it. They were saying the kinds of things that Nancy Reagan's friends and acquaintances were saying to her. These were people trying to grapple with the problem—people who quite frankly needed a champion."

Back at the White House, Wrobleski met with skepticism. "Marijuana? Get a grip!" she was told. Sheila Tate, the first lady's tough-talking press secretary, recalled, "I was worried that 'killer marijuana' would be our focus, and that she'd be made fun of." There were also fears about getting Mrs. Reagan involved in "such a negative subject," Tate said. So she and Wrobleski began considering alternatives.

The parents were not willing to wait, however. With the position of White House drug adviser vacant, they began a campaign to fill it. And there was little debate about who their candidate should be. Dr. Carlton Turner knew as much about marijuana as anyone in the country. The director of the Research Institute of Pharmaceutical Sciences (RIPS) at the University of Mississippi, Turner ran the university's marijuana project, which supplied pot to government-funded researchers. Here, on a ten-acre plantation on the outskirts of the Ole Miss campus, grew some of the world's finest marijuana, tenderly cultivated from seeds imported from Mexico, Colombia, and some fifty other countries.

Carlton Turner, in short, was the government's pot farmer. To the parents, though, he was something more—one of the few scientists in the nation willing to speak out on the perils of marijuana. A Ph.D. in chemistry, Turner had published more than a hundred papers and book chapters on marijuana and the *Cannabis sativa* plant from which it is derived. For the last several years, he had been traveling around the country, testifying against decriminalization, debating Keith Stroup, speaking to parent groups.

With his compact build, neatly combed brown hair, thick glasses, and flat expression, Turner looked like a small-town pharmacist. In fact, his home town, Butler, Alabama, was so tiny that it didn't even have a police department. Raised by his mother (his father died of tuberculosis before Carlton turned four), Turner graduated from high school in 1958, then enrolled at the University of Southern Mississippi. He planned to become premed but had to drop out his freshman year because of a lack of funds. After a stint in the Army, Turner returned to Southern Mississippi, supporting himself by working at a radio station at night. Graduating at the age of twenty-six, he felt he was too old to embark on a medical career and so settled on chemistry. After getting his doctorate at Ole Miss, he stayed on to grow pot.

Turner reveled in his knowledge of the drug. At the 1980 Senate hearings on marijuana, Turner, expressing scorn for his fellow scientists, had lectured Charles Mathias on the drug's properties. Contrary to popular belief, he said, delta 9-tetrahydrocannabinol (THC) was not the only active ingredient in marijuana. Cannabis actually had sixty-one known cannabinoids, all of them active. Unlike other drugs, which passed through the body quickly, Turner stated, cannabinoids "stay in the body for days and are stored in every major organ of the body, particularly in the brain. . . . There is no other drug used or abused by man that has the staying power and broad cellular actions on the body as do the cannabinoids."

In his presentations, Turner could be highly technical, rattling on about chemovariants, cannabinoid ratios, and psychotomimetic effects. The parents, however, exulted in his knowledge. Buddy Gleaton recalled how, at an early stage of his research, he had called the marijuana project in Mississippi and asked "to talk to the person who knows the most in the country about marijuana." "That's me," Turner had replied. "He was real cocky," Gleaton said with admiration.

What some saw as self-assurance, however, others saw as arrogance. "He was such a combative person," said Dr. Coy Waller, who founded the marijuana project in the late 1960s and served as a sort of mentor to Turner. "When you've got the technical facts, you can be domineering and overbearing. Turner could be overbearing. He rubbed some people the wrong way." Even some of the parents found Turner difficult. "Some of the scientists were exploiting the parent movement," said Sue Rusche, one of the Atlanta founders. "They were telling people what they wanted to hear, not what the scientists were saying." Turner, she added, "fed the belief system."

Significantly, Turner was not a psychopharmacologist—a student of the effects of drugs on human behavior. He was not even a pharmacologist—a student of the effects of drugs on the body. He was a pharma*cognosist,* a student of the chemical components of plants from which drugs are derived. When it came to discussing things like potency levels and solubility rates, few could match him. When it came to the psychological effects of pot or other drugs, his knowledge was strictly secondhand.

None of that mattered to the parents, however. Marijuana was their sole concern, and Turner the man best able to articulate it. Giving a demonstration of their ability to mobilize the grassroots, PRIDE and the NFP began flooding the White House with letters urging Turner's nomination as drug czar. Three times, Turner was called to Washington to be interviewed, the last time by Edwin Meese, who was advising the president on domestic policy; the two found themselves in general agreement. In a final snag, it was discovered that

Turner was a Democrat, but at the last moment he was able to produce a Republican membership card. And so, on July 9, 1981, the Mississippi pot farmer was named the president's drug adviser. In effect, the parents had seized control of White House drug policy.

AS HE SETTLED into his office on the second floor of the Old Executive Office Building, Turner was told by one domestic policy adviser that he should not "make any waves." But the parents had not sent him to Washington to sightsee, and he would receive a mandate of sorts from Nancy Reagan. A few days after taking office, Turner was summoned to the White House to talk with the first lady. The meeting was scheduled to last twenty minutes but instead went on for more than an hour as the two traded anecdotes about Ross Perot and other mutual acquaintances and talked about what Turner's role might be if Mrs. Reagan took up the issue. The first lady remained noncommittal, but her repeated expressions of interest in the subject had raised expectations among friends, and so, at the end of the session, she said, "Carlton, we've been here six months now. When are you going to do something?"

That was all the encouragement Turner needed. For, in his view, federal drug policy needed a drastic overhaul. As NIDA's marijuana supplier, Turner had met Jerome Jaffe, Robert DuPont, and the other architects of the national treatment system, and he had concluded that, as he would later put it, "these guys didn't know what the hell policy was." To start, Turner rejected their idea of distinguishing between hard-core and occasional users. In his view, there was no such thing as "casual" or "recreational" drug use. Nor did he accept the distinction between "hard" and "soft" drugs. To his mind, that was "a very smooth public relations ploy to get the American public to accept all kinds of drugs. It was like soft drinks—you can drink them with impunity if you don't mind a few cavities." From now on, Turner asserted, all types of drugs were to be regarded as equally dangerous, and all types of drug use as equally reprehensible.

But the changes Turner had in mind went far beyond terminology. In his view, the foundation on which U.S. drug policy had rested for the last decade —the notion that the government had a responsibility to treat addicts—was completely mistaken: the "New York model," he scornfully called it, adding that it "had gotten us nothing but pain." For Turner, the very idea of treatment was morally questionable. "Under President Reagan," he explained, "I didn't believe that our philosophy should be that it's all right for kids to use marijuana, cocaine, PCP, and Quaaludes, that—'Hey, that's all right, go do it, and then when you wake up and become a heroin addict, we'll put you on methadone.' That's not what this country is all about."

Many Americans, no doubt, would have agreed with Turner's position. But it overlooked one thing: the "New York model" seemed to be working. The nation's heroin problem, once epidemic in scope, had been kept under control for most of the last decade. And maintaining a national treatment system had been critical to that success.

Such details, however, counted for little in the heady days of the Reagan Revolution. Under the direction of David Stockman, the bumptious budget director, the administration was seeking to cut $40 billion from the $700 billion federal budget. With Reagan declaring off-limits the defense budget and entitlement programs like Social Security and Medicare, most of the cuts were to come in discretionary domestic programs. Inevitably, those programs with powerful constituencies were able to rally opposition to the cuts and blunt them. And few constituencies were more powerful than law enforcement. The new attorney general, William French Smith, was a good friend of the president's, and agencies like the FBI and the DEA had their own backers in Congress. As a result, drug enforcement—far from taking a cut in the new budget—would get a 20 percent boost.

Drug addicts, by contrast, had few friends in Washington, and so the treatment budget would be cut a staggering 25 percent. Taking into account the inflation-driven declines of the Carter years, this amounted to a 43 percent reduction in federal treatment funds in just a few years. In real terms, federal spending on treatment was less than one-fourth what it had been in 1974.

Carlton Turner could not have been more pleased. Rather than deal with inner-city drug addicts, the government was now going to get on with its really important business: stopping teenage pot use. To do that, however, he needed an advocate. And he was about to get one. For Nancy Reagan's search for a cause was taking on new urgency. In late July, she had gone to London for the wedding of Prince Charles and Lady Diana. The trip, on which she had taken four hat boxes, twenty dresses, a hairdresser, a photographer, sixteen security agents, and official chaperons Betsy and Alfred Bloomingdale, had been a public-relations disaster. "Queen Nancy," she was dubbed. In an unfortunate bit of timing, news of Mrs. Reagan's decision to purchase $209,000 worth of new china for the White House broke on the same day the Agriculture Department announced it would consider catsup a vegetable in school lunches. "Someone questioned her about foreign policy and whether or not she favored Red China," Johnny Carson joked on *The Tonight Show.* "She said she did, but not with yellow tablecloths."

Clearly, the first lady needed a makeover. In November, her chief of staff, Peter McCoy, was replaced by James Rosebush, an aide to White House adviser Michael Deaver. In addition to eliminating some of Nancy's more visible excesses, such as accepting designer dresses, Rosebush stepped up the effort to find her a project. While the White House staff continued to fret over the drug issue, few other ideas had emerged, and the first lady herself remained drawn to it, and so drugs it would be. To develop a strategy, Rosebush, Wrobleski, and Tate began meeting regularly at the White House. Carlton Turner frequently joined them. Briefing Mrs. Reagan, Turner explained the philosophy of the parent movement and the natural constituency it would provide. And, finally, Nancy was won over.

To highlight her new interest, Mrs. Reagan's staff decided to take her out of Washington and the cynicism that reigned there. Turner suggested a visit to Straight, Inc., a treatment program for adolescents. One of many "tough love" programs springing up around the country, Straight was among the best known, and most rigid. New clients—many of them committed by their parents against their will—were strip-searched on arrival, then placed in the custody of "old-comers" (other teens already in the program), who never let them out of their sight, even when they went to the bathroom. For up to twelve hours a day, clients were required to confess and renounce their habits in front of their peers. Those resisting would be cursed at, thrown up against the wall, and deprived of sleep for days at a time.

To many, Straight seemed little more than a cult, but the parents loved it, and so, on February 15, 1982, Mrs. Reagan, accompanied by Turner, Wrobleski, Tate, nearly a dozen Secret Service agents, and twenty or so reporters, boarded an Air Force plane for a Straight facility in St. Petersburg, Florida. As Wrobleski recalled, there was "enormous anxiety" about the trip, but, arriving at the hall where the event was being held, the first lady was greeted by a vocal crowd of nearly a thousand people, many of them Straight clients and their parents. For nearly three hours Nancy listened as the teenagers told harrowing tales of pill popping and acid tripping, of selling their bodies to support their habits, of turning on younger brothers and sisters. There were cathartic apologies, emotional embraces, and, at the end of each story, tearful declarations of love. When it was her turn to speak, a wet-eyed Mrs. Reagan joined in. "I'm so proud of you, I really am—and I love you, too," she declared. "She cried real tears that night," said Carlton Turner, a fact widely noted in the day's news accounts.

From Florida, the entourage flew to Dallas, where Mrs. Reagan attended a luncheon hosted by Ross Perot. After Perot described how "mother power" had forced the Texas legislature to adopt a tough package of drug penalties, Mrs. Reagan got up to offer some remarks of her own. A woman, she said, "is like a tea bag. You never know her strength until she's in hot water." After lunch, Mrs. Reagan visited a parent group in Richardson, an affluent Dallas suburb.

By the time she boarded the plane for Washington, her staff knew she'd been a hit. "After months of publicity about her tastes in clothes, china and White House redecorating," Donnie Radcliffe wrote in the *Washington Post,* the "first lady's often-stated interest in drug abuse prevention was claiming the headlines."

"The trip to Florida changed everything," Carlton Turner observed, and no sooner had the staff returned to Washington than planning began on the next trip. On April 2, PRIDE was scheduled to hold its annual conference—

an ideal event, it was thought, to showcase the first lady's concern. At the conference, six hundred people cheered as Nancy received an award from Buddy Gleaton for her antidrug efforts. "I'm very happy to be here among all of you concerned parents," Mrs. Reagan said, "because, while drugs have cast a dark shadow in recent years, the parent movement has been a light in the window—it shines with hope and progress." At the end of her speech, members of the audience hoisted her on their shoulders and carried her around the hall as if she had just scored the winning touchdown in a football game.

From that point on, Nancy Reagan would hit the road once every two weeks or so, visiting schools, prevention programs, and treatment centers. "We'd take her to conservative places where she'd have a friendly audience," Turner noted. "Florida, Texas, Alabama, Mississippi, Arkansas—we'd let the local newspapers in these areas see this lady outside of what the national press had painted her as—a bitch." And, everywhere, there were parent groups eager to help.

On the rare occasions on which Mrs. Reagan ventured into the inner city, special precautions were taken. In September 1982, for instance, she was due to visit Central High School in Little Rock, Arkansas, the site of the famous 1957 desegregation crisis. Anticipating a hostile reception, Turner told Wrobleski that they needed a black person "who can go in there and talk to these people." As it happened, Turner had just seen a TV program on which Carl Eller, a former lineman with the Minnesota Vikings, had discussed his successful battle against cocaine addiction. Quickly, Wrobleski tracked him down and added him to the program. Arriving at the school, Mrs. Reagan was greeted by students carrying signs protesting the administration's social policies. Inside, the climate was no less tense. When Eller began speaking about his experience, however, the crowd grew still, and by the end of his presentation he had completely won it over. "We turned a fiasco into a positive event," Turner said.

There was one thing from which Mrs. Reagan could not be shielded, however, and that was questions about the administration's drug policy. The contrast between the first lady's exhortations against drug use and the cuts in the federal treatment budget was so stark that she was constantly asked about it. Carlton Turner coached her on how to respond. "The government is not a panacea," was his mantra. And Mrs. Reagan proved a good student. Appearing on a radio talk show in Des Moines, Iowa, for instance, she was asked what she thought about the fact that the state was about to lose $500,000 in federal treatment funds. "I don't think financing is the real problem," she replied. "Alcoholics Anonymous is extremely successful and it's not federally financed. I never have thought that money is the answer."

Of course, money *was* the answer for many families. Straight, for instance, charged an up-front fee of up to $4,000, plus $1,000 or more per week of residence. Upper-middle-class parents could afford such sums. Inner-city addicts could not, and the administration's cuts in treatment funds meant a drastic decline in the quality of service available to them. It was hard to pursue the matter with the president's wife without seeming a bully, however, and few did.

IN HIS BELIEF that the government should get out of the drug field, Carlton Turner did exempt one area: law enforcement. The government, he believed, could put a real dent in the supply of drugs in the United States—if only it changed its focus. Since the 1960s, U.S. drug agents had concentrated their efforts on fighting heroin. Turner wanted to place the focus on the real threat to the nation's well-being—marijuana. And, backed by the parents, he would quickly expand the war on pot. In 1981, the DEA was eradicating marijuana in seven states; by 1983, it would be active in forty. With more and more marijuana being grown in national forests, both the U.S. Forest Service and the Bureau of Land Management were enlisted in the drug war. Abroad, Turner began pressuring Colombia—now the United States' leading supplier of pot—to attack its crop as Mexico had done its own.

The immediate crisis, however, was in southern Florida. The area had become the main gateway for drugs entering the country, and Dade County had become a free-fire zone, with wild shoot-outs at shopping malls and disfigured corpses showing up on roadsides. Due largely to the drug trade, the homicide rate had jumped 64 percent in Miami in 1980 alone. So much money was being laundered in the area that the Federal Reserve Bank branch in Miami had a surplus in excess of $2 billion—more than the combined surpluses of every other Fed branch in the country.

In the fall of 1981, Carlton Turner went to southern Florida to investigate. In conversations with police officials, prosecutors, and parent groups, he learned how "mother ships" were steaming up from Colombia carrying tons of marijuana. Approaching Florida, the ships would transfer their cargo to speedboats, which would then dash to secluded coves and inlets along the coast. Determined to intercept those ships, Turner helped put together a federal task force to attack the drug trade in southern Florida. More than three hundred agents were culled from the DEA, the FBI, Customs, the Coast Guard, and other agencies and assigned to the region. The U.S. military agreed to provide Navy Hawkeye E2-C radar surveillance planes to locate suspicious craft and high-speed Cobra helicopters to pursue them. To give the operation visibility, Turner recruited Vice President George Bush to head it. And so, in late January 1982, the administration unveiled the South Florida Task Force. It was the most ambitious drug-interdiction effort in the nation's history—all aimed at keeping marijuana out of the country.

In its initial months, the South Florida Task Force did make some impressive seizures. Yet, as the operation unfolded, it became clear that, to avoid detection, the mother ships were simply putting out farther to sea, beyond the reach of U.S. radar. Even more disturbing, U.S. agents, in the course of looking for pot, were finding something else. In one startling incident at Miami International Airport, Customs agents, inspecting a small plane from Colombia, examined some boxes supposedly filled with jeans. Inside, they found cocaine. In all, there was nearly two tons of the stuff—four times as much as the previous record haul. While pleased with their catch, drug agents shuddered to think how much cocaine was actually getting through.

In fact, it was cocaine, not marijuana, that was causing all the turmoil in southern Florida. For the profits to be made from it were immense. In 1981, a kilogram went for $60,000 at the wholesale level, meaning a smuggler could get rich by sneaking a single suitcase through customs. And, whereas marijuana smugglers were mostly aging hippies or laid-back adventurers, the Colombian traffickers were stone killers who thought nothing of wiping out a rival's entire family. None of this was a secret. Hardly a week went by, in fact, that the *Miami Herald* didn't run a story chronicling the exploits of the "cocaine cowboys." With the parents in control of the White House, however, marijuana would remain the administration's main focus in the region. Not until the mid-1980s would the DEA make cocaine a top priority.

Even had it awakened to the problem sooner, though, it's doubtful that the drug agency could have made much difference. For the Colombian *narcos* had developed a pipeline into the United States that, in terms of capacity and sophistication, made the old French Connection look like a capillary. Extending more than 2,500 miles, from the coca-rich highlands of Peru's Upper Huallaga Valley to the dirt airstrips of Florida, the network employed thousands of growers, chemists, pilots, couriers, communications specialists, accountants, bodyguards, spies, bribe payers, and money launderers, all coordinated from the great trafficking centers of Medellín and Cali.

In the face of all this, U.S. drug agents were hopelessly outmatched. The Colombians were so effective at moving cocaine into the United States, in fact, that its price began to drop. And drop, and drop. And, as it did, the market for it would grow and grow. The result would be a dramatic transformation of the American drug world.

13

Storm Warnings

WHAT CAUSES a drug epidemic? A sudden increase in the supply of a drug, creating a new market for it? Or a change in consumer tastes, which calls forth new supplies? As the great American cocaine boom showed, it's usually a combination of the two. In the early 1970s, cocaine was so scarce and expensive (about $1,000 an ounce) that consumption was limited to the mink-and-Malibu set. The "champagne of drugs," the *New York Times Magazine* called it in 1974. In "Hollywood and Hollywood-on-the-Hudson," the *Times* reported, an "after-dinner sniff of the fine white powder—either from a bejeweled coke spoon held to the nostril or through a tightly rolled banknote, the higher the denomination the better—is as common as a snifter of brandy." Such glamorizing accounts only whetted Americans' appetite for the drug, and, to satisfy it, the Colombians began shipping more of it to the United States. By the late 1970s, cocaine had become a staple at bars, discos, and yuppie dinner parties. In the summer of 1981, *Time*, featuring a martini glass filled with white powder on its cover, declared cocaine "the all-American drug." "No longer is it a sinful secret of the moneyed elite, nor merely an elusive glitter of decadence in raffish society circles, . . ." the magazine trilled. "Today, in part precisely because it is such an emblem of wealth and status, coke is the drug of choice for perhaps millions of solid, conventional and often upwardly mobile citizens. . . ."

Adding to the drug's popularity was a belief in its harmlessness. No less than the DEA, treatment specialists underestimated the threat from cocaine. The 1975 *White Paper on Drug Abuse* ranked cocaine down with marijuana in terms of its potential for abuse. "As currently used," it stated, cocaine "usually does not result in serious social consequences such as crime, hospital emergency room admissions, or death." As late as 1980, Dr. Lester Grinspoon (a member of NORML's advisory board) and James Bakalar wrote in the *Comprehensive Textbook of Psychiatry* that "if it is used no more than two or three times a week, cocaine creates no serious problems." "At present," they added, "chronic cocaine abuse does not usually appear as a medical problem, and there is little literature on its treatment."

The same year that textbook appeared, however, comedian Richard Pryor made headlines by setting himself on fire while freebasing cocaine, a messy and somewhat risky process that involved reducing cocaine to a crystalline base and smoking it in a water pipe. Two years later, John Belushi, who had made a career of drug jokes, died after injecting a mixture of cocaine and heroin. NBC anchorwoman Jessica Savitch became so addled by her habit that she once slurred her words on the air, and pro athletes like Steve Howe of the Los Angeles Dodgers and Thomas "Hollywood" Henderson of the Dallas Cowboys found their careers derailed by the drug.

With so many affluent Americans getting hooked, health-care providers rushed to respond. Across the country, private hospitals set up twenty-eight-day rehabs based loosely on AA's twelve-step approach. Many of these facilities resembled resort spas. At the Boulder Psychiatric Institute in Colorado, for instance, residents could take courses in art therapy, yoga, meditation, and aquatic relaxation. At the Betty Ford Center near Palm Springs, California, clients might find themselves taking out the trash alongside Elizabeth Taylor or Johnny Cash. The one criterion for admission was an ability to pay the steep fees, which ranged up to $350 a day. Seeking customers, some of the centers placed ads in entertainment trade journals like *Billboard* and *Variety*.

Even more enterprising was Dr. Mark Gold, a psychiatrist at Fair Oaks Hospital in Summit, New Jersey. In the late 1970s, Gold had made a name for himself by treating celebrity addicts like Mamas and Papas singer John Phillips and his daughter Mackenzie. Seeking more recruits, Gold decided in the spring of 1983 to set up a national cocaine hot line (800-COCAINE). To launch it, he arranged an appearance on the *Today* show. By the time he got back to his office, the hot line had received nearly a hundred calls. Soon, the service was getting a thousand a day, forcing Gold to add new counselors.

A tireless promoter, Gold never failed to present the hot line as a public service. In fact, its main purpose was to recruit potential clients. If a caller had a generous insurance policy, he'd be referred to Fair Oaks or some other plush facility. If he didn't, he'd be referred to Phoenix House or Daytop Village and wished a good day. And, as cocaine slid down the socioeconomic ladder, the number of such callers soared. This occurred just as the Reagan budget cuts were taking effect. A two-tier treatment system was emerging, with a private tier featuring expert counselors, gourmet food, and instant access, and a public one featuring growing caseloads, crumbling buildings, and long waiting lists. A serious crisis was in the making, and members of the treatment fraternity scrambled to publicize it.

Among the most persistent was Karst Besteman. Ten years earlier, Besteman had helped Jerome Jaffe set up the national treatment network. After NIDA was created, Besteman went to work there. In 1980, he was transferred to New York to administer the Public Health Service's programs in the Northeast. Four years later, he left the government to become executive director of the Alcohol and Drug Problems Association of North America, which represented substance-abuse counselors. One of the main problems those counselors faced was the sharp rise in cocaine abuse. "If you looked at the survey data, cocaine was going nuts," he recalled.

Thick-necked, bald-headed, and barrel-chested, Besteman looked as solid as a tree trunk, and, emotionally, he was no less grounded. But the steady breakdown in the nation's treatment network infuriated him. To get a sense of how far things had gone, he sent a survey to state officials, asking them to describe the impact the federal cuts were having on their ability to deliver services.

Things were far worse than he had imagined. In New Jersey, for instance, which had suffered $4.2 million in cuts, the number of slots had gone from 8,000 to 6,100, forcing many programs to operate at 120 percent of capacity. Maryland, by increasing caseloads, had managed to create 360 new slots, but even so the average wait for treatment was up to 47 days. In Minnesota, many counties had had to eliminate transportation to detox facilities—a real hardship in rural areas—while in Louisiana programs were "saturated and operating with a patient to counselor ratio which almost precludes success in treatment. . . . Therapist burnout and employee turnover are increasing at an alarming rate." In Pennsylvania, where more than thirty programs had been forced to close, state officials estimated that between 8,000 and 10,000 people would be refused care in the coming fiscal year. "The system needs a significant infusion of restored federal funds to deal with the uninsured and youth being referred for treatment as a result of prevention initiatives," state officials noted.

On and on the reports went, each recounting its own tale of woe. Having recently left the government, Besteman was free to speak his mind, and he did. "I and several others went to Congress, to the administration, to NIDA, and said, 'For God's sake, look what's going on here,'" he recalled. Testifying before the House Select Committee on Narcotics in June 1984, Besteman declared that, after "eight years of hard effort and a fair Federal investment" in building the nation's treatment system, "we, I think, are at risk right now . . . of having it overwhelmed and having it collapse in the next year or two."

Besteman also took his case to Carlton Turner. Besteman knew Turner from his days at NIDA, when Turner was supplying pot to its researchers. When Besteman approached him at the White House, however, Turner was curt. "He said that I was a Neanderthal from the old heroin days—that I was too tied to treatment," Besteman recalled. "He talked mostly about marijuana." His normally even tone taking on an edge, Besteman observed: "If I wanted to know anything about marijuana, the first person I'd go to would be Carlton Turner. If I wanted to know anything about public policy, the last person I'd go to would be Carlton Turner. He could grow really good pot. But when it came to human behavior, he was out of his element."

Besteman was hardly the only drug-abuse professional to sound the alarm. Dr. Robert Newman of the Beth Israel Medical Center, Dr. Mitchell Rosenthal of Phoenix House, and a host of state and local officials tried to alert the White House. Turner, however, was deaf to them all. By his reckoning, everything was coming along nicely. Across the land, public attitudes toward drugs were hardening, head shops were closing, and state legislatures were enacting tough antidrug laws. Moreover, the University of Michigan's annual survey showed that only 25.2 percent of high school seniors in 1984 had smoked pot in the past month—down from 37.1 percent in 1978. "Every indicator you could look at showed progress being made," Turner said, looking back at that period.

Yet, aside from marijuana, the indicators were anything but rosy. According to that same University of Michigan survey, 5.8 percent of all twelfth-graders had tried cocaine in the past month—*double* the number in 1977. A survey of five hundred callers to the 800-COCAINE hot line found that about half of those sniffing the drug were experiencing feelings of paranoia and panic and considered themselves addicted. "Without question, the number of users of cocaine is escalating with frightening rapidity across the country," Jane Brody wrote in the *New York Times* in May 1984. The administration's own *1984 National Strategy*, drafted by Turner's office, observed that, with prices falling, cocaine use "appeared to be spreading from high-income users to drug abusers in lower socio-economic levels, including narcotics addicts."

Turner, however, felt no need to respond. "If people can afford to go out and buy cocaine," he would later explain, "why should the government pay for their treatment? The government is not responsible for their treatment—*they* are responsible." He added: "This country has a problem accepting the fact that there are really bad people in society. We've got the belief that nobody's bad—that we can rehabilitate everybody."

All the griping from the treatment community irritated Turner. Psychiatrists, in particular, galled him. For years, parents had been taking their pot-addled teenagers to psychiatrists, only to be told, as Turner put it, that "your kids don't have a problem—*you* have a problem." Now it was payback time. "I made a consensus decision," he said, "that we were going to get rid of all the damned psychiatrists." So, even as members of the treatment fraternity were warning the government about the gathering cocaine crisis, Turner was working behind the scenes to isolate them. And, for assistance, he would turn to the most extreme elements of the parent movement.

THE NATIONAL FEDERATION OF PARENTS had two faces. Pat Burch represented the polite one. A master of the inside-Washington game, she and her husband Dean were regulars on the Republican dinner circuit. In recognition of her extensive contacts, the NFP had placed her in charge of its legislative committee. Installing an extra phone line in the living room of her country mansion in Potomac, Maryland, Burch spent up to ten hours a day calling congressmen to solicit their help with legislation. A modest woman despite her rarefied world, Burch would deferentially seek their advice—an effective strategy with ego-driven congressmen.

Just in case they needed prodding, however, Burch could call on the backing of parent groups throughout the country. Within two hours, she could have two thousand telegrams on the Hill in support of NFP positions. And, once a year, when the federation held its annual conference, five hundred parents would swarm through Congress, venting their views with such vehemence that Burch herself sometimes grew worried. "The parents could get so zealous," she said. "A lot of our time was spent calling them off."

This was the other, less genial face of the NFP. From its inception, the parent movement had attracted people of passionate, even fanatical, views. And it was these radical elements that drove the movement. The "shock troops," Buddy Gleaton called them.

Their commander was a middle-aged Massachusetts businessman named Otto Moulton. The NFP's treasurer, Moulton came to wield enormous influence over drug policy during the Reagan years, acting as a sort of ideological gatekeeper. A resident of Danvers, a picture-book town of 25,000, Moulton owned a toolmaking company that manufactured parts for the F-15 fighter, among other projects. The father of four, he coached a girls' high school softball team and had a batting cage installed in his backyard for use by neighborhood kids. With his round belly, fleshy face, and flock of curly locks, Moulton seemed like a giant teddy bear. Whenever the subject of drugs arose, however, he would suddenly flush, grow agitated, and mutter about "druggie bastards" and "assholes." As Moulton saw it, the nation was engaged in an Armageddon-like struggle between upstanding Americans on the one hand and the drug culture on the other; unless the good guys won, America was doomed to third-world status. And no drug threatened the nation like marijuana.

Moulton had been seized by the issue in 1977, when he discovered *High Times* being sold on a local newsstand. Unsettled by this intrusion into his community, he decided to fight back. "When I first got involved in this," he recalled, "I couldn't concentrate on my business. I'd wake up in the middle of the night, trying to figure out ways to help." Using his own money, Moulton began giving speeches around the country, toting two suitcases full of drug paraphernalia and literature. At every stop, he would visit local bookstores, scanning the shelves for out-of-print books on drugs. His basement slowly filled with government reports, congressional hearings, newspaper clippings, scholarly journals, newsletters, NORML literature, and back issues of *High*

Times. Indexing and cross-referencing, he began to discern the existence of one giant, interlocking drug culture.

To monitor that culture, Moulton and his wife Connie set up a network of informants, called the Committees of Correspondence, after the Revolutionary War groups established to track the activities of the British and their traitorous allies. Members would attend meetings, watch television, and read the press in their local communities; if they encountered anyone who seemed the least bit soft on drugs, they would immediately inform Moulton. He, in turn, would dash off an accusatory letter, backed up by a thick packet of documentation from his library. These "Otto Bombs," as they were called, would be sent off to federal and state officials, DEA agents, and congressmen, as well as to dozens of parent groups, who would make their own displeasure known.

As a result of all this, Moulton, who had never gone beyond vocational school, came to exercise a sort of veto power over what people said and wrote about drugs. Nancy Reagan's office, for instance, often sent materials to him for approval. "People would want to put her name on things," Moulton observed. "They would call me up to make sure it checked out." As chairman of the National Federation of Parents' materials review committee, Moulton scoured the publications of the National Institute on Drug Abuse, demanding countless changes in tone and wording. "Dr. Pollin was a real nice guy," Moulton said with a sly smile. "And let's face it—we got some things changed."

But it was not just publications that Moulton monitored. Over the years, he compiled a list of individuals whose views on drugs he regarded as so dangerous that they had to be confronted. In all, about two dozen or so people were on the list—some of them members of the treatment fraternity—and Moulton could make their lives miserable.

Certainly, that was Dr. David Smith's experience. By the early 1980s, the soft-spoken, shaggy-haired doctor had become something of a legend in the treatment field. After receiving the initial grant from the Nixon Administration, his Haight-Ashbury Free Medical Clinic had expanded to the point where it had a half-dozen clinics in San Francisco. Smith personally saw up to fifty patients a week. Long before most, he had recognized the dangers of cocaine; in 1977, for instance, in a monograph for NIDA, he had written that, if cocaine became more readily available at a substantially lower cost, "more destructive patterns of abuse could develop."

On the subject of marijuana, however, Smith's attitudes were more lax. From his work in the Haight, he knew that pot could be abused, but he did not think people should be locked up for it, and so he had joined NORML's advisory board. And, in Moulton's view, that was all that mattered. "This guy wrote more goddamned crap—and lies—in the seventies," Moulton angrily observed. Anytime Smith was invited to speak somewhere, Moulton, hearing of it, would dash off an irate letter. In early 1983, for instance, Moulton, learning that Smith had been invited to address an association of narcotics officers in Hartford, wrote the group's director that "having someone associated with pro-drug forces on programs to fight drug use is like having Adolf Hitler teaching the American Generals how to fight the German Army. The parent movement in the country knows about David E. Smith's activity and associations and are disgusted. . . ."

Moulton was particularly incensed by Smith's presence at events sponsored by Robert DuPont's American Council on Marijuana. By this point, DuPont had become a tireless crusader against pot, but he admired Smith's work with addicts and so would invite him to conferences—to Moulton's great dismay. "I am confused," he wrote DuPont on September 27, 1982. "Why would a prestigious organization like the American Council on Marijuana align itself with . . . individuals like David E. Smith? In my opinion, they have done great damage to our society with their mixed public messages on illegal drugs." The letter went on for five pages, providing examples of Smith's views and those of others associated with DuPont's organization.

DuPont himself was among them. Having once supported decriminalization, DuPont remained deeply suspect in Moulton's eyes. Among other things, Moulton had discovered DuPont's name on some promotional literature for Edward Brecher's 1972 report for Consumers Union, *Licit and Illicit Drugs,* which offered a temperate look at America's drug problem. In his letter to DuPont, Moulton asked if he would consider making "a public statement exposing this book's false information regarding the crude drug marijuana." "You are number one with me!" DuPont wrote back, adding that he did not want to give anyone "any mixed messages" on drugs. "Drugs are bad for people, period," he stated. If Moulton found evidence that he was sounding "pro-drug" in any way, DuPont went on, "let me know." DuPont added that he had sent a letter to Consumers Union demanding that it stop using his name to promote the book. "Is this a satisfactory response?" he wrote. "Or do you want something different?"

Unappeased, Moulton demanded that DuPont fully disassociate himself from Smith. DuPont wrote back that it was not easy to "write off" a long-time friend like Smith. But, based "on the evidence you have brought to my attention," he noted, he was "deeply troubled" by Smith's views. "Keep the messages coming," he added. And Moulton did. Thus was DuPont kept in line.

In his campaign against Smith, Moulton found a ready ally in Carlton Turner. In June 1983, for instance, Turner was invited to attend a conference in Atlanta devoted entirely to cocaine—one of the first such meetings in the country. Among the listed speakers was David Smith. Circling his name, as well as the names of other suspect individuals, Turner sent a copy of the program to Moulton, along with a brief note on White House stationery, asking him to "note the names" he had circled. "They are pro-drug groups of which we should be careful," he wrote.

So, at a time when the nation's public-health experts were meeting to discuss the spreading cocaine epidemic, the White House drug adviser was joining with the parent movement to marginalize them. And this was not an isolated case. "I talked to Otto on a fairly regular basis," Turner noted. "He was very influential."

Using his connections, Moulton tried to get the administration to cut off all federal funds to Smith's clinics. He ultimately failed—Smith had too many friends in high places—but the attacks left him shaken. "Otto Moulton would say the most awful things—things that were total lies," Smith said. "He really smeared me." His campaign, he said, was part of "a very vicious attempt to deny care to addicts and alcoholics who don't have money." Smith, who would weather Moulton's attacks enough to be elected the president of the prestigious American Society of Addiction Medicine in 1994, credited the parent movement with raising public awareness about the problem of pot use among the young; Smith himself would become much more cautious about the drug over the years. At the same time, he faulted the parents for being "very hostile toward treatment, toward people working with addicts at the community level. They were against the whole idea of recovery."

To the parents, the notion of recovery meant that addicts could get well —a message that, they felt, undermined their warnings to young people not to use drugs. They felt so strongly about the issue that they eventually convinced Nancy Reagan not to meet with recovering addicts—a decision that further undermined the public's support for drug treatment.

EVENTUALLY, THE NFP's close ties to the Reagan Administration would prove its undoing, for groups in the field began wondering whose interests it was really serving. "The NFP was a Republican organization," said Buddy Gleaton, who gradually drifted away from it. Tom Adams, a prevention specialist who worked closely with the movement, noted that "a lot of the parent groups wouldn't affiliate with the NFP. They saw it as out of touch."

Adams, a blunt, driven man in his mid-fifties, had a proprietary interest in the movement. During the late 1970s, Adams, as director of the Pyramid Project, a NIDA-funded program to promote drug prevention, had played an important part in putting the various parent groups in touch with one another; it was Adams who had introduced Keith Schuchard to Buddy Gleaton. Since then, Adams, from his base near San Francisco, had watched with pride as the movement had blossomed. Yet, the more powerful the NFP became, the more remote it seemed.

Adams was particularly upset over the federation's failure to reach beyond its white suburban core. "I was very, very concerned over the fact that there were so few black parents in the movement," said Adams, who in the 1960s had worked with juvenile delinquents. "I tried to get them to put more blacks in." Adams had one candidate who seemed ideal, an Oakland-based grandmother and long-time activist named Joan Brann. In early 1984, Adams helped Brann set up Oakland Parents in Action, which quickly emerged as the leading parent group in the black community. Try as he might, however, he could not convince the NFP to add her to its board.

Intent on getting the group some publicity, Adams contacted Ann Wrobleski, with whom he was friendly, and suggested that Nancy Reagan visit Oakland. Throughout 1983 and 1984, the first lady had kept up her antidrug travels. She had steered clear of the inner city, however, afraid of the reception she might get. Adams, though, promised a friendly audience in Oakland, and so on July 3, 1984, Nancy Reagan arrived at the Longfellow Elementary School, located in a rough part of town.

Together with some fifty adults and youngsters, Mrs. Reagan watched a thirteen-minute antidrug film that had been produced by NIDA. In it, a child was asked what he would do if offered drugs. "I'd say no," he responded. The phrase had been coined by the Advertising Council for a NIDA campaign the previous year, but no one had paid it much attention. Now Mrs. Reagan picked up on it. "We only make this trip once," she said. "Let's make it count and just say no to drugs."

Nothing immediately came of the event. But a few months later, when Joan Brann decided to set up a club to keep elementary school kids off drugs, she called it a Just Say No club. Then, in early 1985, Adams learned that the White House was planning an antidrug event for young people, and he got permission to bring several club members from Oakland. He also convinced Nancy Reagan's staff to invite eight-year-old Soleil Moon Frye, the popular star of the TV show *Punky Brewster*. At the meeting, Frye presented Mrs. Reagan with a scrapbook of the Oakland club's activities.

For the first time, Just Say No gained national attention. Back in Oakland, Adams organized a meeting of minority parents from Baltimore, Atlanta, and other cities to encourage them to set up their own clubs. Then *Punky Brewster* devoted an entire episode to Just Say No, and clubs began popping up all over the country. Sensing the movement's potential, Mrs. Reagan began using the phrase in her own presentations. Quickly, the slogan became a national sensation, inspiring thousands of clubs, setting off giant walkathons, appearing on countless T-shirts. Just Say No was on its way to becoming the most remembered phrase of the Reagan presidency.

And the most ridiculed. And, for that, Tom Adams held Nancy Reagan responsible. "Mrs. Reagan never understood that this movement was for little kids," he observed. "She would always use the term with teenagers. It was not for teenagers. People would say, 'Don't you think it's superficial to tell a sixteen-year-old kid "just say no"?' And they were absolutely right." To Adams's chagrin, Mrs. Reagan used the phrase even in treatment centers. "That you could talk to men and women in treatment and tell them that all they had to do was 'just say no'—that was completely ridiculous."

Adams was further irritated by the administration's seeming indifference to the nation's growing cocaine problem. Hoping to sound an alarm, he got an opportunity in October 1985, when Nancy Reagan was scheduled to hold a drug-abuse summit for the first ladies of the world. After attending a series of events in Washington, the women were to travel to New York for a morning-long session at the United Nations. To speak at the event, the White House asked several U.S. officials, plus three specialists—Phoenix House director Mitchell Rosenthal, Keith Schuchard, and Tom Adams.

To introduce his remarks, Adams asked some friends at NBC to produce a videotape that would show various prevention programs in action, including Just Say No. Adams asked the producers to mention survey data showing the severity of the drug problem in the United States. As requested by the White House, Adams submitted his speech for review, and it was duly cleared.

At the last moment, however, Nancy Reagan decided that, instead of the State Department moderator who'd been lined up for the event, she wanted Carlton Turner. At the time, Turner was in Peru, inspecting coca-eradication programs. Rushing back to Washington, he hurriedly reviewed the prepared speeches. When he got to Adams's, with its frank assertions about the rising levels of drug use in the United States, he grew upset. The speech was a "fiasco," he told the first lady. Mrs. Reagan asked if he could clean it up. "I *will* clean it up," Turner promised. Adams was informed that he would not be permitted to speak unless he deleted the negative references. He did.

"You don't embarrass the first lady of the United States," Turner said, explaining his actions. "You don't put the first lady at the United Nations in front of the damned world and have people with a vested interest come up and upstage her." Adams remembered the matter differently: "Carlton said, 'We don't want people to get the impression that there's been a rise in drug abuse during this administration.' Any word that there was more drug abuse, he was nervous about. They didn't want any bad news."

The summit was attended by thirty-one first ladies, from Imelda Marcos of the Philippines to Rosario María Murillo, the wife of Nicaraguan President Daniel Ortega. For two-and-a-half hours, they sat in a U.N. conference room, listening to anodyne speeches about the success the United States was having in combating drug abuse. The conference was so highly scripted that none of the first ladies even got a chance to speak.

The U.N. summit capped a banner year for Nancy Reagan. A one-time political liability for the White House, she had surpassed the president himself in popularity polls. And the press, which had once so reviled her, now had only praise. CO-STARRING AT THE WHITE HOUSE, declared *Time* in a fawning cover story. NANCY REAGAN'S CLOUT AND CAUSES BRING NEW RESPECT. CBS, which had aired some of the toughest pieces about Mrs. Reagan, now offered some of the most effusive. "Even while Mrs. Reagan's critics were accusing her of insensitivity," Lesley Stahl cooed, "she was quietly devoting herself to fighting school-age drug abuse, a cause she says she embraced after raising two children in the 1960s."

So, the strategy that Carlton Turner and Ann Wrobleski had mapped out four years earlier seemed a great success. Certainly, few were challenging the administration's central assertion—that the nation's drug problem was well under control.

14

The Deluge

THE FIRST INDICATION that something awful was afoot in the nation's cities came not from the Drug Enforcement Administration, nor the National Institute on Drug Abuse, nor any other federal agency, but from the *New York Times*. On November 29, 1985, five weeks after Nancy Reagan's drug summit, the paper ran a front-page article headlined, A NEW PURIFIED FORM OF COCAINE CAUSES ALARM AS ABUSE INCREASES. Called crack, the new substance was "spreading throughout the city and its suburbs," Jane Gross wrote. William Hopkins, the director of a street research unit, was quoted as saying that "there's always something new developing, new substances, new ways of using substances. Some of [the] things you hear of die down, but this, I have every reason to believe, is building. This is the wave of the future."

To this day, the origins of crack remain the subject of intense speculation. According to one view, the main culprit was the CIA and the Nicaraguan contra army it backed in the 1980s. "To understand how crack came to curse black America, you have to go into the volcanic hills overlooking Managua, the capital of the Republic of Nicaragua," reporter Gary Webb wrote in his much-publicized series "Dark Alliance: The Story Behind the Crack Explosion," which appeared in the *San Jose Mercury News* in August 1996. According to Webb, right-wing Nicaraguans linked to the contras opened a major cocaine pipeline into the black neighborhoods of Los Angeles, which "helped spark a crack explosion in urban America." The articles fed suspicions—especially among African-Americans—about a possible U.S. government role in spreading the drug.

As an exploration of possible contra involvement in Latin American drug-running, the *Mercury News* series provided some tantalizing leads. As a look at how crack emerged in the United States, it was ludicrous.

By the time crack hit this country, the cocaine trade had become a vast hemispheric enterprise, involving traffickers from every nation from Argentina to Mexico. No doubt Nicaraguans were among them, but, of the more than seventy tons of cocaine being consumed in the United States every year, they supplied but a thimbleful. The great bulk remained in the hands of the Colombian syndicates. It was not Managua, but Medellín and Cali, that controlled the flow of cocaine into the United States.

In New York City, the importing of cocaine was dominated by Colombians living in Jackson Heights, a middle-class section of Queens. Since the Colombians lacked the contacts needed to move drugs on the street, they sold most of their product to Dominicans living in Washington Heights, in upper Manhattan. New York's fastest-growing immigrant group, the Dominicans had both extensive street connections and abundant entrepreneurial skills. Known in the Caribbean as merchants and traders, they had helped turn Washington Heights into a vibrant bazaar full of bodegas, *farmacias,* and bargain clothing outlets. Not a few, however, had applied their marketing talent to the drug trade, and by the early 1980s they had become the city's premier coke dealers.

By that point, many of their customers were freebasing the drug. Because of the hassle involved in producing base, these customers began asking their dealers to convert the powder in advance. Experimenting with various additives, the dealers ultimately found that sodium bicarbonate—simple baking soda—worked best. All one had to do was mix cocaine with Arm & Hammer, add water, and heat to a boil. As it cooled, the compound turned into a hard off-white mass that could be broken into pellets and smoked. Before long, Dominican dealers were out on the streets of Washington Heights, peddling crack in small plastic vials. No longer was it necessary to shell out $80 or $100 for a gram of coke; now a hit could be had for as little as $5 or $10, and in far more potent form. The Moët of drugs had gone the way of McDonald's, helping to turn the Heights into a raucous, roaring Bedlam.

Before long, the Dominicans were supplying cocaine to aspiring crack dealers from other ethnic groups. Certainly, the entry barriers were low. With just a few hundred dollars, an entrepreneur could buy an "eight-ball" (eight grams) of coke, then cook it up in his kitchen and hustle it on the street. Controlled by hundreds of small, faceless organizations and individuals, crack was the most democratic and decentralized drug ever marketed in this country. Within months, sellers were popping up in Spanish Harlem, the South Bronx, and other districts thick with housing projects, abandoned buildings, and overgrown lots.

For that's where the customers were. From the start, crack flourished in the inner city. While plenty of Jerseyites and Long Islanders would try it, most were quickly scared off by its potency. Ghetto residents, by contrast, desperately wanted an escape, and the more powerful the getaway vehicle, the better. Stuck in dead-end jobs, crammed into bleak housing projects, leading lives of quiet desperation, the Yvonne Hamiltons of New York flocked to the curbside markets that were sprouting like boils across the city's face.

In the process, they fed a climate of anarchy and violence that rattled even the most seasoned city dwellers. Hungry for cash, crack users were boosting so many car radios that blaring alarms became a regular nighttime accompaniment. Fighting over turf, Uzi-toting crack gangs were making the city's funeral parlors work overtime. Hospital wards contended with a wave of boarder babies while city caseworkers faced a flood of child-abuse cases.

Most burdened of all were the city's treatment facilities. Given the speed with which crack users crashed, they were soon showing up at rehab centers, desperate for help. DRUG TREATMENT IN CITY IS STRAINED BY CRACK, the *Times* declared in May 1986. According to the paper, "programs in New York City and its suburbs are filled to capacity and are struggling to avoid turning people away as more and more people become addicted to crack." The darkest fears of the treatment fraternity were being realized.

The one bit of positive news was that, thus far, crack was confined to a few enclaves. Aside from New York, only Los Angeles, Miami, and Detroit had developed serious problems. It seemed only a matter of time, however, before the contagion spread. In many respects, the government faced a crisis similar to the one that had confronted the Nixon Administration in the early 1970s, when it had set up the Special Action Office and brought in Jerome Jaffe from Chicago to run it.

As IT HAPPENED, Jaffe was back in Washington at the time of crack's emergence. In 1984, while still in Connecticut, he had been asked if he was interested in becoming the director of NIDA's Addiction Research Center. As a young physician, Jaffe had dreamed of working at the center, and his failure to be assigned to it in Lexington had been a major disappointment. The narcotics farm itself had long since been closed and the center moved to Baltimore. Going to work there would mean both uprooting his family and taking a pay cut, but Jaffe was growing bored in Connecticut and so he agreed to take the job, and he and Faith moved into a townhouse complex in Towson, a suburb of Baltimore.

Then, in early 1985, William Pollin retired as NIDA's director, and, while a search committee sought a new one, Jaffe was asked to serve as acting head. Now in his early fifties, he did not relish the prospect of holding two demanding jobs at once, but his sense of duty prevailed, and in May 1985 he began dividing his time between the research center in Baltimore and the drug institute in Rockville. Twelve years after having left SAODAP, Jaffe was back in charge of the nation's treatment network.

And he was dismayed to see what had become of it. "The programs we funded in the 1970s had no fat," he recalled. "And they had no fat by policy. I knew where the fat was, and I didn't put any in, because I thought we would sell treatment as an alternative to the lock-'em-up-and-throw-away-the-key approach, which even then was far more expensive. Therefore, we tried to keep outlays as close to real costs as possible. That turned out to be a poor judgment politically, because it meant that we trusted the political process to be reasonable and rational—always a mistake. If you take a program that is adequate, but minimally adequate, and cut into it, then the net effect is it's inadequate, and that's what happened." In 1986, the federal treatment budget came to just $190 million—in real terms, barely one-fifth the amount Jaffe had had to work with in 1973. Overall, about 80 percent of the $2.2-billion drug budget was going for the supply side, compared to just 20 percent for the demand side—the reverse of the ratio during the Nixon years.

Jaffe was further distressed to find how little research was being done on treating cocaine addiction. "You had these twenty-thousand-dollars-for-three-week treatments that Mark Gold was purveying, but there was no sense at all of how well these people did, no sense of 'We better learn more about how to treat this,' " Jaffe said. "They were still pretty much interested in PR efforts— the Just Say No kind of thing—plus tough law enforcement."

As the director of NIDA and the Addiction Research Center, Jaffe had frequent contact with Carlton Turner. In their approach to the drug problem, the two men could not have been more different, and their encounters often had a comic edge. Turner, Jaffe recalled, "would open meetings by saying, 'I bring you greetings from the president,' when you were pretty damned sure he hadn't seen the president." Invariably, Turner would discuss the great victories the United States was having against the drug trade abroad. "He would say, 'We captured this many people and destroyed this many clandestine labs in Colombia,' " Jaffe noted. "He had a real enthusiasm for that."

At meetings with NIDA researchers, Turner rarely discussed crack or cocaine. Tobacco seemed his main preoccupation. NIDA was funding several research projects on nicotine, and Turner liked none of them. Jaffe recalled being present at one meeting at which the White House drug adviser "went out of his way to castigate drug-abuse researchers for the silliness and inappropriateness of their interest in tobacco. Given his role, it was sort of a veiled threat—'If you guys continue this research, it might affect your budgets.' " Overall, Jaffe said, Turner "did not have any great respect for the research NIDA was doing, except for its work in marijuana, which he never ceased to see as the central problem."

Through a bizarre turn of events, Jaffe found himself sucked into the marijuana maelstrom. Before rejoining the government, he had agreed to serve as a consultant to a small New York publishing house that was preparing a multivolume encyclopedia on psychoactive drugs. His role consisted mainly of suggesting writers, and, when the work appeared, in 1985, he was listed as a senior editorial consultant. One of the volumes dealt with marijuana, and while the text was fairly balanced, the accompanying photos played up the drug's recreational side. "By the mid-1960s," one caption read, "marijuana had lost much of its stigma as a 'killer drug,' and its widespread use linked American youth of all classes."

The parent groups exploded, and Otto Moulton flooded the publisher with letters demanding changes. Copies were sent to the White House, NIDA, and several members of Congress, including Senator Paula Hawkins of Florida, head of the Senate Subcommittee on Children, Family, Drugs, and Alcoholism. In February 1986, Jaffe appeared before the subcommittee to discuss NIDA's budget. All Hawkins wanted to talk about, however, was the encyclopedia. Reading some sample passages, she fumed, "Those are alarming statements, and the rest of it is like a trip out of reality." Hawkins demanded to know what part Jaffe, and the government, had played in producing the volume.

"This is in no way federally funded," Jaffe quietly replied, noting that he had not seen the material in question prior to publication. "I wrote to the publisher when this was brought to my attention and expressed dismay comparable to yours," he said. "Most of the difficulties were in fact in the captions, and not in the text." Already, Jaffe said, revisions were under way.

Unmollified, Hawkins launched into a rambling monologue about the "fantastic developments" in DNA research that proved that "genetic defects could be passed on to the second generation through the male sperm from heavy marijuana users." Returning to Jaffe's role, she said crossly, "You do not want to be associated with this, but you are. Your name is on there. . . . I was given a copy, and went through it with several parent groups in my State that are outraged by it—not alarmed, not disturbed—they are outraged by it. And I might say that we have probably just heard the beginning of that."

At the end of the hearing, Jaffe was struggling to collect himself when he was approached by Otto Moulton. "God Bless You," Moulton cheerily said. Recalling the incident, Jaffe joked, "It was like something out of Mario Puzo. 'It's nothing personal,' they say as they garrote you."

Eventually, Jaffe decided to take his name off the encyclopedia. "I didn't think it was worth my while to be linked to the project as an editor," he noted. "Look at who was in the White House. There could have been cuts in NIDA's budget. A lot of careers could have been affected." The spectacle of Paula Hawkins lecturing Jerome Jaffe about drug abuse showed how thoroughly the parent movement and its allies had seized control of the drug issue. It also showed how indifferent the federal government was to the rise of crack.

THAT WOULD SUDDENLY change on June 19, 1986. Two days earlier, Len Bias, an All-American forward on the University of Maryland basketball team, had been selected by the Boston Celtics in the first round of the NBA draft. After a whirlwind tour of Boston to meet with the team's management and speak to the press, the six-foot-eight star had returned to his dorm in College Park to celebrate with some friends. By morning, the twenty-two-year-old Bias was dead, the victim of cardiac arrest. Investigating, the police reported that Bias had been using cocaine shortly before his death. Eight days later, Don Rogers, a young defensive back for the Cleveland Browns, died from a cocaine overdose.

That two athletes in top physical shape could drop dead from cocaine stunned the nation. Bias's death in particular would grab the public's attention. Prior to June 19, drugs had been a second-tier issue in Washington; after it, people wanted to talk about little else. The three networks, which had broadcast just a handful of stories on drugs in May 1986, would air more than fifty in June and July. Much of the press coverage dealt with the health risks of cocaine. The "lesson of Len Bias's death," *Newsweek* succinctly stated, is "*cocaine kills.*" Yet, as the weeks passed, the coverage grew increasingly warlike, the health message eclipsed by lurid depictions of a nation under siege. DRUGS: THE ENEMY WITHIN, *Time* declared on its cover, the martini glass of five years earlier replaced by a drawing of a spectral, drug-hollowed face.

Adding to the sense of panic was the sudden spread of crack. By the summer of 1986, the drug was sprinting out from its initial enclaves. From New York City, Jamaican "posses" were moving crack north into Connecticut and south into New Jersey and Pennsylvania. From Los Angeles, street gangs like the Bloods and the Crips were carrying the drug up the coast to Oakland and Seattle and east to Denver and Tulsa. From Miami, traffickers were moving crack up I-95, stopping along the way to supply backwater towns in Georgia and the Carolinas. And, wherever crack struck, crime rates soared. So did the demand for treatment. In Florida's Dade County, programs could accommodate only one of every ten applicants; in Los Angeles's Watts district, two hundred people were waiting to get into one twenty-nine-bed facility.

Against this backdrop, the Reagan Administration's inaction was proving embarrassing. At a July 15 hearing before Charles Rangel's Select Committee on Narcotics, for instance, David Westrate, a senior DEA official, admitted that only in the past week had the agency begun to gather intelligence about the availability, price, and purity of the drug. Edgar Adams, head of NIDA's epidemiological division, confessed that his group had yet to study the prevalence of crack use. "Am I correct, then," asked New York Congressman Benjamin Gilman, "that at this point we really don't have any definitive knowledge of how extensive the use of crack is in our country with all our expertise; is that right?" Adams admitted it was.

On the same day that hearing took place, the White House finally announced its response to the new crisis: it was sending troops to Bolivia. A giant C-5A military transport carrying six Black Hawk helicopters and more than one hundred U.S. Army pilots and support personnel touched down in the city of Santa Cruz, in the heart of Bolivian coca country. Their mission: to help Bolivian security forces attack local coca labs and apprehend those who ran them. Operation Blast Furnace, as it was called, marked the first time that U.S. soldiers were sent into action against drug traffickers. The war on drugs had become a literal reality. Yet, from the start, the operation seemed ill conceived. For, even if the United States did manage to disrupt the drug trade in Bolivia—a remote possibility, given its entrenched nature—Peru, an even richer source of coca, stood ready to make up the difference. And, in a matter of days, the press was declaring Blast Furnace a bust.

Seeking to capitalize, House Speaker Thomas P. O'Neill announced in late July that he was launching a bipartisan effort to draft a comprehensive new drug law. Congressional Republicans, worried about the upcoming November elections, pleaded with the White House to come up with a new program. Thus prodded, it agreed to do so. The job of developing it fell, naturally, to the president's drug adviser. Carlton Turner did not relish his new assignment. For, in his view, everything was coming along nicely, with the University of Michigan surveys showing continued declines in adolescent pot use.

With political realities demanding a response, however, Turner felt he had just the thing. While in Mississippi, he had studied the technology of drug testing, and he had great confidence in its ability to deter drug use—especially in the workplace. Already, an estimated one-fourth of the nation's top corporations were screening job applicants for drugs. Hoping to inspire other companies to follow suit, Turner began drafting a plan to subject the federal government's 2.8 million workers to mandatory drug tests.

Even within the administration, this was controversial. Forcing workers to provide a urine specimen seemed to many a violation of the Fourth Amendment's stricture against unreasonable search and seizure. Reliability was another concern. Cough syrup containing codeine could produce a positive result for morphine; many antihistamines could do the same for amphetamines. Then, too, urine tests were far more effective at detecting marijuana than either cocaine or heroin, since pot lingered in the body longer than either of those drugs. The tests were particularly ill suited to detecting crack. Not only were urine screens unable to distinguish between crack and cocaine, but many crack users were in no position to be tested in the first place. Few worked in the federal government; many, in fact, did not work at all. So, however much workplace testing might help companies weed out drug-using employees, it offered little relief to cities contending with skyrocketing homicide rates, or hospitals with crammed emergency rooms, or treatment programs with long waiting lists.

The White House liked the idea, however, and, with its backing, Turner drafted an executive order mandating federal agencies to develop guidelines for a "drug-free workplace," including testing on a controlled basis. Hoping to get maximum publicity for the program, Turner sent a memo to the White House recommending that President Reagan and other senior officials voluntarily submit to a test. The idea was approved, and in early August the president, vice president, and seventy-eight other White House officials took time out from their jobs to pee into a bottle.

The stunt had little impact, however, for, with the November elections fast approaching, the White House was being overtaken by events. In some races, candidates were challenging their opponents to take a drug test ("jar wars," William Safire called the practice). Both the House and Senate, meanwhile, were preparing huge omnibus drug bills. The long years of work the National Federation of Parents had done on the Hill were about to pay off as antidrug bills that had languished in committee for months were suddenly adopted in a matter of minutes. In one measure that would have lasting consequences, Congress voted to authorize the U.S. armed forces to become more involved in the drug war. In another, it required the president to make an annual determination as to whether source countries were cooperating fully in curtailing production. And, in an effort to seal the Mexican border, Congress approved nearly $300 million for new airplanes, helicopters, radar blimps, and other exotic hardware.

Most significant of all were the changes voted in the criminal code. Since 1970, the federal government had had no mandatory minimum penalties for drug offenses. Led by such hard-liners as Senator Phil Gramm, however, legislators approved a series of whopping new sentences tied solely to the amount of drugs involved. Anyone caught with one or more kilograms of heroin, or five or more kilograms of cocaine, was to serve at least ten years in prison. Specifically targeting crack, Congress voted to impose a mandatory minimum sentence of five years for the sale of just five grams of the drug; triggering the same penalty for cocaine would require five hundred grams—a 100-to-1 disparity that would take on strong symbolic value in the years to come. To make room for new drug offenders, Congress authorized $97 million for new federal prison construction—a small down payment on what was to become a massive prison-building program.

The legislation would not be all stick. At the Democrats' insistence, it would also include $200 million in new funds for drug education and $241 million for drug treatment—the first real increase in such spending in more than a decade. After years of retrenchment, the nation's besieged treatment centers were finally going to get some relief. Nonetheless, most of the $1.7 billion authorized in the bill would go for supply-side programs, thereby reinforcing the lopsidedness of the federal drug budget. With the passage of the Anti-Drug Abuse Act of 1986, the parent model of drug abuse had become, in effect, the law of the land.

SIGNED INTO LAW on October 27, the new drug act left everyone in Washington exhausted, Carlton Turner included. For more than five years, the White House drug adviser had been working sixteen-hour days in the crisis-a-minute atmosphere of the Old Executive Office Building. When a *Newsweek* reporter called him with some questions about drug policy, Turner, disoriented, nattered on about the connection between marijuana and homosexuality. On visits to drug-treatment centers for young people, Turner said, he had been told that

40 percent of the residents had engaged in homosexual activity. "It seems to be something that follows along from their marijuana use," he said. Soon after, his remarks appeared in *Newsweek* under the headline REAGAN AIDE: POT CAN MAKE YOU GAY. Turner's comments drew ridicule from scientists and gay activists alike.

Turner claimed that he had been quoted out of context, but the incident added to his sense that it was time to move on. In December 1986, Turner stepped down as the president's drug adviser. Soon after, he would join a Princeton, New Jersey, firm that specialized in drug testing. As a result of the executive order he had drafted, the drug-testing business was expected to boom, and Turner would be there to share in the profits.

By the time Turner left Washington, the parent movement itself was imploding. From the start, the National Federation of Parents had attracted willful, even mulish individuals, and they were beginning to turn on one another. The catalyst was the eruption of a long-simmering feud between Joyce Nalepka, its executive director, and Pat Burch, the main power on the board. While sparked by personality differences, the fight reflected broader views on how close the organization should be to the Reagan Administration, and a deep schism opened on the NFP board. In December 1986, Nalepka—no match for the well-connected Burch—was forced to resign. Though it would limp along under new leadership, the federation's glory days were over.

It would not really matter, however, for the movement remained strong at the grass roots, guaranteeing its continued influence in Washington. Like everyone else, the parents were worried about crack—not, however, because of the chaos it was causing in the inner city. "Crack was an easy scapegoat," noted Keith Schuchard, who, while retreating into private life, would occasionally reemerge to rally the troops. "Although crack affected just a small part of the population, it allowed the media and others to see the nation's drug problem as a black crack problem." As a result, she said, "people began paying less attention to marijuana and yuppie cocaine use."

The parents were determined to prevent this. And, as usual, the National Institute on Drug Abuse would be a prime target. By the time the Anti-Drug Abuse Act passed, the institute had a new director, Dr. Charles Schuster. A fifty-five-year-old Ph.D. in psychology, Schuster was well known to the treatment fraternity. After earning his doctorate from the University of Maryland and doing research in psychopharmacology at the University of Michigan, Schuster was recruited by Jerome Jaffe to work in the psychiatry department of the University of Chicago; eventually, he would become the associate director of the Illinois Drug Abuse Program. He would remain at the University of Chicago until approached about the NIDA job.

By his own description, Schuster was "much more liberal" in his attitudes toward drugs than most Reagan Administration officials. At one point, however, his son had gotten into trouble with marijuana, and this had earned him the sympathy of the parent representatives on NIDA's search committee. And so, in March 1986, Schuster took over the institute from Jaffe (who resumed his full-time job as director of the Addiction Research Center in Baltimore).

Once at NIDA, however, Schuster quickly ran afoul of the parents. With crack use soaring, Schuster, a thoughtful, straightforward man with a precise manner of speaking, hoped to devote more of NIDA's time to studying cocaine. Like Jaffe, however, he got bogged down in the marijuana issue. One day, for instance, he received a phone call from a senator who said, "We're giving you all these millions of dollars—find something wrong with marijuana." During the 1960s, Schuster said, researchers working on marijuana were mainly interested in finding its "possible beneficial effects"—for example, in easing the impact of glaucoma and chemotherapy. "But," he said, "during the Reagan era, the pressure became, 'Find something wrong with marijuana.'" As a result of such pressure, Schuster went on, NIDA spent a "significant portion" of its budget looking for toxic effects from marijuana. "For many years, we tried to determine whether marijuana produced brain damage. We didn't."

One day, in a talk to some students at the University of Michigan, Schuster remarked that while the idea of a "drug-free America" made for a nice slogan, "in reality we will never have a drug-free society." A member of the NFP shock troops was present, and word of his statement quickly reached Otto Moulton. Moulton proceeded to bombard the administration with letters decrying Schuster's apostasy. "We probably spent thousands of taxpayers' money in an exchange of letters over what I said," Schuster recalled with a sigh. "Mr. Moulton was extremely active in monitoring the public pronouncements of officials such as myself. People around the country would be encouraged to write to their congressman, or to the institute directly, saying, 'How dare you say this?'" As a result, Schuster said, officials "learned to be more circumspect in everything they said in public."

More than statements got affected. "The philosophy that pervaded the Reagan years was one of zero tolerance toward any form of drug use," Schuster said. One result was to "prohibit any kind of public-health type of initiative" that, while seeking ultimately to get people off drugs, recognized that not everybody could do that immediately and so sought to "minimize the harm that drug use caused."

This was nowhere more apparent than with AIDS. By the time Schuster took charge of NIDA, the rate of HIV transmission among drug users was approaching that for homosexuals. Given that drug users were the virus's main route into the general population, reducing the rate of transmission among them would have seemed a top priority. One possible solution was needle-exchange programs, in which addicts could turn in used syringes for clean ones. Schuster thought the concept promising enough to warrant a pilot study. To the parents, however, syringes were just another form of drug paraphernalia, and, as a result, he said, needle-exchange programs "were just out." With zero tolerance, he explained, "you can't allow even for the testing of programs that diminish the spread of HIV infection and hepatitis and so forth. You had to just say no to all of it."

With that path blocked, Schuster turned to another: methadone. If addicts could not receive clean needles, getting them on methadone could eliminate their need to inject altogether. "I had been very active in the use of methadone over the years," Schuster observed, "and felt it was a very, very effective way to help people, especially if you provided them with other kinds of rehabilitative services." By the mid-1980s, however, the Reagan cutbacks had caused a major decline in the quality of methadone treatment. "Those programs lucky enough to still be in business got stretched to the breaking point," Schuster noted, "and many became little more than filling stations."

In his effort to change that, Schuster got a boost from the president's own AIDS commission, set up to study the epidemic and recommend ways of controlling it. Chaired by Admiral James Watkins and including people like John Cardinal O'Connor of New York, the commission created low expectations among AIDS activists. However, its final report, released in June 1988, was remarkably bold, especially in the area of drug treatment. Noting that only 148,000 of the nation's estimated 1.2 million to 1.3 million IV drug users were in treatment, the report stated that it was "imperative to curb drug abuse, especially intravenous drug abuse, by means of treatment in order to slow the HIV epidemic." To that end, it urged the government to adopt a policy of "treatment on demand" for IV drug users, backed by nearly $1.7 billion in new funds.

Endorsed by a respected admiral and a prominent cardinal, such a recommendation could have been expected to impress the White House. It didn't. "There was a very negative feeling on the part of many in the Reagan era about the use of methadone for the treatment of heroin addiction," Schuster noted. As a result of zero tolerance, NIDA was forced to sit idly by while HIV tore through the nation's inner cities.

NO ONE WAS MORE ACTIVE in promoting zero tolerance than Nancy Reagan. The rise of crack had done nothing to diminish her enthusiasm for touring the country and urging people to Just Say No. Only her vehicle would change. Since 1982, Mrs. Reagan had been inseparable from the NFP, attending its annual conferences and helping to raise money for it (including $500,000 donated by the sultan of Brunei). As the infighting at the federation escalated, however, the first lady quietly transferred her loyalties to the Just Say No Foundation, which Tom Adams had set up in 1986 with himself as president and Joan Brann as vice president. By that point there were more than 10,000 clubs nationwide, and the events attended by the first lady were growing ever more extravagant. At a rally at the Universal Amphitheatre in Los Angeles, for instance, Mrs. Reagan was joined by actress Soleil Moon Frye, country-and-western singer Larry Gatlin, two space-shuttle pilots, and 6,000 schoolchildren wearing green JUST SAY NO T-shirts, all swaying together in a noisy two-hour demonstration against drug abuse that at times resembled the halftime show at the Super Bowl.

Overall, Adams appreciated Mrs. Reagan's efforts. "She was very, very supportive," he noted. "She gave a tremendous amount of her time. And she genuinely did like kids." Nonetheless, he became disillusioned over her staff's cavalier attitude toward the kids involved. "Everything was set up for her convenience," he noted. "Her staff was always looking at her image, making sure she looked good. The kids were secondary."

What really soured things for Adams, however, was the growing commercialization of Just Say No. With the phrase branded so deeply into the nation's consciousness, corporations were rushing to join the cause. And, because the foundation was forever low on funds, Adams was open to ideas for joint ventures. The most ambitious came from Procter & Gamble. It proposed underwriting a back-to-school campaign in which millions of youngsters would fill out pledges to Just Say No to drugs. From P&G's standpoint, the campaign offered more than an opportunity to fight drugs, as it made clear in a letter to Adams in March 1987.

"While we are excited about the opportunity to teach kids to stay drug-free, we remind you that our primary objective is to build the business," it stated. Asserting that its relationship with Just Say No "must be exclusive in the packaged goods industry," Procter & Gamble demanded that the foundation "eliminate 'competitive' JUST SAY NO activity" like that of Hill's/Mr. Big paper towels and "minimize the presence" of an already planned Ziploc sandwich bag promotion. "Let's make sure we do everything we can to move millions of Americans to sign pledge cards and buy P&G products," the letter stated.

"The other companies didn't make demands of us," Adams acidly commented. "Procter & Gamble wanted to make money off of us."

The company's efforts did not stop there. With Just Say No fever gripping the land, Adams's foundation was struggling to keep up with the demands being placed on it, and two unsuccessful fundraising events had left it in financial straits. After a March 1987 meeting at the White House, Nancy Reagan, leading Adams to an adjoining room, requested that he hire a Procter & Gamble executive to help manage the foundation. Distrustful of the company's motives, Adams put her off. She pressed the point at a subsequent meeting in May 1987. "If you don't say yes to P&G," Mrs. Reagan said, "I'm pulling out of Just Say No."

Shocked, Adams was nonetheless reluctant to cross the first lady, and a P&G employee was named executive director. And from there things immediately went downhill. "I wouldn't go along with a lot of their stuff," Adams said. "They wanted to get rid of the competition. They didn't want Dow or Clearasil to be involved. I said, 'This doesn't belong to just one group—it doesn't belong just to you.'"

Nonetheless, when the pledge cards went out in the fall of 1987, they included a cover letter from Nancy Reagan and ads and coupons from Procter & Gamble. Eventually, P&G's vice president for marketing was made chairman of Just Say No's board of directors. Amid mounting friction, Adams and Brann resigned. In effect, Just Say No had become a fully owned subsidiary of one of America's leading producers of soaps and detergents.

As a result of Just Say No, Nancy Reagan had by 1988 become more identified with the antidrug cause than anyone else in the world. In the six years since her initial visit to Straight, she had been exposed to literally thousands of people whose lives had been disrupted by drugs. For hours at a time, she had listened to them talk about their painful encounters with cocaine and crack, heroin and alcohol, angel dust and speed. Throughout, however, she remained locked in the initial mindset the parents had instilled in her. "She'd go to these rap sessions and hear all of these kids," observed Donnie Radcliffe of the *Washington Post,* who covered many of the first lady's trips. "She was a good listener. But in the end, her questions would always get around to marijuana. She always thought that marijuana was the culprit that started all these kids on hard drugs. She never went much beyond that in her learning about drugs."

BASED ON THE NUMBERS, Nancy Reagan's crusade against marijuana certainly seemed to be paying off. In 1980, the year before Ronald Reagan became president, 33.7 percent of American high school seniors said they had smoked pot in the past month; by 1988, the number had dropped to 18 percent. The proportion reporting daily marijuana use had gone from 9.1 percent to 2.7 percent. At every age level, in fact, young people were turning away from the drug. From the start, the Republicans had made teenage marijuana use their chief target, and Nancy Reagan's campaign against it no doubt contributed to the turnaround.

Even more credit, however, was due the parent movement. It was Keith Schuchard and her fellow mothers and fathers who provided both the intellectual substance for the antipot campaign and the grassroots troops to carry it out. As Sue Rusche noted with pride, "We stopped decriminalization. We stopped the head shops. We reversed the nation's attitudes about marijuana."

Among middle-class adults, as well, the Reagan years were marked by a sharp falloff in drug use. In large numbers, Americans were giving up not only marijuana but also cocaine and alcohol. And, while this shift may have been hastened by the antidrug actions of the parent movement, a more important factor was the broader changes taking place in American lifestyles. Well-to-do Americans were exercising more, smoking less, and eating broccoli instead of beef, and cocaine simply did not fit with the program. If anyone deserves credit here, it is probably Len Bias. The media avalanche set off by his death constituted the most intensive—and effective—drug-education program in U.S. history. In virtually every drug survey, Bias's death would show up as a fault line, with consumption trends all pointing downward beginning in the summer of 1986.

Except among hard-core users. Here, unfortunately, the trend lines were moving in the opposite direction. In 1980, for instance, the government's Drug Abuse Warning Network had recorded 7,450 drug-related visits to hospital emergency rooms; by 1988, the number had reached 113,000—a fifteen-fold increase. In the same period, the number of annual cocaine-related deaths had jumped from 96 to 1,290. Because of crack, the rate of drug-related HIV transmission, drug use among pregnant women, and drug-related homicides all soared during the Reagan years. Nor had heroin gone away. In the late 1980s, in fact, the country was flooded by a new wave of the drug, resulting in a sharp upturn in heroin-related emergencies.

In a sense, the nation's experience during the 1980s constituted a sweeping repudiation of the gateway theory so beloved by the parent movement. According to that theory, reducing the number of casual drug users should have resulted in less hard-core use; the fewer the number of recreational marijuana smokers and cocaine sniffers, the smaller the pool of candidates for heroin and crack addiction. Instead, in eight years, casual use had declined while hard-core use had soared. In a perverse way, the administration had succeeded in pushing Americans in the aggregate away from softer drugs like pot toward harder ones like crack—the exact opposite of what the gateway theory would have predicted.

It would, of course, be unfair to hold the Reagan Administration responsible for the rise of crack. No more than an outbreak of measles or diphtheria could this virulent phenomenon have been prevented by public officials. Yet Republican policies seem to have guaranteed the worst possible outcome. The administration's decision to slash the federal treatment budget beginning in 1981 effectively destroyed the nation's first line of defense against a new drug outbreak. For the next five years, the White House ignored every warning sign about the impending crisis. Then, when the crisis finally hit, the administration —paralyzed by its zero-tolerance philosophy—refused to take even the most basic countermeasures. The result was the worst drug epidemic in American history. This record of neglect—not the CIA's work in Central America—is the real scandal surrounding the rise of crack.

15

The Philosopher-Czar

BY NEITHER TEMPERAMENT nor philosophy was George Bush inclined to take bold action as president. But drug policy was necessarily an exception. According to one poll, 35 percent of the American people regarded drugs as the nation's most pressing problem. Seeping into towns and hamlets across the country, crack was everywhere setting new homicide records. In the nation's capital, the murder rate jumped a phenomenal 64 percent in 1988, and a local TV station was airing a nightly show, called *City Under Siege,* that documented the carnage. Amid a growing sense that the Reagan drug policy had failed, George Bush promised a new one. "Take my word for it," he declared in his inaugural address. "This scourge will stop!"

In confronting that scourge, the president would have a new weapon at hand. At the end of 1988, Congress, hoping to impose some order on the three dozen federal agencies active in the drug war, had voted to create a new Office of National Drug Control Policy. ONDCP was to have a staff of more than a hundred, be attached to the Executive Office of the President, and have a director with Cabinet-level rank. For the first time since the Special Action Office for Drug Abuse Prevention, then, the government was to have a special office to coordinate national drug policy.

There would be some important differences, however. Unlike SAODAP, ONDCP would have responsibility for not only demand but also supply—a reflection of how important law enforcement had become to national policy. In addition, the Bush White House, in seeking a director, would rely not on a pragmatic aide like Egil Krogh, but rather on Pat Burch. Burch was a close friend of George Bush, and, though she had largely retired from public life, she was intent on influencing his selection of a new drug czar. Among the members of her Bible group was Elayne Bennett, whose husband William had just completed a term as secretary of education. Impressed with Bennett's ability to promote conservative values on a major domestic issue, Burch thought he could do the same for drugs.

Bennett was interested. After leaving the Reagan Administration, he and his friend Allan Bloom, the author of *The Closing of the American Mind,* had set up a think tank called the Madison Center. Named after James Madison, one of Bennett's intellectual heroes, the center was to serve as a sanctuary where scholars could ponder the future of Western civilization. Within months, however, Bennett had grown restless. He missed the heady atmosphere of Cabinet meetings, the glare of television lights, the sparring with reporters.

He especially missed his ability to speak out on the issues of the day. During his time at Education, Bennett had turned one of the most obscure Cabinet posts into one of the most visible. Brash and combative, he took a bad boy's delight in challenging conventions and saying the unmentionable. A former college football lineman who still liked to throw his weight around, Bennett at hearings would blithely contradict senators and upstage congressmen.

Now, ensconced at his new think tank, he found himself mulling Aristotle with a bunch of graduate students. Coveting a broader audience, Bennett felt the new drug office offered an excellent bully pulpit. Meeting with George Bush to discuss the job, he told him that drug abuse was one area in which he, as a conservative, felt comfortable in advocating a strong federal role. Bush agreed, and by the end of the conversation the job was Bennett's.

There was, of course, one small catch in Bennett's becoming drug czar: he knew next to nothing about drugs. Education had been his lifelong concern. Trained as a political philosopher, Bennett had spent most of his early career on college campuses from Austin to Cambridge. In 1981, he had moved to Washington to become director of the National Endowment for the Humanities; four years later he took over Education. There, Bennett had had to deal with the issue of student drug use, and under his direction the department had produced *What Works: Schools Without Drugs,* a how-to guide for principals and parents. He had also attended meetings of the Reagan Administration's National Drug Policy Board, at which he had advocated using U.S. military planes to bomb cocaine labs in Bolivia. Beyond that, however, his experience was scant.

No one was more aware of this than Bennett, and he quickly sought to catch up. In Washington, he held a dozen or so roundtable discussions with experts in law enforcement and treatment, education and prevention. He went to Detroit to ride around with narcotics officers, to Miami to watch a sting operation, to Harlem to hold a crack baby. And, in assembling his staff, Bennett sought out people with expertise. To serve as his associate director for state and local affairs, he hired Reggie Walton, a black judge who, during eight years on the D.C. bench, had seen up close the damage crack was inflicting on the nation's ghettos. To direct the supply side, Bennett chose Stanley Morris, who, since the mid-1970s, had been fighting drug dealers in various posts at the Justice Department, most recently as head of the U.S. Marshals Service.

Bennett took particular care in choosing his deputy for demand reduction. One name that came up in conversations was Jerome Jaffe. Still working at the Addiction Research Center in Baltimore, Jaffe agreed to come to Washington to speak with Bennett. The discussion was friendly, with Jaffe describing his experiences at SAODAP, but the anguish from that period remained fresh in his mind, and, reluctant to risk a reprise, he took himself out of the running.

But Bennett found a worthy substitute. Dr. Herbert D. Kleber, a professor of psychiatry at the Yale Medical School, was just a year younger than Jaffe, and his career had followed a parallel course. Like Jaffe, Kleber had worked at the federal narcotics farm in Lexington. In the late 1960s, while Jaffe was setting up his multimodality program in Chicago, Kleber was creating a similar one in New Haven under the sponsorship of Yale and the Connecticut Mental Health Center. Under his direction, the program grew rapidly, and by the late 1980s it had 1,000 slots and an IDAP-style central intake. Kleber had written more than 150 papers on psychopharmacology, addiction, and cocaine treatment, on which he was a leading expert. With his slight build, glasses, gray wardrobe, and professorial air, Kleber even had the fraternity look.

In one important way, however, Kleber differed from his fellow members: he was a Republican. He prized his establishment credentials and would not think of doing anything to jeopardize them. He also felt at home with terms like drug-free America, zero tolerance, gateway drugs, and the other nomenclature of the Reagan era. Kleber, in short, was a Republican Jaffe—an ideal hybrid from Bennett's standpoint—and so he got the job.

Together, Kleber, Morris, and Walton would provide Bennett an impressive pool of experts on which he could draw. In practice, however, he would rarely do so. For, at the same time as he was hiring these professionals, Bennett was stocking his personal staff with staunch conservatives like himself. Their main qualification for the job was not expertise in drug matters—they had little—but loyalty to William Bennett. They included John Walters, a political scientist who at Education had served as deputy to William Kristol, Bennett's chief of staff. When Kristol went to work for Vice President Dan Quayle, Bennett made Walters his chief of staff at ONDCP. Bruce Carnes, a Ph.D. in English literature who had been the top budget officer at Education, would perform the same role at ONDCP. Also coming over from Education were David Tell, a bright young operative with a caustic sense of humor, and Terence Pell, who had been general counsel at Education and would fill the same position at ONDCP.

At Education, Bennett had relied on this small coterie to wrest control of the department away from the professionals. Every afternoon, the group had gathered in Bennett's office to smoke cigars, plot strategy, and devise ways of riling the old guard. The "A Team," they were called by resentful career officials. At ONDCP, they would be named the "lunch bunch," after the daily midday meetings they held. It was at these informal sessions that drug policy got made. And the experts were rarely invited.

The very layout of the drug office contributed to their exclusion. ONDCP was located in a weather-beaten office building on Connecticut Avenue, just north of Dupont Circle. The drug office occupied two of its floors. The eighth floor was home to the experts. Bennett's office, and those of his cronies, was on the tenth. (The ninth floor was not part of ONDCP.) It was here that speeches got drafted, strategies written, and budgets formulated.

Frank Kalder, who served as Bruce Carnes's deputy, and who had worked on drug issues at OMB during the Reagan years, said, "I think I was the only person of the top twenty people in the office who had any knowledge at all of drugs." An easygoing midwesterner and born-again Christian who had worked as a missionary in Poland in the late 1970s, Kalder considered himself a conservative Republican. Attending sessions of the inner circle, however, he was taken aback by the vehemence of their views. "They were moon howlers, constantly talking about what their driving ideology should be," he said.

"Bennett filled his personal staff with a lot of amateurs," noted Stan Morris, a tall, balding, unpretentious man. "They didn't know anything about drugs. They didn't know about anything other than education." The three deputies, he added, "were expected to bring some degree of credibility, then stay out. We were always sort of outsiders."

Formally, Morris was responsible for all programs aimed at reducing the supply of drugs in the United States. But John Walters became taken with the glamour of the drug war, and, with Bennett's approval, he grabbed control of all international programs. Sandy-haired and boyish-looking, Walters had studied with Allan Bloom at the University of Toronto and was a disciple of the abstruse Plato scholar Leo Strauss. Finding intelligence reports more exciting than the *Republic,* however, he began immersing himself in such arcana as radar capabilities, herbicide potencies, and Caribbean choke points. Every morning, Walters would preside over an intelligence meeting at which agents from the CIA, DEA, Defense Intelligence Agency, and Customs would discuss seizures and arrests. A few months into the job, Walters concluded that the key to winning the drug war was getting the military more involved, and, under his leadership, the Bush Administration would launch a $2 billion, five-year "Andean Initiative" aimed at disrupting the drug trade at its source.

Stan Morris felt he had seen it all before. The Reagan Administration, too, had stepped up military operations in Latin America in the belief that it would reduce the flow of cocaine into the United States. Instead, that flow had only increased. "The idea that we could somehow develop relations with the Peruvian government that were going to reduce the amount of coca being produced in the Upper Huallaga Valley—well, you had to be taking a lot of the stuff to believe it," said Morris. If the goal was to make cocaine scarcer in the United States, he said, "the best place to start wasn't down there, but here, in the United States, disrupting local markets. That has a more direct effect on price and availability than all the various efforts undertaken abroad."

At ONDCP, however, Morris did not get much of a chance to make this case. "The Ph.D.-educated types were more comfortable with the CIA and the generals and the State Department striped-pants-set and less comfortable with foul-talking, blue-collar cops," he observed. "I had been at the Justice Department for ten years, and I think there was a sense that those guys didn't know what was going on, that if only they could get the CIA and Defense Department involved—they did know."

Herbert Kleber was having similar frustrations. In his dealings with the politicos on the tenth floor, he was amazed at how little they knew about addiction. And Bennett was no exception. The drug czar had an open-door policy with Kleber, and Kleber frequently took advantage of it. An avuncular man with bushy eyebrows and an expression that seemed at once wizened and baby-faced, Kleber had a pedagogical manner befitting a Yale professor, and he began an informal tutorial with Bennett, providing him with data showing that treatment was not only effective, but cost-effective.

But Bennett was resistant. The whole idea of treatment made him uncomfortable. Addicts in his view were irresponsible individuals lacking basic levels of self-control. Treatment was a form of "coddling," a term that frequently popped up in his conversation. Bennett was further skeptical of claims that addicts wanted help. "Let's face it," he said in an early speech,

the addict who wakes up one morning and "decides" he's had enough —it's time to enter treatment—is in a very small minority indeed. In the vast majority of cases, the addict is a man or woman whose power to exercise such rational volition has already been seriously eroded by drugs, and whose life is instead organized largely—even exclusively—around the pursuit and satisfaction of his addiction. So it should not surprise us to learn that drug treatment for the most tenacious and intractable addictions—cocaine and heroin dependence—is almost always initiated not by patient choice, but by some external pressure, legal or otherwise.

Only by stepping up that pressure, through an expansion of the criminal justice system, Bennett believed, was it possible to get more addicts into treatment. No matter how much Kleber argued to the contrary, Bennett clung to his beliefs about addiction, with a tenacity his tutor found perplexing.

THOSE BELIEFS, in fact, derived from a broader worldview that Bennett had gradually developed over the course of his life. Raised in Flatbush, Brooklyn, Bennett at the age of thirteen moved with his newly remarried mother to

Arlington, Virginia. After graduating from Washington's Gonzaga College High School, a prestigious Jesuit school, he enrolled in Williams College. Bennett intended to major in English, but, after taking an introductory course in philosophy, he became enthralled with Plato and his teachings about civic virtue, and he decided to devote himself to the big questions about man and society.

First, though, he would go through his own rebellion against society. The sixties were aborning, and Bennett got swept up in them, playing electric guitar in a rock band (called Plato and the Guardians) and opposing the Vietnam War. When Students for a Democratic Society was founded, Bennett gave serious thought to joining but was dissuaded by his brother Robert, who warned of possible career consequences.

After Williams, Bennett entered graduate school at the University of Texas, whose philosophy department was chaired by the then-liberal John Silber. Bennett remained deeply involved with the antiwar and civil rights movements. And, in a cosmic brush with the counterculture, he had a blind date with Janis Joplin. (There was no chemistry.) During a year as an instructor at the University of Southern Mississippi, Bennett led a teach-in after the assassination of Martin Luther King, Jr.

Bennett's views began to change in 1969, when he entered Harvard Law School. Harvard was still reeling from the takeover of University Hall by antiwar students the previous spring, and Bennett shared in the shock many faculty members felt. Drugs, meanwhile, were sweeping the campus, and Bennett, serving as a proctor in a freshman dorm, was disgusted to find students spending their afternoons getting high and watching TV rather than taking advantage of a Harvard education. One day, he found two freshmen kneeling on the floor of their room, selling prescription drugs to kids in their early teens. When Bennett demanded to know what was going on, the students scrambled out the window and down the fire escape. Bennett filed a written complaint with the university. Senior faculty members were inclined to let the matter drop, but Bennett persisted, and Harvard eventually suspended the students for a year—a scandalously lenient penalty in his eyes.

After receiving his J.D., Bennett took a job at Boston University as an assistant to John Silber, who had become the school's president. Silber was embroiled in a bitter dispute with campus radicals over military recruiting, and on several occasions Bennett escorted recruiters through crowds of taunting demonstrators. Alienated by such excesses, Bennett, like Silber, was drifting into the camp of once-liberal intellectuals known as neoconservatives. The neocons believed that America's mounting social problems were due not to any socioeconomic factors but to a decline in cultural standards and a rejection of traditional values. Urging a restoration of individual responsibility and civic duty, the neocons provided for Bennett the intellectual home he'd been seeking since his initial exposure to Plato.

They also helped him land his next job. While at BU, Bennett had met

Irving Kristol, the godfather of the new movement, and his wife, the historian Gertrude Himmelfarb. They recommended Bennett to Charles Frankel, the director of the National Humanities Center in North Carolina, who was looking for an assistant. Bennett took the job, and the two became close friends. One day in May 1979, Bennett arrived at Frankel's home in Bedford Hills, New York, intending to stay for several days. Before he had a chance to unpack, however, he was summoned back to North Carolina on urgent business. Hours later, Frankel and his wife were murdered by intruders seeking money to support their drug habit. The shock of the experience deepened Bennett's disgust at the growing breakdown in American values, and at the contribution drugs were making to it.

After Reagan's election, Kristol led a campaign to get Bennett appointed chairman of the National Endowment for the Humanities, and after a bitter fight he was confirmed. Displaying his flair for ideological combat, Bennett denounced an NEH-funded documentary on Nicaragua as "unabashed socialist-realist propaganda" and awarded $30,000 to the right-wing Accuracy in Media to produce a rebuttal to Stanley Karnow's middle-of-the-road PBS series on Vietnam.

It was as secretary of education, however, that Bennett made his mark. The decline in American education, he felt, was due to a retreat from traditional standards. Rather than have to master history and math, students were being allowed to take all kinds of trendy courses. Discipline was seen as reactionary and homework assignments as oppressive. The major culprit, Bennett believed, was the liberal education establishment. To get this message across, Bennett and his aides hit on the idea of traveling to schoolrooms across the country. From the South Bronx to Osburn, Idaho, Bennett was busy awarding certificates of merit, issuing reading lists, teaching *The Federalist Papers*. The press often went along, and Bennett—tie loosened, chalk in hand—seemed always in the news, preaching to anyone who would listen the need to return to basics and instill moral values in the young.

From these travels grew Bennett's broader vision of what was ailing America. Values like hard work, public service, and family devotion were being undermined by Ivy League professors, Hollywood producers, media pundits, and other members of the liberal elite. Particularly galling to Bennett was the way these liberals arrived at their views—"not, ironically, through intellect, through open-ended, disinterested thinking and inquiry, but through disposition, sentiment, bias, and ideology," as he put it in his book *The De-Valuing of America*. For them, Bennett wrote, the "starting point is not evidence but ideology." Through his own open-ended thinking, Bennett had come to see the nation as engaged in a culture war pitting the liberal elite against the American people. And that war was being fought not just in education but among the broad array of issues facing the nation, including the family, race, and drugs.

In Bennett's view, the crack and cocaine epidemics were not a public-health crisis but a moral one, traceable back to the counterculture and its nose-thumbing attitude toward authority. "Somewhere along the way, in the late 1960s and 1970s, part of America lost its moral bearings regarding drugs . . . ," Bennett wrote in his book. "It was the collapse of institutional government authority, essentially giving permission to take drugs, that was largely responsible for the epidemic that eventually hit us."

Combatting that epidemic, then, would require a reconstitution of that authority. In his maiden speech as drug czar, delivered on May 3, 1989, to the United Hebrew Congregation in Washington, D.C., Bennett declared that "the idea that breaking the law is wrong, even when the lawbreaking goes unde-tected, has lost its power to deter." His response, he said, could be summed up in two words: "consequences" and "confrontation." "Those who use, sell, and traffic in drugs must be confronted, and they must suffer consequences," Bennett asserted. This, he added, applied to not only the addict but also the "so called 'casual user' ":

> Casual use is not just a matter of personal preference. It has costs—wide, horrible social costs. The suburban man who drives his BMW downtown to buy cocaine is killing himself—of course. But he's kill-ing the city at the same time. And his "casual" use is best deterred not by empty threats of long, hard punishment, but by *certain* pun-ishment.

Hostility for the casual drug user was nothing new, of course. It had been a pillar of the parent movement and of the Reagan Administration's drug policy. For Bennett, though, it fit nicely with his notion of a culture war, and he incorporated it into his analysis of the nation's drug predicament.

By law, ONDCP was required to prepare a national drug strategy. Bennett hoped to make it a grand summation of his philosophy, a sweeping Magna Carta of national drug policy. And attacking casual drug use would be at its core.

YET, BY 1989, there was overwhelming evidence that casual drug use was already falling. According to the University of Michigan's annual survey, for instance, high school seniors were shunning not only marijuana but other drugs as well. In 1988, for instance, just 3.4 percent of those polled said they had used cocaine in the last month—down from 6.7 percent in 1985, the year before Len Bias's death. Similarly, the typical profile of callers to the 800-COCAINE hotline had shifted from the affluent college-educated cocaine sniffer of the early 1980s to the unemployed, undereducated crack smoker of the late 1980s.

Indeed, even as casual drug use was falling, hard-core crack use was continuing to soar. A 1988 report by NIDA's epidemiology division provided a grim catalogue of the effects crack was having around the country. In New Orleans, it stated, "crack use has increased, with prices down to $10–$20 a rock. A 20-percent rise in violent crime is attributed to cocaine trafficking." In Philadelphia, it noted, "crack sales and use have increased significantly" and "trafficking-related violence has escalated," while in Washington "an unprecedented number of homicides and violent incidents have been associated with the crack market."

The press was giving ample coverage to these contrasting trends. THE AMERICAN DRUG PROBLEM TAKES ON 2 FACES, the *New York Times* declared in July 1988. "It is a tale of a nation with two drug problems," Peter Kerr reported, "one that may be getting better for the more affluent, and one of accelerating despair and social disintegration among the poor." "TWO-TIER" DRUG CULTURE SEEN EMERGING, the *Washington Post* reported in January 1989. Among the experts cited by Michael Isikoff was Dr. David Musto, a professor at the Yale Medical School and one of the nation's leading drug historians. "You have a fundamental change of attitudes among the middle class and a growing bewilderment that anybody still uses drugs," Musto said. ". . . But then you have the world of the inner city where there isn't the education, the jobs or the other kinds of things that give people a reason to stop using drugs."

Virtually every expert in the country was saying the same thing: it was crack use in the inner city, not casual use in the suburbs, that was driving the nation's drug problem. The tenth floor of ONDCP did not agree, however. "Our office was created not because of the hard-core user problem, but because of concern about exploding drug use in the suburbs and among young people," said Bruce Carnes, giving his own view of ONDCP's origins. "It was not directed at hard-core addicts. They consumed the vast bulk of the drugs, and contributed a significant part of the crime, but they weren't the main threat to your kids becoming drug users."

As ONDCP's head of budget and planning, Carnes was in charge of the team drafting the national strategy. With his receding hairline, narrow ties, and white shirts, the forty-five-year-old Carnes seemed the consummate bureaucrat. In fact, he burned with a sense of mission. His astringent bearing, inexhaustible work habits, and taste for intrigue inspired comparisons to Cardinal Richelieu. An ardent Republican who sometimes rode to work on a Harley-Davidson, Carnes liked to boast that he once dated the woman who would become Oliver North's wife. And his views were, if anything, even fiercer than Bennett's. Among other things, he wanted to hold addicts responsible for the cost of their treatment, requiring them to pay back the government once they got better. "Bruce would say that the most effective treatment program cost fifty cents—a bullet," said Frank Kalder, quickly adding that he was joking.

Carnes's views were no laughing matter on the eighth floor, however. "We had to fight like bloody murder to get into the strategy views we thought important," noted Linda Lewis, one of Herbert Kleber's two deputies and the former director of drug treatment programs for the state of Florida. "There were critical meetings we weren't allowed to attend, and endless rewrites of policy documents where the flavor of what we were trying to communicate was not only not used but was purposely changed in the opposite direction." She added: "We tried to be straightforward. We would say, for instance, that not every addict off the street wants treatment." This, she said, would "get twisted" into the belief that few addicts want help.

AIDS was a particular sore point. "The data on AIDS were overwhelming," Lewis observed. "The number of cases was going up, especially among minority women. I sent memos to Herb, and he'd try to argue it with the folks upstairs. We wanted resources for training, outreach, and treatment for substance abusers with HIV." The memos died in Carnes's office.

By mid-July, the strategy was nearly complete. The one missing piece was the results of NIDA's 1988 National Household Survey on Drug Abuse. It was the first such survey in three years, and the tenth floor was eagerly awaiting the results. Finally ready at the end of July, they were rushed over to the drug office. Carnes was stunned. The number of casual drug users (those who'd used an illegal drug at least once in the previous month) had fallen 37 percent, from 23 million in 1985 to 14.5 million in 1988; the number of casual cocaine users had plummeted 50 percent, to 2.9 million.

By contrast, those who used cocaine once a week or more had jumped 33 percent, while those using on a daily basis had increased 19 percent. In short, the survey confirmed what all the drug experts had been saying—that casual use was plunging while chronic use was soaring.

On the tenth floor, the news was received "like a punch to the stomach," Frank Kalder recalled. "It just took our wind away. We were all geared up for the release of a big strategy with big budget increases by a new office. And suddenly, on the eve of its unveiling, the problem was disappearing before our eyes. People were saying, 'Oh my God, there goes our issue!' "

Bill Bennett was off in North Carolina with his family when the news arrived, and, when the staff called him about it, he was not happy. "He panicked," David Tell recalled. "He wanted to be J. Edgar Hoover and save the country. Now he felt there was no problem anymore."

Over the next few days, some thought was given to rewriting the strategy, but this was ultimately rejected. "We didn't significantly change course," Frank Kalder recalled, "and the reason we didn't was that we didn't know what to change it to." Eventually, the tenth floor decided simply to acknowledge the reality of the crack crisis while leaving the rest of the document unchanged.

The result was a grand muddle. On the one hand, the *National Drug Control Strategy*, released in September 1989, eloquently summarized the nation's current predicament. "We are now fighting two drug wars, not just one," Bennett wrote in a signed introduction. "The first and easiest is against 'casual' use of drugs by many Americans, and we are winning it. The other, much more difficult war is against addiction to cocaine. And on this second front, increasingly located in our cities, we are losing—badly." The nation's "most intense and immediate problem," Bennett went on, "is inner-city crack use. It is an acid that is fast corroding the hopes and possibilities of an entire generation of disadvantaged young people. They need help. Their neighborhoods need help. A decent and responsible America must fully mobilize to provide it."

Having so trenchantly described the problem, however, the document offered few ideas for resolving it. Instead, it served up nuggets of Bennett's culture-war philosophy. The drug problem was a "crisis of national character," the strategy stated, adding, "We declare clearly and emphatically that there is no such thing as innocent drug use." The document went so far as to assert that casual drug users are more dangerous than hard-core ones. "A true addict's use is not very contagious," Bennett explained.

> The non-addicted casual or regular user, however, is a very different story. He is likely to have a still-intact family, social, and work life. He is likely still to "enjoy" his drug for the pleasure it offers. And he is thus much more willing and able to proselytize his drug use—by action or example—among his remaining non-user peers, friends, and acquaintances. A non-addict's drug use, in other words, is *highly* contagious.

Bennett provided no data to back up this contagion theory. In fact, it was flatly contradicted by all the surveys showing increased hard-core use and falling casual use. Nonetheless, the theory provided a rationale for keeping casual users at the center of the strategy, and for recommending a battery of penalties against them, including "dramatically increasing" the number of drug arrests and rapidly expanding the nation's prison system. By contrast, the strategy's discussion of treatment was grudging and dismissive. While acknowledging that the nation suffered from a lack of capacity, the document asserted that "too many people who use drugs—including many with severe drug dependencies—do not want to be treated. For a variety of reasons, they prefer life with drugs to life without them." Consequently, it noted, "it is time to reexamine the premise that voluntary drug treatment should continue to be the mainstay of our treatment system."

The strategy's budget numbers faithfully reflected Bennett's worldview. Overall, it proposed increasing federal drug spending by 39 percent, to $7.9 billion. The largest single item—$1.6 billion—was to go for the federal prison system. Spending on international programs was to rise 80 percent, to $449 million, while aid for state and local law enforcement was to increase 133 percent, to $350 million. Drug treatment, meanwhile, was to get $925 million, a 53 percent increase. This was not an insignificant sum; nonetheless, it would make only a small dent in the nation's waiting lists. Overall, the Bennett strategy proposed spending 73 percent of the drug budget on supply programs and 27 percent on demand ones. In effect, Bennett and the lunch bunch had produced a document that, in most key respects, recapitulated the same Reagan policy that had been so widely viewed as a failure.

ONCE THE STRATEGY was released, Bennett decided to hit the road. As he explained in *The De-Valuing of America,* "I've never liked being desk- or Washington-bound; as in the education job, I could find out more by going to where the action was and talking to the people. . . . I needed to see *with my own eyes* what was happening." Ultimately, Bennett would visit scores of communities. In speeches and interviews, he would frequently mention the people he met on these trips—the "real drug experts," he called them—and cite them as confirming the wisdom of his strategy. In fact, their views often conflicted sharply with his own.

One raw morning in December 1989, for instance, Bennett visited Women Inc., a treatment program in the low-income Dorchester section of Boston. He arrived in a six-car motorcade led by a police car with whirring siren and flashing lights. Accompanying him were a speechwriter, press spokesman, advance man, personal aide, and two bodyguards, plus Senators Edward Kennedy and John Kerry, Governor Michael Dukakis, and about forty journalists. Waiting in the library of the three-story clapboard building were twenty-five women seated in rows of plastic chairs; about half of them were black and half white. Bennett and his fellow politicians took seats at a rectangular table in front while the journalists jockeyed for position in the aisles.

When everyone was settled, Candice Cason, the center's director, explained that most of the program's clients were single mothers who had lost their children as a result of their addiction; the facility sought to ease their recovery by allowing them to be with their children. The program had twenty-four residential and fifty outpatient slots, plus day-care facilities for their kids. "We've survived basically by the skin of our teeth," Cason said. "The funding has not been consistent, and I do hope that the gentlemen here will consider making sure there's more money for programs like this that have a track record of success."

"Can I ask a question?" Bennett said, moving to take control of the meeting. "There are twenty-four women here? Does it work?"

"Yes!" the women shouted in unison.

"Did you come voluntarily?" Bennett continued.

"No!" came the chorus, amid much laughter.

"Were you referred by the courts?"

"I was involved in a house raid," said a black woman with braids, who explained that she had been assigned to treatment as an alternative to prison.

"So some of you came here not entirely wanting to," Bennett said, satisfying his belief that most addicts do not seek treatment voluntarily. Next, he asked what the rules were at Women Inc.—no drugs, violence, or sex, he was told—and what a typical day was like. Bennett earnestly scribbled notes as the women told of rising early in the morning, taking showers, and preparing breakfast.

Senator Kennedy then took the floor. It was Kennedy who had invited Bennett to visit Women Inc. He had done so because the program was one of the few in Massachusetts that allowed women to have their children with them in treatment, and he wanted to make sure that this feature did not get lost. "One of the aspects of our whole substance challenge in our country is the fact that many of those who are addicted are women expecting children," he mumbled. "About 380,000 children are born to addicted mothers every year. We have not devised a system to help those expectant mothers, or single mothers who have children. This program has been really remarkable. Perhaps you could tell Dr. Bennett a little about that aspect of your life here."

The women suddenly stirred to life. One graduate of the program who was now counseling pregnant women said that she tried to encourage her clients to enter treatment but was stymied because they first had to go to detox, and detoxes would not accept them. And, because these women were homeless, she said, "they go back on the street."

Governor Dukakis asked why the detoxes wouldn't accept them. "Because there are no beds," the woman said. "I've been in my position three or four months and only once have I been able to find a bed."

A heavyset white woman introduced her teenage daughter, who was seated next to her. Twice, she said, she had been in prison, but that had given her "no incentive to get clean." Only by entering treatment had she learned to "accept responsibility" for her behavior and "be a mother" to her daughter. Fortunately, she said, she had been able to find a detox when she needed one. "That's not the case now," she added, "with detoxes closing left and right."

"So what funding is going to be available for more beds and treatment?" one woman loudly demanded. "Building more jail cells doesn't help women." There was loud applause.

Bennett frowned. "If we turn this into a political rally, I'm going to walk out of here," he said, his voice low and tight. "I want to ask questions and get your answers. If you have questions at the end, I'll be very happy to answer them."

There was a moment of stunned silence. "Mr. Secretary," boomed William Owens, a black Massachusetts state senator who was standing in back, "if people are asking you about funding, that's not a political rally. Please don't insult the integrity of folks in here. More money for beds and treatment— that's all they asked you about."

Bennett was unmoved. "There'll be more money," he said. "But the reason we're here is to find out what works—why this program is good."

This seemed to incite the women further. One sitting in the front row said, "Before I came here, the message I got was, 'If you do drugs, you're *bad.*' But it's not true. Before I came here, I heard no message about drug programs. When I did hear there was help, I ran to get it." Challenging the four dark-suited men at the front table, she said, "I want to ask all of you, Do you believe that people addicted to drugs or alcohol are bad?"

"I believe some of them are," Bennett coolly replied. "With some people, if they become addicted, I don't think they're in control of themselves. The drug is ruling their lives. But I do think there are people who get into drugs and do it because they don't exercise responsibility, because they care more about themselves than their kids and other people. You've got to accept responsibility."

The room was tense for the remaining twenty minutes of the meeting, with Bennett and the women sparring over the nature of addiction and what the government should be doing about it. When the meeting was over, the four politicians strode from the room and reassembled on the driveway outside, where, bundled against the cold, they faced a knot of TV cameras. Asked what he had learned from the meeting, Bennett replied:

I was struck by people talking about their day here—about getting up in the morning, coming downstairs, and cooking breakfast. People here are learning about good habits. They're learning about punctuality, they're learning about neatness, they're learning about personal responsibility. Isn't it interesting that the way out of drug addiction is to relearn this lesson about personal responsibility?

No doubt most of the residents at Women Inc. would have agreed with that statement; learning to behave responsibly was a major goal of their program. Yet there was so much else that they had wanted to convey—about the superiority of treatment over prison as a place to learn about responsibility; about the many barriers they faced in getting into treatment; and, perhaps most important, about how poorly the treatment system was serving women's needs. Yet Bennett had seemed indifferent to it all. Faced with an opportunity to learn from these "real drug experts," the drug czar had instead retreated into the comfortable womb of his ideology, with its preconceptions about addiction and treatment.

IN THE SPRING OF 1990, ONDCP moved into a new office building on 17th Street, a block from the White House. It was not only better located than the old office but plusher as well, with soft lighting, sleek furniture, and handsome carpeting. The old physical divisions remained, however, with the lunch bunch housed on the eighth floor and the experts on the sixth and seventh. With Bennett on the road so often, Herb Kleber had fewer chances to stop by his office, but Bennett sometimes invited him on his trips, and on them Kleber would continue his tutorials. And, as the months passed, he felt he was making progress. Bennett was talking less and less often about coddling and coercion and addicts' reluctance to seek help. He even agreed to sign his name to a white paper on treatment that Kleber had prepared.

By the summer, however, Bennett no longer seemed interested. In Washington, the drug issue was losing its luster, and Bennett was less often in the news. He became so distracted that, on the rare times when he was in town, the lunch bunch found his presence an intrusion. Increasingly, Bennett seemed preoccupied not with drugs but with money. Around the office, he talked about his desire to buy a house in the suburbs. With his national stature, Bennett knew that the speeches he was giving for free as drug czar could earn him $25,000 apiece as a private citizen. And so, in November 1990, after just nineteen months on the job, he decided to call it quits. "People were shocked," Frank Kalder recalled, adding that he had been among them. In retrospect, though, he said, Bennett's departure should not have been so surprising, since he "had been so uninvolved from the get-go."

Bennett's hasty departure dealt a major blow to the prestige of the drug office. THE SKIPPER QUITS, stated the headline atop a critical column by A. M. Rosenthal of the *New York Times,* previously a strong Bennett backer. Yet ONDCP's image would sink even further under his successor. Bob Martinez had just been defeated in his bid to be reelected governor of Florida. Feeling sorry for him, George Bush, a good friend, offered him the drug-czar job as a sort of consolation prize. And, from his first day in office, Martinez treated it like one. Inarticulate, stiff in public, lacking in political acumen, and unversed in the subject matter, Martinez became almost invisible in Washington. And, seeing the vacuum at the top, John Walters and Bruce Carnes moved quickly to fill it. "As Martinez's light-weightedness became apparent, Walters and Carnes just started running the place," Frank Kalder observed.

Under the new regime, Herb Kleber was having more trouble than ever getting a hearing. Far more formal than Bennett, Martinez would see him only by appointment, and even then he seemed little interested in what he had to say. Meanwhile, Walters and Carnes were preparing a new strategy that, while requesting more money, would allocate it in the same old ways. With uncharacteristic boldness, Kleber in mid-1991 sent Martinez a memo suggesting a major new presidential initiative. It would be aimed at what he called "the new reality"—

that casual drug use has fallen off dramatically [while] hard-core use among our urban and working class populations is still a serious problem that must be addressed. Unless a concerted effort is made to target these populations with increased resources in the areas of both supply and demand, our nation's cities will be dominated by drugs and the resulting crime for years to come.

Kleber proposed spending $1 billion to address the problem, some to beef up law enforcement but most "to expand the availability of comprehensive treatment programs for the many individuals who can benefit from treatment, but have not had access to it." Pregnant addicts and high-risk youth would get top priority.

Full of hope, Kleber sent the memo to the eighth floor. There it died. "An utter non-starter," Carnes sniffed. Kleber—finally getting a feel for how the game was played—enlisted some friends of George Bush to bring his proposal to his personal attention. And the president expressed interest. Thus encouraged, Kleber shepherded the proposal through the Office of Management and Budget, where it eventually landed on the desk of OMB director Richard Darman. Unfortunately, Darman was no more sympathetic to treatment than Bruce Carnes, and Kleber's initiative met its final demise.

At that point, Kleber felt that the chance to make any real change was gone. And so, in the fall of 1991, he left ONDCP to take a job as a professor of psychiatry at Columbia University. A week later, his deputy Linda Lewis was asked to leave. With both Stanley Morris and Reggie Walton also departing, the purge of the professionals was complete. Over the remainder of Bush's term, ONDCP would become a dumping ground for Republican loyalists, among them Richard "Digger" Phelps, the former Notre Dame basketball coach, who was named to a senior post. His only recommendation for it was his friendship with George Bush and Dan Quayle. "The symbolism of his appointment was unreal," Frank Kalder said. "The office became a joke in Washington."

In the spring of 1992, John Carnevale, a senior budget analyst working under Bruce Carnes, sat down to assess what if any progress the nation had made over the previous year in its fight against drugs. A career official who shared none of Carnes's ideological fervor, Carnevale summed up his findings in a four-page internal memo, and it was remarkably frank. On the demand side, it noted, the most recent National Household Survey showed a large increase in the number of regular cocaine users. Similarly, the Drug Abuse Warning Network showed sharp increases in the number of cocaine-related visits to hospital emergency rooms. On the supply side, the memo went on, the price of cocaine had fallen in the previous year—an indication that the flow of the drug into the country had increased.

From all this, the memo stated, it was clear that "in 1991 both the supply and demand for cocaine increased from 1990—precisely the opposite outcome expected by the President's drug control Strategy." The data, the document added, reveal the two-front nature of the war against cocaine use in America. One front challenges wide-spread, casual use, and is the area where we are having great success. The other is hard-core, frequent cocaine use, where the going is slower.

This was precisely the situation William Bennett had faced on becoming drug czar in March 1989. So, after three years of unrelenting culture war, the nation's drug problem had not abated; the "scourge," as George Bush had called it, had not stopped.

16

An Officer
and a General

FOR ALL THOSE LABORING in the trenches of drug treatment, the election of Bill Clinton seemed a cause for rejoicing. Aside from being the first Democrat to occupy the White House in twelve years, Clinton had had to face the problem of drug abuse in his own family. In the early 1980s, Clinton's half-brother Roger had become addicted to cocaine and was dealing it as well. As governor of Arkansas, Clinton, informed by the state police that Roger was under surveillance for selling drugs, had authorized a sting operation that resulted in his arrest. While awaiting disposition of his case, Roger received counseling for his addiction, and Bill and his mother Virginia sat in on some of the sessions. For the first time, Clinton had an opportunity to talk about his alcoholic stepfather and the ways in which dealing with him had shaped his own personality. With characteristic zest, Clinton plunged into the twelve-step literature, and terms like codependency and denial began popping up in his conversation.

Eventually, Roger was sentenced to two years in prison, and during the 1992 campaign Clinton would cite his experience as an argument against legalizing drugs. "If drugs were legal," he said in one of the presidential debates, "I don't think he'd be alive today." But he also cited the episode as evidence that treatment works. While Clinton's touchy-feely recovery-movement comments evoked ridicule from the press, they showed treatment counselors that he was no stranger to their world.

They took further encouragement from *Putting People First,* the Clinton-Gore campaign manifesto. "Thousands of addicts," it stated, "have volunteered to take themselves off the streets, only to hear the government tell them that they have to wait six months. In a Clinton-Gore Administration, federal assistance will help communities dramatically increase their ability to offer drug treatment to everyone who needs help."

The task of carrying out that promise would fall to the new drug czar. As a Democrat determined to make treatment a priority, Clinton could have been expected to select someone from the treatment fraternity. But, just as Nixon had defied expectations by choosing a psychiatrist, Clinton felt the need for a tough-minded individual who could sell treatment to a skeptical public. A cop with a conscience was the ideal, and, after much sifting of candidates, the administration felt it had just the man. Lee Brown had recently stepped down as commissioner of the New York City Police Department. In that job, he had helped implement David Dinkins's Safe Streets, Safe City program, with its unprecedented expansion of the city's police force. And, under his direction, crime had gone down in the city two years in a row. It was the latest in a string of successes for the fifty-five-year-old Brown, a record that had won him election as president of the International Association of Chiefs of Police. At six feet three and 230 pounds, with a large, regal head, the shoulders of a blocking back, and dark eyes peering out coolly from behind gold-rimmed glasses, Brown looked as imposing as his résumé.

But Brown's experience extended far beyond the squad car. One of the first African-Americans in the country to earn a Ph.D. in criminology (from Berkeley), he preferred the title "doctor" to "chief." Brown had taught at Portland State University, helping to set up a department in criminal justice there, and served as associate director of the Institute for Urban Affairs and Research at Howard University. In the early 1990s, he had participated in an elite seminar on policing at Harvard's Kennedy School, using the forum to push his belief in the need for cops to work with citizens and become their partners in problem solving.

Even by noncop standards, Brown's views were quite liberal. He supported affirmative action, opposed mandatory minimum sentences, and lamented the number of black men in prison. After leaving the NYPD, Brown had returned to his home in Houston to direct the Black Male Initiative at Texas Southern University. In a statement to Congress in 1991, Brown had stressed the need to "find long-term, permanent remedies" to the drug problem, "whether they involve education or employment or something that we have yet to focus on."

Such views reflected Brown's own trials as an African-American. In 1942, when he was five years old, his parents, sharecroppers in Oklahoma, loaded all of their possessions on the back of a truck and headed for California in search of work. Growing up poor outside Fresno, Brown spent his summers pitching watermelons and sacking potatoes in the San Joaquin Valley. Attending California State University at Fresno on a football scholarship, he intended to become a high school coach, but, after taking a course in criminology, he switched to law enforcement. In 1960, Brown went to work for the San Jose police department. Only the second black on the force, he became an undercover narcotics cop, posing as a junkie. "I saw firsthand what addiction can do to people," Brown recalled of that period. Ever after, he would feel a visceral disgust for drugs.

But he would also feel compassion for the victims of drugs, many of whom were blacks facing the same barriers as himself. Still, as a narc, Brown had no choice but to arrest them. Struggling to make sense of such contradictions, he enrolled as a part-time graduate student in criminology at Berkeley. Even in the people's republic atmosphere of the school, the criminology department was known for its radicalism, and Brown was exposed to a Marxist-inflected curriculum that stressed the discriminatory aspects of the nation's justice system. Brown's own life seemed to offer corroboration. Because of his skin color, he realized that he would never rise above the rank of captain in San Jose, and so in 1968 he left to teach at Portland State University. While there, he got his first taste of politics, becoming the president of the Oregon Black Caucus, which sought to redress problems of racial discrimination.

His great leap forward came in 1978, when he became head of the Atlanta police force. Soon after his arrival, the city was jolted by the disappearance of more than two dozen black children and young men, and Brown led the investigation that eventually solved the case. Four years later, he moved to Houston, where his success in transforming the police force won him praise from groups ranging from the Chamber of Commerce to the NAACP. From there it was on to New York. Arriving in the midst of the crack epidemic, Brown needed little convincing about its role in driving up the city's crime rate. From his experience, though, he believed that simply rounding up low-level dealers was not the answer, and so, with the support of David Dinkins, he had decided to deemphasize street-level arrests and go instead after higher-ups. In the end, Brown believed, the only long-term hope for resolving the nation's drug problem lay in reducing demand.

Brown's time in New York was marred by the Crown Heights riots, in which the police seemed to hold back as black demonstrators attacked local Orthodox Jews, resulting in the stabbing death of a rabbinical student. An investigation into the incident criticized Brown for not having acted decisively enough to quell the disturbance. The episode pointed up one of Brown's chief weaknesses—his disengaged style. An aloof, brooding man who nursed his many wounds in private, Brown had little of the human touch commonly associated with leadership. In New York, he had rarely come down from his aerie at One Police Plaza to appear in the ranks. He was, in cop vernacular, a "suit."

After heading the NYPD, the administration's offer to run the gnatlike ONDCP seemed almost an insult. To add injury to it, the White House had pared the office's staff from 146 to 25 as part of its downsizing campaign. Still, Brown had the mix of brawn and benevolence that the administration wanted in its drug czar, and, to sweeten the deal, Clinton promised to make him a member of his Cabinet. And, with that, the philosopher-cop signed on.

Soon after taking over, Brown sat for a detailed briefing on the state of the nation's drug problem. "What jumped out was the fact that the number of chronic, hard-core addicted users hadn't changed," Brown said in his clipped manner. "They were the individuals who were committing most of the crime, who were causing our health-care costs to soar, who were spreading disease. It became quite clear that if we really wanted to make a dent in the drug problem, we had to do something about these hard-core users."

And that something was *not* law enforcement, Brown believed. "From my background, it was clear that we couldn't arrest our way out of the problem," he observed. The very term "war on drugs" made Brown uncomfortable. "A country shouldn't declare war on its own people," he said. "We had to look for a different way. And my conclusion was that that way was treatment. All the empirical research told me that treatment works." According to a study commissioned by ONDCP, the number of people on the nation's waiting lists had reached a whopping 200,000. Getting rid of those lists became Brown's top priority.

Since there was a limit to how much new money the treatment system could absorb at once, Brown asked John Carnevale, now ONDCP's budget director, to come up with a realistic spending goal. After polling various experts, Carnevale proposed a one-year increase of $355 million—enough to fund 74,000 new slots. In contrast to past increases, which were made in the form of general block grants that the states could use as they saw fit, the new funds were to be aimed specifically at hard-core users. And, in a sign of his own commitment to treatment, President Clinton personally approved inclusion of the money in his budget over the objections of OMB.

As BROWN was attempting to boost spending on the demand side, the National Security Council was trying to reduce it on the supply side. There, a DEA detailee named Richard Cañas had embarked on a personal mission to deescalate the drug war abroad. A short, peppery, tough-talking man who had joined the NSC staff in 1990, Cañas had watched as the Pentagon's antinarcotics budget went from virtually nothing in 1988 to $1.1 billion in 1993, much of it for detecting cocaine smugglers in the transit zones of Central America and the Caribbean. Despite these efforts, the United States had remained awash in cocaine.

In an early conversation with Anthony Lake, the new national security adviser, Cañas described these shortcomings. "I told him that there were twenty-eight agencies all vying for attention," recalled Cañas, whose penchant for candor compensated for a fondness for drug-war jargon. "There were five air wings, and five CINCs [commanders in chief]. Each had its own rice bowl. Everybody was feeding off the billion-dollar-a-year funding." When Lake asked what should be done, Cañas suggested a zero-based review. Agreeing, Lake got Clinton to sign a presidential directive authorizing a full assessment of U.S. counternarcotics programs abroad. Working out of his office in the Old Executive Office Building, Cañas demanded from each agency a full report on how it had spent its drug funds and what it had to show for them. Invariably, the reports came back full of self-serving generalities. Cañas sent them back with a demand for a detailed accounting of every dollar spent.

"We went after Customs, the Coast Guard, and especially the Pentagon," he recalled with a gleeful chuckle. "We really got into their knickers. It became the NSC versus the world." From the reports, Cañas found that the Defense Department was spending $700 million a year on "detection and monitoring," most of it in the form of Air Force surveillance flights and Navy cruiser patrols aimed at identifying suspicious-looking boats and planes. Unfortunately, the Pentagon had no way of telling if those craft had drugs on them, and no real capacity for going after them if they did.

In the end, the most damning document came from the CIA. Drawing on both human and electronic sources, the agency developed a national intelligence estimate of the amount of drugs produced, seized, and sold in the United States. According to the estimate, worldwide seizures of cocaine had increased from 321 tons in 1991 to 342 in 1992 and a projected 375 in 1993. But the level of cocaine production had kept pace. "We were seizing more, and they were producing more," Cañas said. "The margin of profit was so great that they could take those kinds of hits." Based on the continuing drop in the prices of cocaine and heroin, and the continuing increase in their purity levels, the CIA concluded that all the seizures and arrests of the last four years had done nothing to reduce the supply of drugs in the United States.

By September, the NSC review was complete. With the interdiction strategy of the Bush years judged a failure, the administration decided on a "controlled shift" in focus away from the transit zones and toward the source countries. Instead of seizing the drugs as they were shipped north to the United States, the administration would attempt to smash the drug syndicates on their home turf in Colombia, Peru, Bolivia, and Mexico. In reality, of course, such an approach was not new. For twelve years, the Republicans had been trying to disrupt cocaine production at its source, without much to show for it. In effect, the controlled shift was a cover for reducing the overall spending on international programs. In total, more than $200 million was to be trimmed from the Pentagon's $1.1 billion budget.

Overall, the administration's 1994 *National Drug Control Strategy* proposed a 9 percent increase in federal drug spending, to $13.2 billion, with the funding for treatment jumping 14.3 percent and that for interdiction falling 7.3 percent. If enacted, the budget would mark an important turning point in national drug policy, a move away from the parent model of the 1980s and back toward the public-health model of the 1970s.

There remained one last obstacle to making that happen: Congress. It had a tradition of chopping treatment requests sent over by the executive branch. To pass, the hard-core initiative would need strong leadership from the White House. And that, Lee Brown felt sure, he would get. Indeed, Bill Clinton had personally promised him that he would participate in an event to mark the release of the strategy, scheduled for February 9, 1994.

THE FIRST SIGN of trouble came in late January, when the University of Michigan released the results of its latest high school survey. Of the twelfth-graders polled in 1993, 26 percent said they had smoked marijuana in the previous year, up from 21.9 percent in 1992. Past-month use had risen to 15.5 percent, up from 11.9 percent. It was the first increase in the marijuana numbers in fourteen years, and the fact that it had occurred on a Democrat's watch spelled trouble for Bill Clinton.

No one was more aware of this than Ricia McMahon, ONDCP's acting chief of staff. A stout, steely-eyed woman in her fifties, McMahon was intensely loyal to Bill Clinton. At the drug office, she was known as "Ms. New Hampshire" for her role in driving Clinton around that state during the primary. McMahon was rewarded with a high-ranking job at the drug office. Having worked in the prevention field in New Hampshire, she knew how intently people followed the University of Michigan survey, and, with the marijuana numbers ticking up, she quickly alerted the White House.

There, in a reflection of the low priority drugs had for the administration, the issue was being tracked by two junior assistants—Jose Cerda, a former congressional aide who was so fresh-faced that he seemed too young to have even tried drugs, and Liz Bernstein, a tall, brassy, wisecracking woman who had worked on the campaign. Immediately grasping the potential peril in the new survey, they notified Mark Gearan, the White House communications director. In an effort to preempt possible criticism, the White House decided to release the results of the survey at a press conference at the Department of Health and Human Services. To highlight its concern, it arranged for the presence of three Cabinet members—Donna Shalala, the secretary of health and human services; Richard Riley, the secretary of education, and Lee Brown. More than fifty journalists showed up. Lloyd Johnston, the director of the survey, told them, "We have the unenviable role of informing the country that drug use is making a comeback, that the epidemic could be reemerging."

In the inner city of course, the epidemic had never disappeared. But no one at the press conference wanted to talk about that; rising pot use among teens was the theme of the day. And the press duly went along. STUDY FINDS MARIJUANA USE IS UP IN HIGH SCHOOLS, the *New York Times* declared on its front page on February 1, 1994. The new numbers, the paper reported, were "another indication that after more than a decade of decline, drug use may be on the upswing." The article went on to implicate Bill Clinton, noting that he had "scarcely mentioned drugs as President."

In case Clinton needed any more prodding, he got it that same day in a meeting with two powerful figures in the drug field, James Burke and Joseph Califano. At first glance, they seemed an unlikely pair—the one a former chairman of Johnson & Johnson and a prominent Republican, the other a former secretary of HEW and a well-known Democrat. But they had developed a symbiotic relationship in the world where drugs and corporate America intersect. After leaving Johnson & Johnson, Burke had become head of the Partnership for a Drug-Free America, the consortium of ad agencies and media companies responsible for all those this-is-your-brain-on-drugs TV commercials. As its name implied, the Partnership saw the problem much as the parent movement did, and its commercials sought mainly to prevent adolescent pot use.

A grandfatherly man who asked everyone to call him Jim, Burke was nonetheless used to being listened to, and, in speeches and interviews, he would stress how casual drug use was at the core of the nation's drug problem. Between 1990 and 1992, when his good friend George Bush was president, Burke had secured more than $1 billion worth of donated time for the Partnership's antidrug commercials. Since then, however, the level of donations had fallen off, and Burke felt certain that Bill Clinton's low profile on the issue was responsible.

Joe Califano agreed. A forceful and pugnacious attorney, Califano had recently set up the Center on Addiction and Substance Abuse. Affiliated with Columbia University and located in a glittering office building next to Carnegie Hall, CASA had put together a blue-chip staff of experts pulling down corporate-level salaries. (Among them was Herbert Kleber, now serving as CASA's medical director.) Califano could not have started CASA without the assistance of Burke, who had helped arrange a huge start-up grant from the Robert Wood Johnson Foundation, on whose board he sat. CASA, in turn, produced a study on gateway drugs (marijuana as well as cigarettes and alcohol) that backed up the Partnership's prevention messages.

For weeks, Burke and Califano had been pushing for a meeting with the president to discuss their concerns, and on February 1 they got it. Lee Brown sat in on the session, held in the Oval Office. Burke did most of the talking. Owing to the White House's lack of leadership on the issue, he said, the antidrug message that had been transmitted so strongly during the Republican years was getting blurred. And the fallout was apparent in the recent University of Michigan numbers. Though couched in the politest terms, the message to the president was unmistakable: either become more active in publicizing the evils of drugs or face the political consequences.

AS IT HAPPENED, the pressure for a new stance on drugs came as the White House was staking out a new position on crime. During the 1992 campaign, Clinton, casting himself as a new type of Democrat on the issue, had promised to put 100,000 new cops on the street. Once in office, however, he had paid scant attention to that pledge, absorbed as he was in cutting the deficit and reforming health care. And no one had seemed to care—until November 2, 1993. In elections held that day, Republicans scored an impressive hat trick:

Rudolph Giuliani became mayor of New York, Christine Todd Whitman became governor of New Jersey, and George Allen, Jr., became governor of Virginia.

The press wasted little time in proclaiming the meaning of it all. "Crime is this year's anti-incumbent issue," wrote William Schneider in a much-echoed analysis in the *Washington Post*. The message of the election, he asserted, "is that crime-obsessed voters are looking for candidates who show toughness and discipline. That doesn't sound much like Bill Clinton." The claim of such a mandate was odd, in that the nation's crime rate had fallen by 5 percent in the first half of the year. Nonetheless, by the end of the week, the networks were airing stories about the new crime wave gripping the land. And, in a frenzy recalling the period after Len Bias's death, panicked legislators in the House and Senate were voting to spend tens of billions of dollars on new prisons, police officers, and boot camps.

If the Democrats were ever to redefine themselves on crime, now was the time. In his State of the Union address, delivered on January 25, 1994, Clinton, in addition to reiterating his 100,000-cop pledge, declared that "those who commit repeated violent crimes should be told, 'When you commit a third violent crime, you will be put away and put away for good. Three strikes and you are out.' " It was a draconian proposal, but the public response was favorable, and the White House began holding daily crime meetings to devise ways in which it could outflank the Republicans on the issue.

It was in this climate that the White House prepared to mark the release of Lee Brown's drug strategy. The task of selecting a site fell to Ricia McMahon, Jose Cerda, and Liz Bernstein. With the hard-core initiative at the heart of the strategy, visiting a treatment center would have seemed a logical choice. Given the mood in Washington, however, that was out of the question. As Liz Bernstein recalled, "Treatment was seen as squishy. Pushing it was seen as making the president vulnerable on crime." Still, with treatment the strategy's main news, it could not be totally ignored, and, after much mulling, the group arrived at what seemed the perfect solution—the president could visit a treatment program *in prison*. "We decided to go to a prison because Newt Gingrich likes treatment in prison," recalled Bernstein.

It was Bernstein's job to find the right prison. Visiting several facilities in the Washington area, she was impressed with the jail in Maryland's Prince George's County, which had a model ninety-day treatment program. Hoping to find a recent graduate to speak at the event, Bernstein drove around the area with a social worker, interviewing ex-cons. After several misfires, she came upon Joseph Mundo in a 7-Eleven. A forty-two-year-old former junkie who had been clean for eleven months, Mundo agreed to participate, and in the remaining two days Bernstein worked feverishly to prepare him. Meanwhile, the White House, anticipating a giant photo op, was arranging for half the Cabinet to attend.

And so, on the morning of February 9, 1994, in an event that showed how twisted the drug debate in America had become, the Democratic president of the United States, seeking to promote a drug strategy with treatment at its core, arrived at the Prince George's County Correctional Center in Upper Marlboro, Maryland. Traveling the fifteen miles from the White House in a motorcade, Clinton was accompanied by Al Gore, Lee Brown, Janet Reno, Donna Shalala, Henry Cisneros, Federico Peña, and Richard Riley. Passing through a chain-link fence topped with coils of barbed wire, the entourage headed for the building's gym, an airy space packed with about three hundred people, including congressmen, law-enforcement officials, and state legislators, plus some forty inmates dressed in bright-orange jump suits.

Looking sharp in a gray suit, Joseph Mundo, who not long before had been shooting up in the streets, stood before the sea of dignitaries and, in a halting voice, praised treatment in prison as the "best thing that could have happened to me." When it was his turn, Bill Clinton, looking out at the sea of dignitaries, singled out two for acknowledgment—Jim Burke and Joe Califano. In his speech, the president called for more cops, boot camps, drug courts, "drug-free" workplaces and schools, attacks on the drug cartels, personal responsibility, bipartisanship, and, finally, drug treatment—a subject that took up no more than two minutes of his twenty-minute address.

TO ANYONE BETTER ATTUNED to the political cadences of Washington, the president's performance would have raised immediate questions about the depth of his commitment to drug treatment. On that score, however, Lee Brown was nearly deaf. Despite a career spent in the hurly-burly world of big-city policing, he was remarkably untutored in the nuances of politics. And so, despite the militant mood in the capital, and the president's own hard-line rhetoric, the drug czar remained confident that he had Clinton's full backing for the hard-core initiative. All that remained was making the necessary rounds on the Hill.

During his appearances in Congress, however, Brown was treated like a human punching bag. "I tell you, I am very worried that your strategy to shift the focus . . . toward treatment and education will allow more drugs to come into this country," Senator Christopher Bond, a Republican from Missouri, told him at a hearing in late February 1994. Treatment, he said, was a "revolving door" that had "not seen a great deal of success. . . . I am very much concerned that we are seeing a strategy of retreat." Senator Dennis DeConcini, an Arizona Democrat and ardent friend of the Customs Service, decried the administration's intention to cut the federal interdiction budget. Brown's responses were tentative and perfunctory.

His speeches were not much better. In March, for instance, he visited the District of Columbia General Hospital. The District's lone public hospital, D.C. General was being overrun by addicts, and Brown, in visiting it, hoped to dramatize their plight. Arriving at the sprawling medical complex with a body-guard and a press aide, he was led upstairs to a special ward set up to treat drug abusers with mental disorders. Seven sad-eyed patients, all black, sat at a table stitching together leather wallets. Towering over them in his gray suit and crisp white shirt, Brown ham-handedly described his efforts to help people in their situation. "Five weeks ago," he stammered, "the president released the national drug control strategy. It's different from past strategies. It puts more emphasis on drug treatment."

Brown expanded on the point in a speech to one hundred or so staff members gathered in the hospital's auditorium for their grand rounds. "The drug problem," he declared, "will not be solved by tougher law enforcement alone. We must pay just as much attention to medical, as well as educational and prevention, solutions. That is why the new strategy places greater emphasis on—and more resources in—programs that reduce the demand for drugs."

Overall, the speech offered much for these health workers to cheer. Yet their applause was distinctly muted—a reflection, no doubt, of Brown's wooden speaking style. He had read the entire speech in a monotone, and, even with the words in front of him, had stumbled repeatedly. He was quickly upstaged, in fact, by former mayor Marion Barry, who, hot on the comeback trail after his own brush with crack, hopped up uninvited on the podium and roused the crowd with his revival-like style. In the end, Brown's visit to D.C. General would gain little public notice.

And so it went throughout the spring. A subdued, even shy man who had trouble making small talk, Brown was not good copy, and so few reporters bothered to cover him. That spring, Brown's name would barely appear in the *Washington Post*. Yet the fault was not his alone. Whatever his public awkwardness, Brown's efforts to change the direction of U.S. drug policy seemed a good story by any journalistic standard. Clearly, editors disagreed. The decrepit state of the nation's treatment facilities, the existence of long waiting lists, the frequency with which addicts seeking help were turned back onto the street—all this was "old news" as far as journalists were concerned. By contrast, every time the University of Michigan reported an upturn in teenage pot use, it was front-page news.

The ultimate responsibility for Brown's invisibility, however, lay with the White House. Throughout the spring, as the drug czar was struggling to pro-mote the 1994 strategy, the administration remained silent. Not once after his visit to Prince George's County did Bill Clinton speak out about the hard-core initiative. Liz Bernstein, seeing the trouble Brown was in with Congress, ap-proached her superiors at the White House and begged them to send someone over to ONDCP to coach him. They could not be bothered.

Brown's moment of truth came in July 1994, when the Senate Appropria-tions Subcommittee on Labor, Health and Human Services, and Education was preparing its final budget decisions. With so many different programs competing for funds, the White House handed over a secret list of its priorities for the three departments. In all, there were some ten items on the list, and the hard-core initiative was not among them. As a result, the subcommittee felt free to ignore it.

"I was very naive," Liz Bernstein said, looking back on the episode after leaving the White House. "I thought it was going to be great: After twelve years of Republican rule, we were going to have a treatment initiative—a breath of fresh air." In the end, however, she said, "the initiative was not well regarded at the White House." Ultimately, Congress would approve only $57 million in new funds for treatment—none of them earmarked for hard-core users.

EVEN AS the hard-core initiative was going down to defeat, the administration was preparing a new one. And, significantly, the task of developing it fell not to the drug office but to the White House communications office and its deputy director, Rahm Emanuel. A thirty-four-year-old political operative—or, in his own more piquant description, a "fucked up Jewish kid from Chicago" —Emanuel had almost no background in public policy. Through sheer chutz-pah and tenacity, however, he had become an important presence in the White House. A dapper, smooth-faced man with modishly cut brown hair and the sleek build of a ballet dancer—he took lessons twice a week—Emanuel had first displayed his drive during the 1992 campaign, when, as finance director, he had amassed a huge war chest. As a reward, he was made White House political director. His abrasive style earned him numerous enemies, however, and he was subsequently assigned to the White House team pushing NAFTA. There, he found his calling. Tracking votes and twisting arms, Emanuel helped engineer the administration's narrow victory. Afterward, he was made second-in-command at communications. In that capacity, Emanuel, restlessly sifting through polling data and focus-group reports, worked hard at his overriding goal—boosting the president's approval ratings.

Emanuel had shown his talent at that during the crime debate in early 1994, helping to define a New Democrat stance on the issue. He now hoped to do the same for drugs. The past strategy of helping inner-city addicts typified the old Democrat approach. From now on, the administration was going to focus on teenage pot use, an issue popular with middle-class voters. To that end, Emanuel pressed ONDCP to come up with a plan.

As a first step, the drug office contacted Lloyd Johnston of the University of Michigan and asked him to convene a group of prevention experts to discuss the recent rise in pot use. Over a day and a half, seventeen of them met in Ann Arbor to ponder the latest survey numbers and what they meant. As the report on the meeting noted, "There was consensus about one thing: These changes are real and constitute a wake-up call for the country. There was genuine concern that the reversal of the downward trend in drug use could signal the emergence of a new epidemic of drug use." As to why more young people were using drugs, the report offered a grab bag of hypotheses, including a "general rise in deviance," a "seeming increase in the number of pop songs which glorify drug use," a "steady erosion in the influence of parents and teachers," and a "decline in the motivating force of executive leadership."

Yet there were some alternative conclusions the Ann Arbor report did not consider. For all the hoopla over rising pot use, the actual numbers remained quite low. The rate of monthly marijuana use, while up some, was still less than half what it had been in the late 1970s. The rate of daily use—2.4 percent —was not even one-fourth the peak level. As for harder drugs, consumption rates remained negligible, with just 1.3 percent of all high school seniors saying they had used cocaine in the last month and a mere 0.2 percent saying they had used heroin. In many ways, the most striking numbers in the survey concerned not pot or heroin, but alcohol. Fully 27.5 percent of the seniors polled said they had had five or more drinks in one sitting during the previous two weeks. In other words, one in every four twelfth-graders was getting smashed on a regular basis. The health risks from this seemed much greater than anything associated with illegal drugs. To point this out, however, would have been politically inconvenient, for the alcohol industry was a major backer of the Democratic Party. And so, in a glaring omission, the Ann Arbor report did not even mention alcohol and the dangers it posed to young people, reserving its ire exclusively for illicit drugs.

Released in June 1994, the report became the basis for a series of brainstorming sessions at ONDCP (or "group gropes," as one senior staff member disdainfully called them). "We were trying to focus on issues that would grab people's attention," said Charlotte Hayes, a participant in the sessions. A tall, self-assured black woman given to frequently checking her watch, Hayes had been sent over to ONDCP from the White House to help formulate a plan. "People didn't give a hoot about the drug problem unless it affected them personally," she observed. "Americans didn't care about hard-core addicts. They felt they were at fault for their problem. So we made a concerted effort to refocus the drug office on what Americans were focused on—kids using drugs."

By the fall, an action plan was ready and sent to Rahm Emanuel, who approved it. Lee Brown, who had previously visited treatment centers and hospital emergency rooms, would now attend staged events publicizing the evils of pot. Signaling the change, the drug czar in October 1994 joined with Buddy Gleaton to release the results of PRIDE's own alarmist survey on rising drug use. Soon after, he went to New York to help the Partnership for a Drug-Free America launch a new media campaign against marijuana. In Washington, Brown participated in a special Marijuana Conference attended by angry antipot activists from around the country. And, in Kentucky, he ventured into a marijuana field to chop down cannabis plants for the benefit of local camera crews. "I am on a crusade for no drug use, especially among young people," Brown declared. "My message is simple and clear. Marijuana is not benign, it is not harmless and should not be legalized. It's a very dangerous drug that can cause you to fight for your health and your life in a hospital emergency room."

The extent of Brown's transformation became most apparent on June 20, 1995. During ONDCP's group gropes, it had been decided that Brown should lie in wait for an opportunity to attack a celebrity drug user. "Our strategy," Charlotte Hayes recalled, "was that the next time a high-profile guy who had been involved with drugs came into the news—someone getting millions of dollars—we would respond." The opportunity finally arose when the New York Yankees announced they were signing Darryl Strawberry to a $2-million-plus contract. Strawberry had been through repeated bouts with drugs and alcohol, but he now said he was clean, and Yankee owner George Steinbrenner was desperate for some left-handed hitting. On cue, Brown exploded. "The Yankees have struck out by signing Darryl Strawberry," he fumed in a press release. "They are sending the worst possible message to the youth of America that if you use drugs, you can be rewarded with big money in big-time sports."

Brown's comments rankled many in the treatment field. For, viewed another way, the Yankees, in signing Strawberry, were giving work to a recovering addict—a key component in the rehabilitation process. Lee Brown himself had frequently talked about the importance of work as part of treatment aftercare. One did not have to like or admire Strawberry to feel that he deserved another shot at surmounting his troubles. Such considerations counted for little, though, in the White House's push for middle-class votes. And so Brown kept up the pressure on the Yankees, demanding a meeting with Steinbrenner. Eventually, the Yankee boss talked with him by phone, but, to no one's surprise, refused to budge. Brown had considerably more success with the news media. In addition to being quoted in papers across the country, he was asked to appear on *Nightline* to discuss the issue. At long last, Lee Brown was in the news. It was for very different reasons, however, than those that had driven him when he first took the job.

To those who knew Brown well, his crusade against marijuana did not seem out of character. Having seen the devastation drugs had caused in the black community, he was deeply intolerant of them. Youths in the inner city seemed at particular risk, so the idea of launching a campaign aimed at teens held great appeal. Yet, by engaging in such lush rhetoric, Brown was helping feed the same war-on-drugs excesses that he had initially so opposed. And, in focusing so narrowly on marijuana, he was neglecting the hard-core heroin and cocaine users whom he had earlier singled out as the real core of the nation's problem. By the time he stepped down as drug czar, in December 1995, only 35 percent of the federal drug budget was earmarked for treatment and prevention—exactly the same proportion as in the final year of the Bush Administration.

THE TASK OF REPLACING Brown fell, naturally, to Rahm Emanuel. As usual, he was guided more by political than programmatic concerns. With the Republicans continuing to pummel the administration over teenage drug use, Emanuel drew up a list of four categories of candidates—soldier, cop, prosecutor, and inner-city leader—and presented it to the president. As he expected, Clinton picked the first. And Emanuel was ready with his candidate. General Barry R. McCaffrey was one of the brightest stars in the U.S. military. A 1964 graduate of West Point, he had served two tours in Vietnam, where he was wounded three times, one of which nearly cost him the use of his left arm. During the Gulf War, McCaffrey, as the commander of the 24th Infantry Division, had led the famous "left hook" maneuver that trapped Iraq's forces inside Kuwait. In 1992, he had served as an assistant to Colin Powell, and in 1994 he became commander of the U.S. Southern Command in Panama. Over the years, McCaffrey had been awarded two Distinguished Service Crosses, two Silver Stars, and three Purple Hearts. With the 1996 election looming, who better to shield the administration against attack than a certified war hero?

Yet McCaffrey was hardly a typical military man. His father—Lieutenant General William McCaffrey, a veteran of World War II, Korea, and Vietnam —was a liberal Irish Catholic who had instilled in his son a belief in civil rights and social justice. The holder of a master's degree in civil government from American University, McCaffrey was an early proponent of bringing more women into the military, and in 1991 he received an award from the NAACP for his efforts to recruit minorities.

On the drug issue, too, McCaffrey was something of a maverick. While at SouthCom, he had overseen many of the Pentagon's antidrug programs in Latin America. The most notable was Green Clover, a radar-and-intelligence-gathering operation that sought to intercept the small planes that flew coca paste from the jungles of Peru to the processing labs of Colombia. Tactically, the operation was a great success, rupturing the air bridge between the two countries. As always, though, the traffickers quickly adapted, using boats to move their cargo by river and ocean, and the flow of cocaine into the United States had not ebbed. In a speech to the Heritage Foundation shortly before his nomination as drug czar, McCaffrey frankly noted that "there's been no diminishment at all in the price or availability of cocaine on the streets of America in the time we've been working at it." Rejecting the idea of a war on drugs, McCaffrey said that he regarded the drug problem more as a "cancer" that required a "holistic approach," including "a renewed commitment on the domestic front to reducing demand."

Shortly before taking office, McCaffrey met with treatment providers at a reception hosted by Tipper Gore at the vice president's sumptuous office in the Old Executive Office Building. McCaffrey impressed the crowd with his knowledgeable comments about the physiology of addiction and the effectiveness of treatment. Providers took further encouragement from his confirmation hearing, held on February 27, 1996. "We must focus as a priority on reducing consumption among the three million hard-core users who consume 75 percent of the total tonnage of illegal drugs," the general said. Asked by Senator Arlen Specter how he felt the federal drug budget should be divided up, McCaffrey said, "Our treatment and education programs, my gut tells me, are the heart of this entire effort. I told the President I thought this was three-quarters of what I was supposed to do."

McCaffrey would get an early opportunity to move policy in that direction. In agreeing to become drug czar, McCaffrey had wrangled from the White House a promise to put at his disposal $500 million (later reduced to $250 million) in funds reprogrammed from the Pentagon. How McCaffrey chose to spend that money would set an early tone for his term, and, to advise him, he appointed a large interagency task force. After weeks of study and consultation, the general arrived at his decision: $202 million of the $250 million would go for increased interdiction efforts in Latin America. The largest single item— $98 million—would go for upgrading two Navy P-3B airplanes. The main purpose of the package, McCaffrey wrote Congress, would be "to disrupt the cocaine airbridge in Peru and Colombia"—the same program that had proved so ineffective while he was at SouthCom.

McCaffrey's staffing decisions were equally mystifying. To help him carry out his mission, McCaffrey had obtained the White House's permission to expand ONDCP's staff from the 40 people then serving on it to the 150 it had had under George Bush. As an initial step toward reaching that goal, McCaffrey had arranged to bring over 30 detailees from other government agencies. He chose to bring all 30 from the Pentagon. To handle sensitive tasks within ONDCP, McCaffrey set up a new Office of Strategic Planning and stocked it with active and retired military personnel. The crucial job of drafting the annual strategy was taken out of the hands of John Carnevale—one of ONDCP's most experienced officials—and placed in those of Pancho Kinney, a lieutenant colonel in the Army who had no prior experience in drug matters. And, in place of the elegant supply-demand divide that had so dependably guided national policymakers since the Nixon days, McCaffrey instituted a military-style "systems" approach that splintered drug policy into a complex array of five goals, thirty-two objectives, and ninety-four performance targets.

McCaffrey's militarization of the nation's drug policy would become most apparent in the fall of 1997, when ONDCP was preparing its 1998 strategy. As part of that process, every department with a role in the drug war had to submit a proposed antidrug budget for the coming year. The Pentagon's submission came to $809 million—about $35 million less than it was currently spending. This reflected the Pentagon's growing awareness of its limited ability to keep drugs out of the country, and its sense that the money could be spent better elsewhere. Notwithstanding his many comments about the need to focus on demand, McCaffrey insisted that the Pentagon add $141 million to its budget request. When a meeting with Secretary of Defense William Cohen failed to resolve the matter, McCaffrey took the rare step of decertifying the Pentagon's budget request. Eventually, a compromise was worked out in which the Pentagon agreed to add nearly $80 million to its request, most of it to fight coca production in Peru, patrol transit routes in the Caribbean, and strengthen interdiction efforts along the Mexican border.

Mexico was, in many ways, the linchpin of McCaffrey's strategy. By the mid-1990s, Mexico had emerged as the main conduit of drugs into the United States, and as the level of trafficking there increased, so did the violence and corruption. And McCaffrey was determined to stop it. In December 1996, he went to Mexico to meet with top law-enforcement and military personnel. When Mexico named Jesús Gutiérrez Rebollo, an army general, to be its new antidrug chief, McCaffrey praised him as "a guy of absolute, unquestioned integrity." Weeks later, Gutiérrez was arrested on corruption charges.

Such a public humiliation might have chastened a less determined man, but the general plunged on, returning to Mexico in May 1997, then visiting the Southwest border in October. McCaffrey spent a full week on the border, examining points of entry, meeting with Customs officials, and watching truck inspections. He was struck by how little impact U.S. efforts were having. Of the 900,000 U.S.-bound trucks inspected for drugs in 1996, just 16 were found to contain cocaine. An ONDCP memo, summing up the findings from the trip, noted that "our current interdiction efforts almost completely fail to achieve our purpose of reducing the flow of cocaine, heroin, and methamphetamine across the border." Drug trafficking and violence, it added, "remain persistent and growing threats to border region residents."

One plausible conclusion to be drawn from this, of course, was that Washington's ongoing efforts to keep drugs out of the country were futile. Since the mid-1970s, when the Ford and Carter administrations tried to squelch the Mexican drug trade, there had accumulated a vast storehouse of think-tank studies, internal government documents, General Accounting Office reports, intelligence assessments, newspaper articles, and congressional reports chronicling the failure of U.S. efforts to seal the nation's borders. None of this would daunt McCaffrey, however. Much of his time in office would be spent conjuring up ways to escalate the drug war in Mexico. Under his direction, the United States would provide that country with seventy-three Huey helicopters, four fixed-wing turboprop planes, and two U.S. Knox-class frigates for use in counternarcotics operations. It would also train hundreds of Mexican soldiers and sailors and assign new National Guard units to the border. In his most cherished project, McCaffrey would push for the installation of new X-ray units along the border that would allow Customs inspectors to peer into the holds of container trucks.

In an interview over breakfast in his office in the Old Executive Office Building, McCaffrey offered a staunch defense of his strategy. "If you want to

stop drug abuse in Baltimore, with its thirty-five thousand heroin addicts staggering around the city, then the place to do it ain't El Paso," the trim, tough-
minded general said as he struggled with his disabled left hand to cut into a
Danish. "But, having said that, I would argue that we can and should implement a security system at our thirty-nine border crossings with Mexico which
models itself on air travel, in which millions of Americans a year fly on planes
and put up with a modest cramp in their movement, but with a high probability
of screening out guns and bombs. We can do the same thing on the Southwest
border." If the drug smugglers could be forced away from the border and out
to sea, McCaffrey said, "there'll be less murder and corruption of democratic
institutions in Mexico and the United States." But would there be any reduction in the amount of drugs coming into the country? "No," McCaffrey frankly
acknowledged. "We won't stop heroin addicts in Baltimore from getting access
to drugs. But we'll lower the violence and corruption that impacts these two
societies."

In short, under Barry McCaffrey, U.S. drug policy had reached the point
where it seemed directed more at achieving a foreign-policy goal—bolstering
democratic institutions in Mexico—than at reducing the level of drug abuse in
the United States.

To be fair, McCaffrey's 1999 budget did offer some succor to those addicts
in Baltimore, in the form of a $143-million increase in the federal block grant
for drug treatment. Yet, when compared to the crushing need in the nation's
cities, it was a trivial sum. Indeed, it came to barely a third of the amount Lee
Brown had requested in 1994 for his hard-core initiative. For all his promises
to address the demand for drugs, McCaffrey by his actions showed that his
real preoccupation was cutting the supply. Given that he had spent his entire
career in the military, this should have come as no surprise. With a former
four-star general now in charge of U.S. drug policy, the war on drugs had
reached its logical culmination.

BY THE TIME Barry McCaffrey became drug czar, Jerome Jaffe was working
at the Center for Substance Abuse Treatment in Rockville, Maryland, a unit
created by Congress in 1992 to improve the quality of drug treatment in the
United States. As CSAT's associate director, Jaffe, now nearing retirement age,
was involved in much the same kind of work he had done while director of
SAODAP. In many cases, in fact, he found himself fighting the same battles.
Whereas before, though, he could pick up the phone and make Cabinet secretaries jump, he was now left to fight rearguard actions in a bureaucratic backwater.

His main preoccupation was methadone. Among Jaffe's most satisfying
achievements while at SAODAP had been making methadone available to
heroin addicts around the country. In the years since, study after study had
confirmed methadone's effectiveness in reducing drug consumption, cutting

crime, and boosting employment. With the public's toughening attitudes toward drugs, however, national methadone capacity had become frozen at 115,000 slots—not quite 15 percent of the nation's estimated 810,000 heroin addicts. As a result, most cities had long waiting lists for methadone, and eight states had no clinics at all.

Even those clinics that did exist had become so run-down that they were having trouble retaining clients. The problem was aggravated by the intricate web of federal regulations that governed every detail of the clinics' operations, from acceptable dose levels to the frequency of urine tests. Particularly onerous was the requirement that methadone be dispensed only in a clinical setting. Even clients who had been on the drug for years and were doing well had to keep showing up at the clinics to get their medication. "There are a lot of people who are working, who've turned their lives around, but who are still required, because of the obsession with diversion, to come back to the clinic and line up once a week with people who are just off the street," Jaffe observed. And many of those people eventually dropped out as a result.

Jaffe was intimately familiar with the methadone regulations; he had written them himself while at SAODAP. The provision requiring clients to pick up their drugs at clinics had been included to allay fears about diversion. But, expecting this problem to be quickly resolved, Jaffe had also inserted a provision allowing the director of a methadone program to designate a nearby pharmacy to dispense the medication to patients who were doing well. At CSAT, Jaffe had embarked on a personal crusade to get this section implemented. At every point, however, he was blocked by the DEA. "There will always be some diversion," Jaffe noted, "but we have to balance that against the need to make medication available. It's like when somebody escapes from a concentration camp and the guards say, 'We're going to shoot everyone in the barracks.' If three or four percent of all methadone clients sell methadone, they say, 'We're going to make everyone come back every day.' "

Recalling how, at Albert Einstein, he used to send his patients to a pharmacy around the corner to get their prescriptions filled, Jaffe said with a sigh, "It's depressing that we can't get back to where we were thirty years ago."

Sometimes, Jaffe, listening to the harsh pronouncements being made in Washington, felt that he was back in the days of Harry Anslinger. "We know that you can deliver good treatment in a therapeutic community for less than half of what it costs to keep someone in prison," he said, his wryness undiminished by time. "Yet people keep advocating the building of more and more prisons." Congress, he added, "wants to mandate people to treatment through the courts when in fact you have people pounding on the door for treatment and can't get it. They say, 'Let's force treatment on people who don't want it,' at a time when people who want it can't get it." A quarter-century after he first came to Washington, Jaffe found himself having to preach the same message he had back then—that many addicts do want to get well, and that treatment can help them do it.

PART THREE

THE STREET
1993–1997

17

Rise and Fall

ATTENDING CHURCH a few days after the community meeting at which he had exploded, Raphael Flores ran into the woman whose door the police had broken down. An elderly, gray-haired Puerto Rican immigrant, Anna McLaughlin told Raphael how happy she'd been on hearing that he had spoken up for her. Remarkably, the police department's policy was that it had no responsibility for replacing doors that it had destroyed in the course of botched drug raids, and for two months Anna's had gone unrepaired. Inspired by Raphael, however, she had gone to the Del Toro brothers to complain, and they had put her in touch with the precinct to see about compensation. As for Raphael, the Del Toros were predictably displeased with his performance, and, as a result, his grant application with the state's AIDS Institute was all but dead.

Raphael's other fundraising efforts were faring no better. Even people who'd faithfully supported Hot Line Cares in the past seemed indifferent to his pleas; he'd simply cried "wolf" too many times. For the addicts of Spanish Harlem, however, Hot Line's financial problems were of no moment, and they continued to besiege the center. And, more and more, they seemed to be women. Eight years into the crack epidemic, the many inner-city women who had been swept up in it all seemed to be burning out at once. And the treatment world was not prepared for them. Having come into being in the 1960s, when most addicts were men, that world remained strongly oriented toward them. Most counselors were men, and a disproportionate number of slots were reserved for them. Few programs would accept pregnant addicts, and even fewer had provisions for child care. As a result, the ongoing decline in the nation's treatment system was hurting women the most, and every day at Hot Line brought another tough case.

One afternoon, it was a thirty-five-year-old black woman who was seven months pregnant with her first child. A sniffer of cocaine, she had stopped using as soon as she discovered she was pregnant, but, two weeks earlier, she had again picked up. Horrified at what she might be doing to her baby, she desperately wanted help in stopping. Since she was pregnant, Marvin told her, it would be hard to find a detox willing to take her. Making a stab at it, he called a hospital in Beacon where Hot Line had had some luck in the past. Due to the crushing demand, however, the hospital said it would not have an opening for two weeks. "That's too long!" the woman cried. She had no choice but to wait, however.

A few days later, Raphael became involved in the case of a Puerto Rican woman who was not only addicted to various drugs but who also had a history of mental problems, including several suicide attempts. Many hospitals were reluctant to accept patients with psychiatric conditions, but Raphael, working with the woman's mother, managed to find a detox in Brooklyn willing to take her. Certain that the woman would relapse once she left, he arranged to send her to Ellenville for a piggyback detox. While she was there, he reserved a bed at New Hope Manor, and, like Yvonne Hamilton before her, she was taken there by bus.

The Ellenville–New Hope connection became a common one for Hot Line as it contended with its many female clients. The combination of a quiet detox in a community hospital far from the city followed by an intimate, all-women's residential program seemed to work well with these hard-core women. Or so Hot Line assumed. For it was having a hard time getting information out of New Hope. In the months since Yvonne's arrival there, for instance, Marvin had sent her several letters asking about her progress but had received none in return. Yvonne's mother had spoken with her several times, but the conversations had been so brief, and Yvonne so close-mouthed, that she had been unable to glean much beyond the fact that her daughter was dutifully making her way through the program.

Then, one warm day in May 1993, Yvonne suddenly showed up at Hot Line. Marvin was struck by the change in her appearance. Instead of the hunted, frazzled look she had had a year earlier, she now seemed self-confident, even serene. In place of the smudged, ragged clothes she had worn then, she now had on a freshly laundered shirt and jeans. And, from her ample waistline, it was clear that she had been eating well. Puffing on a Newport, Yvonne apologized to Marvin for not answering his letters. The program, she explained, would not let residents write anyone outside their immediate family —one of many odd restrictions, she said, that the nuns at New Hope enforced.

IN FACT, Yvonne's year at New Hope had been full of both frustration and growth. Her experience there provides a look at why treatment works—and how it could do better. During her first few months away, Yvonne had felt like an inmate in a remote prison camp. New Hope was located in tiny Barryville, at the western end of the Catskill Mountains. Once known as the Borscht Belt, the Catskills had become a sort of Rehab Ridge as treatment programs— unable to obtain sites in New York City—bought up the roomy old resorts that had once catered to vacationing Jews. New Hope was in a former hunting and fishing lodge. Its four clapboard buildings included a schoolhouse crammed with books and computers, a crafts building full of hobby supplies, and a two-story dormitory with the type of dowdy furniture one might expect to find in the home of an aging aunt. There were also three greenhouses, a volleyball court, and a creek, all set on one hundred acres of meadows and woods.

Inside, however, the atmosphere was anything but vacationlike. Of New Hope's five counselors, three were nuns. Yvonne was assigned to Sister Pat Conway, a tight-lipped, gray-haired woman in her late forties whose no-frills wardrobe of pale shirts and dark pants added to her austere air. Like most residential programs, New Hope featured a ladderlike approach, with clients working their way from one rung to the next. Along with other recent arrivals, Yvonne was placed in Level I, a month-long orientation session. For six hours a day, the women met in the dining room to listen to Sister Pat discuss the rules and regulations of the program.

They were endless and arcane. Every day, residents were required to read the *New York Times*—except for Section B, which was prohibited (too much distracting metro news). Both the *Daily News* and the *Post* were strictly off- limits (too racy). At night, residents could watch television, but only CNN and history programs. At meals, residents were required to eat everything on their plate; once a month, they were allowed a soda. Phone privileges were limited to one five-minute call a week, and letters could be sent only to "positive" family members (after being vetted by the staff). Rule breakers were subject to strict penalties, called "restrictions," ranging from extra dish duty to enforced isolation.

Listening to all this, Yvonne could only sneer. For the last eight years, she had done nothing but break rules, and she had no intention of stopping now. Sitting through the orientation sessions, she would frequently interrupt Sister Pat with wisecracks and complaints. Despite her best efforts, though, she could not ruffle the nun. "I'm going to break you before you break me," Pat said after one outburst.

Things got no easier on Level II. Here residents were expected to master basic values like self-control, respect for others, and acceptance of authority. After rising at seven and eating breakfast, the women got an inspirational reading and a rundown of the day's news, followed by chores like bathroom cleanup. From nine until three (with a break for lunch) they were in school, taking classes in subjects like American history and computer programming. From three until four-thirty, they had recreation—itself highly organized— then an hour of "quiet time" devoted mostly to studying and reading. After dinner, the women were required to attend two or three hours' worth of study groups or group therapy. The rest of the night was given over to homework and writing assignments, with lights out at eleven-thirty.

Like every other client, Yvonne had trouble keeping up. Forced to sit through lengthy lectures, she developed excruciating back pains. Working her way through the endless writing exercises, she found her hands cramping up with fatigue. At night, she would collapse into bed, numb with exhaustion, only to be kept awake by her cravings for crack. During the day, she fought constantly with the counselors and shunned the other residents as beneath her. "Your attitude is *fundamentally* and *constantly* disrespectful," a counselor wrote on one of her papers.

Yvonne gave vent to her despair in a letter written to her mother in the early summer of 1992 (but not sent because it contained a reference to a nonfamily member):

> I am not having the best of times here. I don't like the place or the people, there are two [sic] many rules and two many you can't do this or that. I want to come home with a passion, but in reality it wouldn't be the best place for me now. . . . Just to think of the streets is very scary. . . . My dearest sweet mother I have done you so wrong thru the years. So many painful memories, I cry so many days and nights. . . . You stuck with me you have one hell of a love for me may you live and never die. . . . On the day I came here, I took $50 in food stamps from you, but I didn't enjoy the high at all. Sorry I took your stamps. . . .

Three months into her stay at New Hope, then, Yvonne's alienation seemed complete.

Yet, as the contrite tone of her letter suggests, the program was beginning to take hold. Gradually emerging from her crack fog, Yvonne was showing some tentative interest in her classes. As strict as the counselors were, most were good teachers. Each had at least a bachelor's degree, and, with five counselors for forty women, each resident was assured abundant attention. Attending lectures on subjects like self-esteem and ego gratification, Yvonne almost involuntarily found herself listening in.

The turning point came, oddly enough, after one of her most wrenching episodes. One August afternoon, while looking through a bookshelf in the main building, Yvonne came upon a volume called *Black Rage*. The title seemed to sum up her feelings about New Hope, and, eager to learn more, she began reading. While she was at it, however, Sister Pat passed by and, glancing at the title, told her that the book was off-limits. Scowling at her, Yvonne said that she had found the book on the shelf, so why couldn't she read it? She just couldn't, Sister Pat replied. Exploding, Yvonne began shouting profanities at the staff and the program and all the white people who ran it. She became so agitated that other staff members had to come help restrain her. As punishment, Yvonne was placed in isolation. For the next four days, she had to sit all day in a corner with a partition separating her from the rest of the residents, and she was barred from talking to anyone.

"Found a good book to read, Black Rage, but it was taken away from me," Yvonne confided in one of her assignments. "I thought I had the right to read any book of literature within the house, but it was not proven so. Why would you have books within my reach, and then snatch them away? I guess I must deal with life from the white man's point of view." She continued: "I am at a low point in my life, I find it scary. My urges are kicking up, but I don't have the strength to walk." Then, almost against her will, she added: "Class on self esteem really opened my eyes to a lot of things. I opened up and spoke a little more than I normally do."

Soon after, she went a step further. Every Wednesday afternoon, the residents were required to attend a lecture by Father Aquinas, the elderly director and patriarch of the center. For three or four hours, Aquinas—tall, gray, and ecclesiastical—would discuss some aspect of personal development, and the women were expected to sit quietly and take notes. Most dreaded the experience, and for months Yvonne had, too, shifting uncomfortably in her chair as the "Pope," as she called him, droned on. Gradually tuning in, however, Yvonne was impressed by his observations. How to control one's temper, how to rein in one's impulses, how to draw up an emotional balance sheet—these were tools she could use in her own life. After one session, Yvonne wrote, "I made a choice to stop alienating myself from others. Aquinas seminar on Problems and How to Prevent Them. A lot of girls find his seminars boring but to me I look forward to them." Not completely reformed, Yvonne could not help adding that the "pork chops at dinner could have been cooked a little longer." She also complained that "work is beginning to pile on—I don't have time to do too much reading."

Yet read she did. Residents were routinely assigned chunks from *Reader's Digest*, and Yvonne, who in the past had regarded them as chores, began devouring them. Reading the *Times* and *Newsweek*, she developed an interest in national and international affairs. For her psychology classes, she delved into Freud and Abraham Maslow, the father of self-actualizing psychology. And, while the endless writing assignments remained a burden, Yvonne began using them to explore her behavior. After another round of restrictions, Yvonne, writing in her neat, childlike script, described her conflicting emotions about New Hope:

> I find the girls here very negitive, which I try to avoid. . . . I accept my punishment of doing the dishes. . . . What I dislike is if your policy says avoid negitive people and conversations, what am I doing

in isolation? . . . I understand I am bullheaded. . . . The realness of
my dilima is I need the tools of this program. . . . With all honesty I
have grown a little to realize I owe the house an apology. . . . I apolo-
gize for my childish, rude behavior. . . . I am not out for revenge, I
have nothing up my sleeves, I honestly want to work my program.

In February 1993—more than eight months into her stay—Yvonne was
finally ready to acknowledge New Hope's hold on her. "Today," she wrote, "I
realize that New Hope Manor is my focal point, this program is playing a major
role within my life. I now value and respect all aspects of this program. I
choose no longer to be defiant."

In response, Yvonne was promoted to Level III. This brought many new
privileges, including the right to make additional phone calls and to go off the
premises two nights a month. But it also brought new duties. Yvonne became a
"coordinator," with responsibility for supervising other, less advanced residents.
Now, in addition to having to master the usual mix of classes, groups, homework, and writing assignments, she was expected to manage the activities of
dozens of other women, many of them as unruly as she had once been. From
seven in the morning until eleven at night, she had barely a moment to herself.
And, no matter how much she did, it was never enough.

In one writing exercise, Yvonne, asked to "make a searching and fearless
moral inventory" of herself, poured out a highly detailed and graphic account.
"I stole from the cash register at Pathmark," she wrote,

> stole a letter with $100 from a blind man. Stole three cars, stole
> clothing and jewelry from Bloomingdales, stole credit cards, stole my
> mother's wedding rings, wrote checks in her name forged on her
> bank accounts. Spent her rent money, robbed her home of televi-
> sions, radios, food, cameras, VCR, camcord, fur coats, asthma ma-
> chine, pills, stole my mother's clothing, stole her bible watch, stole
> my children's money from public assistance, forged Medicaid cards.
> I stole my father's $10,000 hidden in his drawer, his car, credit cards,
> I robbed his store countless times. . . . I slept with Jimmie for
> drugs, I slept with Lenora for her money, I slept with Gloria to have
> a place to stay. . . . I sometimes slept in my car, I wore clothing for
> days on end, I went off with strangers on out-of-state trips for drugs.
> I left my children with my mother and didn't return for days . . .

. . . and so on, for fourteen meticulously written pages. In response, Yvonne
received only a grudging "OK" scribbled at the top of her paper. It was typical
of the nuns' stinginess with praise, a quality that struck Yvonne as downright
unchristian.

As winter dragged on in the Catskills, the atmosphere at New Hope grew
increasingly cheerless. And, to make matters worse, the nuns were giving no

indication of when she might be able to leave. Then, as spring approached, she learned that her mother had suffered a heart attack. Frantic to learn more, she begged the nuns to let her call New York, but they refused. Disgusted, Yvonne announced her intention to leave. The counselors were not supportive. "I'll give you six months before you're back," Father Aquinas chided her. Yvonne was willing to take her chances, however, and in May 1993—thirteen months after her arrival at New Hope—she boarded a bus back to the city.

YVONNE'S EXPERIENCE at New Hope Manor faithfully mirrors the research on drug treatment. Over and over, studies have found that one variable, and only one, correlates with success in treatment. It's not a client's race, sex, or age, nor the type of drug or length of habit, but the amount of time spent in treatment. The longer the stay, the greater the benefits. In Yvonne's case, it took her three months simply to overcome her cravings for crack and start paying attention to the program. It took another three for the program's teachings to begin to sink in. By the end of her first year in treatment, Yvonne's entire outlook on life had changed.

"I have to hand it to them, they broke down a lot of my attitudes," she observed soon after her departure. "I went in there being a bullshit artist. I was very rebellious. They pushed me to do better. They said, 'Yvonne, you can become anything you want to. Stop shooting for the basement when you can shoot for the stars.' " Before treatment, she went on, "I had no sense of right and wrong. New Hope changed that. It taught you how to maintain your dignity and increase your self-esteem. I fought them, but I'll be eternally grateful to them."

Unfortunately, most of the residents at New Hope did not stay long enough to reap those benefits. About 40 percent left during the monthlong orientation phase and another 20 percent in the two months after that. Only a quarter or so made it to Level III.

The numbers are similar in most residential programs. With few exceptions, they have high dropout rates. Of course, given the hard-bitten nature of the population involved, some attrition is inevitable. Yet the programs themselves must bear some of the responsibility. At New Hope Manor, for instance, Yvonne felt the staff went out of its way to alienate residents. "As much as I liked New Hope, I felt they beat people down, telling them they're no good," she said. "A lot of the residents couldn't take it, especially the weaker ones. There's a way to demand respect without belittling people." The work schedule was a good example: "You had to work from seven to nine in the morning, attend school from nine to three, then work three to eleven, with an hour or hour and a half off to do homework. In between, they wanted me to assign people jobs. It was too much. And when I accomplished this, they didn't even offer praise. Even a dog needs that." For all its positive qualities, then, the program at New Hope at times seemed unnecessarily severe.

It's a problem common to many drug-treatment programs—one that's been present, in fact, since the very first one. Synanon practiced a strict form of behavior modification that attempted to break down an addict's personality through a regimen of confrontation and intimidation. The encounter groups at Synanon's core could be quite harrowing, with rule breakers subject to head shavings and other humiliating penalties. Eventually, Synanon collapsed under the weight of its own harshness. (In the late 1970s, it was investigated by the California attorney general's office for alleged complicity in more than a dozen assaults, including one involving a rattlesnake placed in the mailbox of a Los Angeles lawyer.) Nonetheless, the concept of using a small, self-contained community run by ex-addicts proved popular, and today there are hundreds of such therapeutic communities across the country.

To prevent a repeat of Synanon's excesses, TCs have eliminated some of its more draconian features. Clients who want to leave are allowed to do so, and head shavings have been transformed into verbal scalpings. Nonetheless, therapeutic communities continue to use Synanon's "tough love" approach. Encounter groups remain a central tool, and infractions are still punished with stringent "contracts." A recalcitrant resident might be required to rise at dawn to clean bathroom floors with a toothbrush, or to pick up garbage thrown on the floor by a counselor.

Such rigor can be effective with hard-core users, especially those caught up in the criminal justice system. In New York, for instance, nonviolent drug offenders are frequently mandated to therapeutic communities as an alternative to incarceration. Since these offenders face going to prison if they bolt, they tend to stay for long periods, and many benefit as a result. By contrast, voluntary enrollees—facing no such sanction—are usually much less willing to stick around. On the street, in fact, therapeutic communities are so feared and disdained that many addicts would never dream of entering one. Even many criminal offenders, faced with choosing between a therapeutic community or prison, select the latter.

"I'll never forget the first defendant who asked for that," said Rhonda Ferdinand, the head of alternative sentencing for the special narcotics prosecutor in Manhattan. "He was very polite. He called and said, 'I'm very sorry, you spent all this time trying to arrange this program for me, but in jail I don't have to get up at five-thirty every morning. I can watch TV and play basketball there. I can't do that in a TC.' I almost fell out of my chair." Ferdinand, who has seen many drug offenders thrive in therapeutic communities, admires them, but, she observes, TCs "are very tough. I couldn't make it in one."

Even within TCs, there is a growing tide of criticism. "TCs are hostile and barbaric," noted Dr. Stephan Sorrell, a 1983 graduate of Daytop Village who went on to sit on its board of directors. "TCs work on humiliation. They are too long. They're homophobic. And they're prejudiced against blacks and Hispanics." Sorrell expressed particular concern about the quality of the counselors in TCs. "They should have more training," he said. "And they need to be better supervised. It's unheard of for a counselor to be called into a meeting and asked about what he's doing with a patient to effect change." Therapeutic communities, Sorrell added, "are very good for people who are unemployed and homeless—people who have long histories of drug addiction and criminality. If you go to a TC, they give you meals and a place to live." For others, he said, the programs could do much better.

Women have an especially hard time in therapeutic communities. Most are dominated by men, which helps to explain the stress they place on intimidation. Recognizing this, some programs have attempted to soften their approach. "Modified TCs," they're called. And New Hope Manor is one. "Most programs are heavily confrontational, and that's difficult for women to handle," Father Aquinas said in his office at New Hope amid piles of newspapers, magazines, and books. A towering, square-jawed man with a low, deep voice that exuded authority, he said, "We have some level of confrontation, but mostly we're into motivational counseling, which tries to get the women to draw up their own plan of action and otherwise get them motivated." That, he added, was why New Hope placed so much emphasis on education and writing, and why it required counselors to have at least a college degree.

Still, New Hope retained many TC features. The heavy workload, the many sanctions, the endless lectures, the rigid rules—all seemed designed to make people drop out. If New Hope, and other residential programs, were to show less toughness and more love, they would undoubtedly retain more clients. As Yvonne succinctly put it, "If you treat people nice, they'll respond that way."

BACK IN SPANISH HARLEM, Yvonne felt oddly disoriented. On the one hand, 110th Street seemed as downtrodden as ever. The blowsy crowds of hustlers and dope fiends were still out, and Yvonne could barely take a step without running into an old crony. She struggled to be polite, but she could not suppress the stirrings of contempt in her stomach. For, if the neighborhood had not changed, Yvonne certainly had, and what before had seemed all energy and excitement now seemed only degradation and despair, and the realization that she had once been part of it made her shudder.

To keep out of trouble, Yvonne, who was staying at her mother's apartment, had taken to attending services at a Pentecostal church on 111th Street. A pale-beige brick on the outside, Greater Highway to Heaven seemed afire within. From the walls to the carpet to the robes of the women jammed into the front pew, everything in the boxy sanctuary seemed to glow cardinal red. Taking a seat in the third row, Yvonne watched intently as the all-black congregation rocked through the service, belting out hymns, shouting praise for the Lord, twisting frenziedly in the aisles. Only rarely did Yvonne herself join in. Recalling how she used to laugh at her mother's church-going, she remained self-conscious about such overt displays of faith. Nonetheless, the Lord's presence seemed palpable in the church, and she took great comfort in it. "I have an opportunity to start up life again, with new people," she observed brightly.

Still, she felt unsettled. Going to Metropolitan Hospital to see her mother, Yvonne was shocked at how shrunken and shriveled she looked. Talking with her daughter, Nancy expressed pleasure at the evident progress she had made. Nonetheless, she warned her against getting too comfortable in her apartment; the memories of Yvonne's tantrums remained too fresh. Yvonne got a further dose of reality upon seeing her kids. Both had been taken in by young women who had relatives living at Clinton, and while Nancy Lee seemed to be thriving, Gerald, now in elementary school, was causing all kinds of havoc—the result, Yvonne felt sure, of her neglectful behavior. Yvonne desperately wanted her kids back but knew that she would first have to find a way to support them. And, despite her soaring self-esteem, she felt she was not quite up to the task. Father Aquinas had been right—she did need more treatment.

And so, late on a Friday afternoon, she had returned to Hot Line. There she told Marvin of her desire for another residential program, adding, however, that she did not want to go too far away because of her mother's condition.

"What about a program in the city?" said Raphael, who had been listening in. Looking even more frazzled than usual, Raphael had spent most of the morning trying to find a detox bed for an elderly Puerto Rican man with a drinking problem; coming up empty, he had told him to return on Monday. Then, in the early afternoon, a hospital in Westchester had called to say that a bed had opened up—did Hot Line have anyone to fill it? Recalling that the Puerto Rican had told him where he liked to hang out, Raphael dashed out of the building to look for him. A half-hour later he returned, the man in tow. "I found him in the park on a bench," Raphael said, out of breath. "He even had his bag with him. It was an act of God."

After finding a volunteer to take the man to the hospital, Raphael, still giddy from his triumph, turned his attention to Yvonne. Hearing her describe the progress she had made at New Hope, he said that perhaps it was time to test herself in the city. And he had just the place: the Salvation Army. Though known mostly for its thrift shops and Christmas appeals, the Army was in fact the nation's largest provider of drug and alcohol treatment, operating 112 adult rehabilitation centers (ARCs) throughout the United States. One of them was located on West 48th Street in Manhattan. As a religious institution, the Salvation Army offered Christian instruction along with its therapy, Raphael explained. With her newfound sense of spirituality, Yvonne approved. She was further encouraged to learn that the ARC was not a therapeutic community. Instead of contracts and encounter groups, it offered "work therapy," in which clients literally worked their way toward recovery. At the mention of work, Yvonne perked up, and Raphael, phoning the center, arranged an interview for the following week.

Located in an aging seven-story building in a bleak industrial section of Hell's Kitchen, the ARC on the outside looked like a throwback to the industrial revolution; inside, though, it was bright and clean if somewhat spartan. During her interview, Yvonne attested to her interest in the Bible and to her regular attendance at church. She also showed that she was able-bodied and ready to work. For her part, Yvonne, having thrived in the all-women environment of New Hope, was troubled by the center's gender ratio—120 men to 12 women. Once again, women seemed to get the short end. On the other hand, the women had an entire floor to themselves, and, unlike the men's quarters, it was air-conditioned. Checking out the rest of the facility—the cheerful chapel, the comfortable cafeteria, the spacious meeting rooms—Yvonne pronounced the place up to her standard, and in mid-June 1993 she moved in.

While not as strict as New Hope, the ARC unfortunately had some problems of its own. Like most new arrivals, Yvonne was put to work in the Sally's clothing warehouse, located two blocks south, on 46th Street. All clothing donations made to the Salvation Army in Manhattan were trucked here to be sorted before being sent back to the thrift shops for sale. After being unloaded from the trucks, the clothes were sent upstairs to an open area filled with tables and bins. Together with scores of other residents, Yvonne spent eight hours a day sorting shirts, pants, and coats. For someone like Yvonne, who had already spent months in treatment, the work, while tedious, was not particularly strenuous, and the days passed quickly.

Not so for more recent addicts. Many of them—fresh from binging on crack—were overcome by cravings for the drug. The simple sound of a lighter being flicked or a cigarette being inhaled could trigger an overpowering desire for crack. As a further handicap, many new arrivals had not worked in years and so had limited stamina. Yet, from the day of their arrival at the ARC, they were required to put in eight hours a day, five days a week. And the pay—$5 a week—seemed a joke. "People work forty hours a week, and they can't even afford a pack of cigarettes," Yvonne complained at the end of one work day. "They feel taken advantage of."

The lack of counseling made matters worse. In contrast to New Hope Manor, with its high counselor-to-resident ratio, the ARC had but three counselors to serve its much larger clientele. Overwhelmed by cases, counselors were barely able to remember their clients' names, let alone their histories. Moreover, the counselors tended to be ex-alcoholics with little clue as to what heroin and crack users were going through. Frightened and frustrated, many of those users sought out Yvonne, who became a sort of impromptu counselor. "I'm working with people who are having dreams about crack in which they can actually *taste* the drug," she said wearily. "I tell them that it's normal to have these feelings and that the cravings will pass. The Army's not doing any of this. Their counselors are outdated."

For all that, Yvonne felt she was benefiting from the program. The sleeping quarters at the ARC were comfortable and the food nourishing. While putting in her eight hours of work and attending the mandatory classes on the New Testament, Yvonne was quietly pursuing her own course of study based on the techniques she'd learned at New Hope. She assigned herself frequent writing exercises, did her own Bible readings, and perused the newspaper. Strolling down Tenth Avenue, a seedy strip of tenements, bodegas, and carry-out restaurants, Yvonne would frequently pass crack dealers, but they simply strengthened her resolve. Accosted by a peddler one night, she said mockingly, "You expect me to walk around looking like you—a space cadet?"

Yvonne's greatest test, however, came over the summer, when her mother passed away. Yvonne had come to regard Nancy as her best friend, and her pain at her death was deepened by the knowledge that she had probably hastened it. A loss of this sort has pushed many a recovering addict over the edge, but Yvonne drew on the reserves she'd developed at New Hope, and a few weeks after the funeral she joined her sister Joyce at Apartment 4H to sort through their mother's belongings. With its smudged walls, battered doors, and kitchen ceiling speckled with grease, the apartment seemed a glum memorial to all the emotional travails Nancy's family had endured over the past three decades. "When my mother moved in here, this place was so beautiful," Joyce fumed as she inspected the apartment. "I couldn't wait to get off work to come here. I'd rush here to have a meal. My mother was such a good cook. And now look at it!" Examining a still-gleaming washing machine in the kitchen, she hollered, "I gave this to Mother, and it didn't even last a year! Nothing that I gave my mother is here. Everything is either broken or gone." Yvonne, who was wearing a T-shirt stamped THERE'S A BRAND NEW ME INSIDE, looked sheepish.

Despite the tension between them, the two sisters managed to spend several hours sifting through piles of clothes, photos, toys, and family memen-tos, sorting out the keepsakes and putting the rest in brown garbage bags, which were then carried out to the street. After finishing, they decided to reward themselves by getting a bite on Third Avenue. As they passed the C-Town supermarket on 110th Street, Joyce glanced at the meager items a homeless man had spread out on the sidewalk. "Look, there's mother's sugar pot!" she said, pointing in disbelief, and the two sisters shared a melancholy laugh at how fast the junkies of 110th Street worked.

They would share much more that summer. For Joyce could sense the changes coming over her sister, and, eager to encourage them, invited her to dinner several times at her home in the Bronx. Reminiscing over various family exploits, the sisters comforted one another over their mutual loss. One Sunday morning in August, Joyce, in a further show of support, attended the chapel service at the ARC. After the psalms were sung and the thirty-day sobriety cards handed out, the floor was opened to visitors, and the normally reticent Joyce stood up. "I have so much to give thanks for," she said, her voice trembling. "I speak for my mother. We lost her a little while ago. And she would be so happy with my sister Yvonne. I'm *so* proud of her." When the collection plate was passed, Yvonne, dropping a dollar bill into it, whispered to her sister, "They say you get double what you put in." Joyce took out a five and placed it on the plate, then took Yvonne's hand and squeezed it.

Eventually, Yvonne's progress became evident to the ARC as well, and she was assigned to work in the director's office. The center was managed by a team of husband-and-wife "majors" (the Salvation Army uses military ranks), and Yvonne became the wife's administrative assistant. Though pleased with the promotion, she was rankled by her pay—now all of $12.50 a week. "I'm so sick of being broke," she complained soon after starting the new position. "I can't even afford deodorant." The two majors, who had previously run an adult rehabilitation center in Cleveland, seemed forever flustered at the pace of life in the Big Apple, and much of Yvonne's job consisted of calming her boss down. Yvonne was so good at it that the woman kept saddling her with new tasks, such as walking her dog Fluffy.

From her perch in the front office, Yvonne got a close look at how the ARC was run, and the more she saw, the less she liked. Every Wednesday, the staff met to decide which residents to eject from the facility. Every week, two or three people were singled out, and while some were clearly deserving, others were seemingly booted solely for not being productive enough. "The Salvation Army has good intentions, but they have lost their focus," she observed. "It's a business. If you can't produce, they have no use for you. There's not genuine concern for people."

Yvonne's assessment is disputed by Captain John Cheydleur, director of all adult rehabilitation centers in the eastern United States. "People in their first month of recovery are pretty fuzzy," he noted. "If we got rid of all the residents and hired a few part-time housewives, we could raise a lot more money in one of these centers. For a guy in a ninety-day program, we put about ten thousand dollars into him in supervision and get about two thousand dollars back in labor." Even Cheydleur, however, acknowledged that the level of counseling in the ARCs was not always what it should be. "There's supposed to be one counselor for every fifteen men and one for every twelve women, but there are times when some of the centers are more shallow than I'd like," he said. "That's budget-dictated." When it came to work therapy, then, the Salvation Army seemed more interested in work than therapy. And, as a result, it suffered from the same high dropout rates as other residential programs.

As 1993 was nearing an end, so was Yvonne's patience. Her boss was dumping so many niggling chores on her that she was devising elaborate schemes to avoid her. And she was so low on cash that she was unable to buy her kids Christmas gifts. Having gotten her six-month sobriety card in November, Yvonne was focusing her energy on finding a job. The Salvation Army was not much help in this, offering little more than a "transition group" that coached residents in writing résumés and preparing for interviews. Worse, residents wanting to look for work could take off only one day a month to do so. "The Army has no program to get people jobs," Yvonne said with disgust. "It just wants you to work for free." Fortunately, Joyce invited her to come stay with her in the Bronx until she could get her feet on the ground. And so, in mid-January 1994, Yvonne, full of anticipation and trepidation, notified the ARC of her intention to leave in two weeks. Her posttreatment life was about to begin.

FOR RAPHAEL FLORES, who had done so much to get Yvonne to that point, things were not going so well. The campaign to save Hot Line Cares was foundering. Hardly a day went by that Raphael didn't call at least one potential funder, but he usually came up empty. Personally, he was faring no better. Over the summer, he received his final eviction notice, and city inspectors came to board up his front door. They did leave a window open, however, and Raphael, sneaking in through the fire escape, would stay there at night. Soon after, however, Con Edison turned off his electricity, and so, after more than twenty years in the same cramped apartment, Raphael finally had to leave it. Fortunately, his mother, who lived in a modest apartment in the Bronx, agreed to take him in for a while.

The loss of his apartment was a real blow, however, and Raphael, straggling into the office at ten or eleven in the morning, his face unshaven and his eyes bloodshot, seemed strangely disoriented. He also seemed obsessed with money. With his daughter's wedding set for September 1993, Raphael, now resigned to the event, desperately wanted to help out, but his penurious state precluded it. Loudly lamenting his inability to be a good father, he was spending hours on the phone, hitting up everyone he could think of for cash. Once, the staff heard complaints that Raphael had solicited bus fare from a client's family to send him upstate, then changed his mind and referred him locally—without, however, returning the money.

Well aware of his own deteriorating condition, Raphael enlisted the help of a former Hot Line employee named Martina Coriano. A slender twenty-five-year-old with long brown hair and intense dark eyes, Martina was well acquainted with Spanish Harlem's drug problem. She had been raised on 110th Street, by a pharmacist father and a junkie mother, and might well have followed in her mother's footsteps had she not gone to work at Hot Line as a teen volunteer and come under Raphael's wing. Sensing her promise, Hot Line had arranged for her to attend a private high school on a scholarship; she went on to college and to the Columbia School of Social Work, where she earned a master's degree. After graduating, Martina—hearing of Hot Line's plight—had volunteered to help out around the office, and Raphael, seeing her ability to work with the staff, agreed to let her handle all administrative matters while he tended to clients.

As in the past, however, Raphael found it hard to give up control, and in August 1993, the staff, tiring of his outbursts, met in Hot Line's back room to discuss what to do. "We're getting so much stress from Ralph," said Marvin, using Raphael's familiar name. "We have to deal not only with clients but with Ralph's problems. Unless things change, this will be the last year I'm here. Ralph helped me in the past, so I feel some commitment. But you get to a point. . . ." He was so worked up that he couldn't continue. Ethel said that at times she got so angry that she worried she might "go get a bottle. It's hurting Ralph that he can't provide for his daughter's wedding, but we've got to tell him that he's got to get his own head on straight if he wants to keep working here." At the end of the meeting, it was decided to confront Raphael with an ultimatum on ceding control to Martina.

While the meeting was taking place, Raphael was out on the street, talking with a Mexican who'd arrived in the city only three days earlier. "There are so many Mexicans coming in, and I don't know how to work on their situations," he observed back in the office. Seeing Ethel emerge from the meeting, Raphael asked if she knew anything about helping immigrants. "Damn, we can barely help people who have no ID," she snapped. "Now you want to help somebody who's just arrived here?"

"So the answer is no, I assume," he responded coolly. "You don't know how to help him. That's all I want to know."

When the staff told Raphael that Martina had to take over, he did not resist. Trying, instead, to take his mind off the impending transfer, he threw himself into his client work with ever more abandon, often working two phones at a time while tending to the never-ending flow of walk-ins.

A surprising number of those walk-ins were coming from Apartment 17E. Seeing the progress Yvonne had made, regulars from the drug den were coming by to inquire about Hot Line's services. One day, it was a heroin-injecting woman in her forties who worked at a psychiatric hospital in Rockland County. She had private health insurance, so Raphael was able to place her in a thirty-day rehab. Next, a young crack user who supported his habit by begging on the subway came by looking for a detox bed; Raphael found him one at Metropolitan Hospital. A few days later, a middle-aged man who used to smoke crack with Yvonne stopped by for a detox. When Raphael raised the idea of a long-term program, the man balked. Discovering that he had kids, Raphael took him into the back room and, talking father to father, impressed him with how much it would mean to his children if he got clean. Ten minutes later, the two men reemerged, both of them teary. "He's agreed to go away to Syracuse," Raphael announced, choked up.

Even in a drug den, it seemed, there was latent interest in treatment. By offering trust and quick service, Hot Line was able to bring it to the surface. Had Raphael been able to keep at it, he might have managed to put a real dent in the business in 17E. But his own problems kept getting in the way.

Martina, who had worked closely with Raphael in the 1980s, was struck by the changes she saw in him. "Back then, he would never curse in front of young people, or say things to the staff in front of clients," she said, struggling to control herself. "Now, he's disrupting volunteers and employees, and he's not following up on the things he said he would. Even his appearance has gotten worse. He's not taking care of himself. He's at the point where he doesn't trust anybody. He thinks everyone's out to get him." She was particularly upset over Raphael's preoccupation with money. "So many people have told me that Ralph was asking them for money," she said. "They're asking, 'Is he on drugs?' "

Marvin was asking the same question. "When I first came here," he said, "I saw Ralph as a sort of big brother, a role model. But two years ago, things started changing. He would tell little lies, like he was going to Philadelphia with a client and would be back at such and such a time, then not show up. And he'd have such mood swings, snapping at me and Ethel." As for Raphael's attitudes toward money, Marvin said, "He'd ask people for donations. But we're supposed to be a nonprofit organization."

For Marvin, the moment of truth came at the end of the summer, when he took a weekend off to visit some friends. While he was away, Raphael, wanting to give his mother a break, stayed in Hot Line's back room. When Marvin returned and went into the room, he saw a strange-looking object on his cot. Examining it more closely, he saw to his shock that it was a crack pipe. Quickly searching the room, he found two lighters of the type favored by crack smokers. At long last, Marvin felt, he had found the cause of Raphael's erratic behavior.

Jerry Frohnhoefer, a college teacher in Manhattan who had worked at Hot Line Cares in the 1980s and stayed on as an adviser, said he had seen Raphael undergo a steady decline since the late 1980s, when crack caused Hot Line's caseload to soar. "Raphael became overextended," Frohnhoefer recalled. "His temper got short. He got upset with volunteers. He burned bridges to funders. He became quasi-suicidal." Along the way, he added, "he started dipping and dabbling in drugs. He might have been using pot and hash— maybe even crack. We confronted him on it a number of times."

While at the rehab in Arizona, Frohnhoefer said, Raphael had sought to "face up" to his substance abuse. On his return, however, his therapist put him on a potent stew of medications, including Prozac and Halcion (a strong sleeping pill). "He got overloaded on that," Frohnhoefer said. "And he was drinking pretty heavily." By 1993, he added, Raphael had "begun to understand that Hot Line was eating up his life. His daughter had grown up and he regretted the years he had missed being with her. He felt bad that he had nothing to offer her, that he couldn't help pay for her wedding. He felt guilty, depressed, and angry at himself." And, despite his best efforts, he continued to use intoxicants. "It was a back-and-forth struggle," Frohnhoefer said. "And he never got a handle on it."

The subject was not one Raphael himself liked to discuss. One afternoon, while hunched over a plate of rice and beans in a three-table *lonchería* in Spanish Harlem, he was asked if he was using drugs. He admitted to taking large doses of sleeping pills for his insomnia, which, he acknowledged, sometimes caused him to behave erratically. When pressed about reports that he was using street drugs, Raphael exploded. "I'm not going to respond to that!" he shouted, his fleshy face reddening. "I'll never, never address rumors! For years I've been dealing with rumors. I have no tolerance for that."

By the fall, Raphael's presence at Hot Line had become so disruptive that he was informed that he was no longer welcome there, and on October 1, 1993, Martina officially took over as director. With Raphael out of the picture, the gloom in the office immediately lifted, and Martina set about developing a recovery plan. To survive, she believed, Hot Line had to redefine its mission. If it continued to serve mainly as a drug referral center, she felt, it wouldn't be able to make it; addicts were simply too tough a sell. Instead, she wanted Hot Line to return to its glory days, when it served as a drop-in center for young people. For that the funding potential was great.

As for Raphael, even his mother was losing patience with him. With him one step from the street, Jerry Frohnhoefer, making some inquiries on his behalf, found out about a residence for homeless veterans that had recently opened on East 119th Street. Raphael sneered at the idea of living in such a place—an SRO (single room occupancy), he called it—but, with few remaining options, he agreed to check it out. To his surprise, it was clean and comfortable, with a brightly painted cinder-block lobby that seemed right out of a college dorm. A room became available in late December, and soon after Raphael moved in.

The room was barely large enough to accommodate a bed, desk, and chair, but, with his radio and Bible to keep him company, Raphael quickly settled in. On the wall over his desk, he arranged several photos of his daughter, most from when she was a toddler. Seeking spiritual guidance, he pored over the book of Revelation and Harold Camping's latest book, *Are You Ready?* As much as he tried, he could not poke any holes in Camping's dark vision for 1994. Sitting in his cubicle, inspecting his daughter's pictures and pondering the coming apocalypse, Raphael dolefully asked, "Is this where I end up, given everything that's happened? Does God want me here, in an SRO?"

18

The Mayor

THE SAME WEEK Raphael moved into the veterans residence, Rudolph Giuliani became mayor of New York. During the campaign, Giuliani had repeatedly referred to the corrosive effect drugs were having on the city. "If there's one problem, and only one, that you had to say is harming the city the most—the one problem that's made us most depressed about our future, that's robbing us of a generation of children—it's the problem of illegal drugs," Giuliani told a cheering crowd at the Sheraton New York Hotel in October 1993. That problem had gotten much worse in the previous four years, he said, and the reason was clear: a "deliberate policy" by the Dinkins Administration of "not arresting street-level dealers." Summing up his own philosophy, the former prosecutor said that "there should be no group of drug dealers—at the highest or lowest levels—that should believe it has immunity from being prosecuted, arrested, and sent to prison. Our message to buyers and dealers alike will be, 'We can't catch all of you, but we will begin to catch most of you, and you will go to prison.' "

During David Dinkins's four years in office, the number of drug arrests in the city had indeed fallen. And, as Giuliani had noted, that had been by design, for neither Dinkins nor his police commissioner, Lee Brown, had believed in the utility of mass drug arrests. Unfortunately, Dinkins had at the same time done little to address the demand for drugs in the city. During his term, the city had created about 10,000 new treatment slots—far more than under Ed Koch, but still only a fraction of the need. In a sense, New York under Dinkins had had the worst of both worlds—a falloff in enforcement with little expansion in treatment. The result was a boom in the city's open-air drug markets.

Now Giuliani was intent on crushing those markets. To help bring that about, he turned to his new police commissioner. At forty-six, William Bratton was charismatic, flamboyant, unashamedly ambitious, and supremely self-confident. Interviewed by Giuliani during the campaign, Bratton had impressed him with his sharp analysis of the NYPD. The department, he argued, had become too flaccid, too restrained, too top-heavy. Above all, he said, it had become too soft on crime.

Bratton was a proponent of the "broken windows" school of policing. Inspired by a 1982 *Atlantic Monthly* article by James Q. Wilson and George Kelling, this school maintained that seemingly minor acts like prostitution and public drunkenness fostered a climate of disorder in which more serious crimes could flourish. "If a window in a building is broken *and is left unrepaired,*" Wilson and Kelling wrote, "all the rest of the windows will soon be broken." By paying more attention to smaller violators like panhandlers and drunks, they asserted, the police could reduce serious offenses like muggings and robberies.

In their article, Wilson and Kelling did not say much about drugs, but their theory clearly applied to it. In cities like New York, few conditions promoted a sense of disorder more than street-level drug dealing. To design a remedy, Bratton enlisted two of his top aides. John Timoney, the department's second-in-command, was a trim, voluble, gung-ho native of Ireland who had spent twenty-five years on the force, five of them in Narcotics; highly respected by beat cops, he was widely viewed as a potential commissioner himself. Jack Maple, Bratton's top crime-control strategist, was a rotund, Runyonesque figure who wore a homburg, bow ties, and two-toned shoes; a walking compendium of crime stats, he prided himself on his understanding of the criminal mind, and he relished an opportunity to take on the city's dealers.

As a first step, Timoney and Maple sat down to assess how the department had been fighting those dealers in the past. What they found seemed worthy of the Keystone Kops. The department's tactical narcotics teams (TNTs) had basically adopted bankers' hours, limiting their raids to the time between 9 A.M. and 6 P.M., Monday to Friday. The dealers had quickly caught on and set their own hours accordingly. In addition, TNT officials often held advance meetings with neighborhood residents to publicize their operations, and the dealers, themselves sitting in, would learn what to expect. To make matters worse, cops at the precinct level had essentially been barred from making drug arrests. The reason was fear of corruption, but the result was blatant dealing in front of cops, which paradoxically fed the impression that the police were on the take.

Furthermore, under the community policing regimen introduced by Lee Brown, the police were attending too many meetings. There were meetings with tenant groups and community groups, business groups and school groups. There were so many meetings that the police had little time left for the dealers themselves. The Drugbusters program, meanwhile, was a complete fiasco, with so few volunteers signing up that cops had to pad the lists.

"People don't want to be the eyes and ears of the cops," said John Timoney, describing the department's thinking in those early days under Bratton. A ruddy, restless man who spoke in excited bursts of brogue, Timoney said, "I don't want to help the sanitation people pick up the garbage. It's the cops' job to fight crime. Community policing said that the cops can't do it alone. Our answer was, 'Yes, they can.'" The only meetings cops should be attending, Timoney said, were "meetings of criminals."

Politically, the department could not simply jettison community policing; in Washington, President Clinton was extolling it, and the public liked the idea of cops talking to kids. At One Police Plaza, though, use of the term was forbidden. While continuing to walk the beat, cops were going to drop all pretense of reaching out to the community. Instead, they were going to earn their money the old-fashioned way—by arresting dealers. And, to do that, the department was going to rely not just on undercover cops but on precinct ones as well. Each precinct was to set up street narcotics enforcement units (SNEUs), teams of cops assigned to observe drug deals and arrest those involved. And those arrests were not going to be limited to a particular time of day; the cops, like the dealers, were going to operate around the clock. Moreover, the police were going to hit buyers as well as sellers, not to mention smoke shops, head shops, nightclubs, and any other establishment that sold drugs or paraphernalia. In all, the police calculated, there were 12,526 sites in the city where drugs were sold, and the goal was to shut them all down. "The policy of the New York Police Department will be one of No Tolerance for drug sellers and buyers," the department declared in a strategy paper titled "Driving Drug Dealers Out of New York." The police's ability to quash the city's drug trade was going to get its clearest test yet.

WATCHING ALL THIS UNFOLD at the 23rd Precinct, Sergeant Steve Ringe was wary. On the one hand, he had voted for Giuliani and liked his new police commissioner. Bill Bratton had a quality that officers everywhere looked for in a police chief: he was procop. But, hearing the tough pronouncements coming out of headquarters, Ringe was worried about the future of his beloved community policing.

Deep down, though, he had to admit that the Sunshine Project was not going very well. The operation had continued throughout 1993 and into 1994, with the police making about a hundred arrests a month in the six-block target zone. With the dealers moving around the corner, from 110th Street to Lexington, the police had shifted their attention accordingly. After they began hitting Lexington, however, the dealers had moved once again, this time to Park, one block to the west, and the normally tranquil sidewalk in front of Clinton Building Number One had become a teeming, grasping bazaar. At the January 27, 1994, meeting of the Sunshine Project, held at the Clinton community center, the handful of community residents in attendance had complained bitterly about the situation. "From eleven in the morning until one-thirty in the afternoon, there are so many sellers and buyers that you have to push your way through them," a Clinton tenant said. "You have to ask, 'Can I get through, please?' "

In response, Sergeant Ringe said that the police had done all they could. "We have come to the end of the law-enforcement phase of the project," he declared. "When we started, we said that flooding the area with police officers would cause displacement of the dealers. That has happened. Now that we've made a vacuum in the area, we have to revitalize the neighborhood. We need input from merchants, residents, and city agencies. We have to make the area more presentable for people coming into it." Unfortunately, he said, attendance by local residents had remained sparse. He hoped to see a change at the next meeting.

There would not be another meeting, however. For, with community policing dead, the Sunshine Project was, too. "They want the police to make more arrests and do less social-service-type work," Ringe glumly noted in his office in February 1994. On 110th Street, of course, the police *had* been making plenty of arrests. Under the new regime, however, they were going to make even more. Rather than rely on undercover cops from the Narcotics Division, Ringe was now expected to set up his own street narcotics enforcement units. In them, cops from the precinct, working in plainclothes, would stand on rooftops with field glasses or sit in unmarked cars, trying to catch dealers in the act. Once they did, they would communicate via walkie-talkie with the "catch team" (usually two uniformed officers), who would rush in to make the collar. By the spring of 1994, Ringe was deploying SNEUs on a near-daily basis, and the number of drug arrests in the area around 110th Street soared.

Meanwhile, Bratton's efforts to streamline the NYPD were taking hold. A teleconferencing system was installed in each precinct, allowing arresting officers to discuss their cases with prosecutors on a video monitor rather than having to make the trip to Central Booking; thus freed, cops were able to spend more time on the street. An on-line warrants system was set up, allowing officers to check if the recipient of a summons had any outstanding warrants; if he did, he would be immediately booked rather than released, as in the past. In addition, each precinct was outfitted with new computers into which arrests and complaints could be logged, allowing commanding officers to see new crime patterns at a glance. Once a week, every precinct commander had to attend meetings at One Police Plaza to be questioned by senior officers. These "Compstat" sessions, as they were called (after "Computer Statistics"), could be quite cruel, with officers mercilessly grilled about crime trends in their area, but the precincts were becoming more accountable as a result, and, whenever the Two-Three came in for criticism, line officers like Steve Ringe would hear about it.

For Ringe, the new accountability meant more work, but he didn't mind, for that work was becoming more interesting. Under the old regime, he had had to spend hours every day writing up complaints and filling out beat books. Now, with paperwork being reduced, he was able to spend more time on the street, participating in SNEUs, raiding buildings, making collars. And, by late May 1994, Ringe had been won over to the new approach. "With community policing, you often felt you were just filling out papers," he observed. Bratton, he said, "is very results-oriented. We're learning how to do cases instead of just avoiding getting sued. I see more effectiveness. And morale is definitely changing for the better."

Initially, the impact of all this was hard to see. Patrolling 110th Street, Ringe saw pretty much what he had under Sunshine: displacement. While 110th and Lex remained quiet, the dealers were continuing to fan out, to Third, Park, and Madison. But the precinct was not letting up. When a drug gang was taken out, the police, rather than wait for local residents to step in, were continuing to pound its turf. To prune the foot traffic in the area, officers were slapping beer drinkers with summonses and pressing loiterers to move on.

And, as 1995 began, Ringe noticed a change. The hordes of customers that for so long had streamed out of the subway were beginning to thin out. The derelicts and hustlers who normally lingered about the intersection—tired of being hounded—were taking their loitering elsewhere, and the steps in front of the Clinton community center—long a rest stop for junkies—were suddenly clear. Most impressive of all, the dealers themselves appeared to be scattering. Walking up and down Lexington, crossing 110th from Third to Park, Ringe was struck by how much scarcer they seemed.

Of course, the sales volume on 110th Street always dipped during cold weather. Yet, even as the temperatures rose, the level of activity did not. On a given afternoon, there would usually be a few hustlers hanging out on the corner and a junkie or two selling boosted items in front of the supermarket, but the sidewalks no longer teemed with layabouts, and discarded syringes were harder to find. "We're having a real effect," Ringe said with satisfaction in his office on a steamy afternoon in August 1995. "There's been a definite change on 110th Street." And the reason, he said, was simple: "We're rounding up more people than ever." And, Ringe felt sure, the attack on the drug trade was contributing to the drop in crime that was taking place in Spanish Harlem, as in the rest of the city.

It was a heady time to be a New York cop. THE END OF CRIME AS WE KNOW IT, *New York* magazine declared on its cover, atop a photo of a strutting Giuliani and Bratton. TV shows like *NYPD Blue* were touting the exploits of New York's finest, and twiggy young women in the city were wearing NYPD T-shirts as a fashion statement. Ringe himself was sporting new designer glasses—a bit of flair in keeping with the department's new cool. "They've changed the whole way the department treats crime," said Ringe, who rarely mentioned the community anymore. "Before, there was tolerance of crime. Now, we're being much more aggressive."

THE JUNKIES on 110th Street readily acknowledged the effect of that new aggressiveness. "There used to be people selling from here to there," said Luisa, indicating the largely deserted stretch of 110th Street between Lexington and Park. She was wearing the same bright-red nail polish and lipstick she had when encountered two years earlier (see Chapter 5), but her drawn face showed the toll her drug use had taken. Back then, Luisa said, it rarely took her more than five minutes to cop; now, it could take up to an hour. "There's so much paranoia out here," she said. "If a person sells something, they're taking a very big risk." While talking, she was nervously scanning the street, looking for a familiar face. "Oh my God," she exclaimed, looking at her watch, "it's five to three. It's getting late." And with that she scurried off toward 109th Street, hoping to find a connection.

Even when addicts were able to find dope, its quality was often poor. "I feel like not copping because of all the shit around here," moaned Bettina, a pallid twenty-five-year-old woman. "When I first began coming around here, it was like a *marqueta*"—a market. "Now it's much harder to cop. Last week it took me three hours. You had to know somebody who took you to somebody else." Conditions were not much better elsewhere. "I went to 138th and Brookhaven in the South Bronx, and Avenue D on the Lower East Side—it's dead all over the place."

As Bettina's comments suggested, the trough in New York's drug trade was not limited to Spanish Harlem. Citywide, the NYPD in 1995 made 78,977 cocaine and heroin arrests—41 percent more than in 1993. The police were closing bodegas on the Lower East Side, seizing cars off the George Washington Bridge, busting pot dealers in Washington Square Park, and dismantling gangs in Manhattan Valley. And the results were apparent everywhere. From Spanish Harlem to the Lower East Side, from the South Bronx to Bedford-Stuyvesant, the city's open-air drug markets were finally beginning to recede. The great Giuliani drug offensive seemed a resounding success.

Yet, even before 1995 was out, some troubling signs were emerging. One came from the federal government's Drug Abuse Warning Network. DAWN provided an annual tally of drug-related visits to hospital emergency rooms— a good measure of trends in hard-core drug use. If, as a result of the police crackdown, people were turning away from drugs, the DAWN numbers would be down. In 1995, however, the city's hospitals registered 20,013 cocaine-related visits—virtually unchanged from the year before. Similarly, heroin-related visits remained stuck at about 11,000. Drug mortality figures, meanwhile, were actually moving upward. In 1995, for instance, the city recorded 906 cocaine-related deaths, up from 755 in 1994, while heroin-related deaths went from 612 to 751.

The data on the supply side were no more encouraging. The main numbers here came from the Drug Enforcement Administration, which monitored the availability of drugs in the city by tracking the price and purity of under-cover buys. Given the many drug arrests being made in the city, plus the federal government's ongoing efforts to arrest international traffickers and seize drugs at the border, the police department fully expected to see drugs becoming more expensive. Most of the time, however, agents were able to buy cocaine at the same low $20,000-a-kilo price it had been for years. Occasionally, when a major shipment was seized, the price would spurt up to $30,000, but invariably it would slip back to its customary floor.

The data for heroin were even more dismaying. Back in the early 1990s, it was rarely possible to find a kilogram of heroin in the city for less than $200,000; by 1995, agents seldom had to pay more than $100,000. Over the same period, purity levels increased from 30 percent to 65 percent. Clearly, supplies were soaring, and the reason could be found in Colombia. As late as 1991, that country had no heroin industry. But, with cocaine sales flat and consumer tastes changing, Colombia's traffickers had decided to diversify into heroin. Quickly planting poppies and importing Chinese chemists, they were soon producing tons of the stuff, and by the mid-1990s they were challenging Asian traffickers for control of the New York market. "With the competition among Southeast and Southwest Asian, and Colombian traffickers, New York City has more heroin on the street than ever before," the DEA noted in an October 1995 internal report. So, despite the Giuliani crackdown, the city remained awash in drugs.

Nor was there any lack of hands to distribute them. Slowly but relentlessly, the city's dealers were adapting to the police department's new tactics. Rather than assign pitchers to an exposed patch of sidewalk, many drug gangs were moving their operations indoors, away from police scrutiny. Others, while remaining outside, were becoming floating dispensaries, with sellers constantly on the move. More generally, organizations were shrinking so as to reduce their visibility. "The drug trade is going from the supermarket to the bodega, to a more individual type of operation," observed John Galea, director of street research for the state's Office of Alcoholism and Substance Abuse Services. Whatever form their operations took, dealers were becoming much more cautious in whom they would sell to. "The sellers—especially the more rational ones—will no longer sell to people they don't know, especially if they look like a cop," observed Bruce Johnson of the National Development and Research Institute in Manhattan.

On 110th Street, these changes were exemplified by Khamillo Parker. A short, stocky forty-year-old native of Queens, Khamillo (pronounced "Cameo") had been active on 110th Street since 1992. A longtime user of heroin, he had enrolled in a methadone program in the neighborhood. Every morning, before entering it, he would buy a bag or two of heroin and sniff it; the stuff was so powerful that, even with the methadone, he would get high. To help finance his habit, Khamillo went to work as a pitcher for an organization on 109th Street that sold a brand of dope called "9½." "I would stand on the block and sell drugs all day without being bothered by the police," he recalled.

Then Giuliani became mayor, and everything went to hell. "Before, you only had to worry about getting arrested by undercover cops," Khamillo said, sounding like an analyst from the Kennedy School. "The city police saw what was going on, but they didn't do anything. Under Giuliani, you had to worry about the uniformed guys, too. That made a hell of a difference." So did the merger between the NYPD and the Transit and Housing police. "There's much better coordination now," he noted. Eventually, the organization Khamillo worked for was busted and its top members sent to jail. Khamillo managed to hook up with another group but was arrested three times over two years. The last time, in November 1994, he had six bundles on him. He was let off with three years' probation, but, if picked up again, he faced doing serious time—a risk he was unwilling to take.

"I said, 'Fuck this,' and basically got out," Khamillo said. Still, he continued to hang out on 110th Street, dabbling in dope. And, over time, he saw the drug trade there slowly rebound. By the fall of 1995, the dealers were again out in force, though far more covertly than in the past. By the summer of 1996, Khamillo himself was back at it, signing on as a tout, or steerer, with a local drug gang. Every day around noon, a hustler would approach him on 110th Street and whisper a two-digit number keyed to the city's zip codes. "Two-Nine," for instance, signified the northeast corner of Central Park. When approached by customers he considered legit, Khamillo would lead them to the park, where two or three dealers would be waiting on benches inside the entrance. After making sure Khamillo was not being followed, one of the dealers would quietly raise a finger to indicate that he had the goods. And the deal would quickly go down. Tipped a couple of dollars by both parties, Khamillo on a good day could make $20 an hour. "Demand," he observed one afternoon as junkies buzzed around him, "is as great as ever."

Khamillo may have been exaggerating some. The number of buyers in neighborhoods like Spanish Harlem had no doubt declined some since the peak of the crack epidemic in the late 1980s and early 1990s. Some users, like Yvonne Hamilton, had entered treatment. Others had gone to jail. Many more had burned out, gotten sick, or died. And few young people were taking their place. Having seen the damage crack had done to their parents, they wanted little part of it.

Even so, the demand for crack remained enormous. The introduction of the drug in the mid-1980s had set off such a boom in consumption that, even with the ebbing of the epidemic, the market for it remained vast. "Crack use has leveled off, but at a very high level," observed John Galea. "It's still the number-one drug on the street."

Heroin, meanwhile, was quickly gaining on it. The sudden availability of

high-quality dope on the street was giving rise to a new cohort of users. Some
of them were lawyers, stockbrokers, and other members of the middle class,
attracted to a grade of heroin that could be sniffed rather than injected. Most
of the dope flooding New York, however, ended up in the inner city. There,
many long-time crack and cocaine users were adding heroin to their repertoire
as a means of taking the edge off their high. Some liked to mix the drug with
crack and smoke it (chasing the dragon); others injected it together with cocaine (speedballing). One way or another, the new heroin surge was being
fueled by the usual coterie of hard-core users. And, until something was done
to reduce their number, the city's drug trade would continue to flourish.

During the 1993 campaign for mayor, Rudolph Giuliani had acknowledged the need to address this aspect of the city's drug problem. In the same
speech in which he had lambasted street-level dealers, Giuliani had said that
"there must be a recognition by the city's mayor that we can reduce the
demand for drugs at the same time as we are reducing the sale of illegal drugs.
We need equal emphasis on both sides of the problem." Giuliani praised
"community-based" efforts to reduce demand and said that "sustaining and
strengthening such efforts will be the cornerstone of my administration." He
also promised to create "neighborhood-based centers" to serve as an entry
point for addicts and to expand the city's treatment capacity by 5,000 slots a
year, with a special focus on "high-risk groups" like pregnant women and the
homeless.

As mayor, however, Giuliani would deliver on none of these promises. He
would create no neighborhood-based intake centers, nor provide much new
funding for community-based programs. As for new treatment slots, Giuliani
would create virtually none during his first four years in office. And, reflecting
this, the number of people on treatment waiting lists at the end of his first
term—about 3,500—would be as high as at the start.

Actually, when it came to high-risk groups, the mayor, far from creating
new services, would cut them. A good example was the Family Rehabilitation
Program. This was created in 1991 to address the problem of drug addiction
among low-income parents—a major factor in the city's high rates of child
abuse. The FRP provided drug-abusing mothers and fathers an intensive mix
of parenting classes and outpatient drug therapy. Of the several hundred families enrolled in the FRP's thirty-one units, only 4 percent had children placed
in foster care. The city's share of the program's cost came to just $4.8 million a
year. (The state provided $13.3 million more.) Even this, however, was too
much for the mayor, who in 1995 ended the city's contribution to the drug
treatment component of the program. As a result, many of the units were
forced to close.

As it happened, in November of that same year, the city was rocked by
the case of Elisa Izquierdo, a six-year-old whose broken body was discovered
by police in a rundown apartment in Brooklyn. Elisa, it turned out, had been

repeatedly beaten by her mother, Awilda Lopez, a heavy user of crack and alcohol. In response, the city launched an investigation into its Child Welfare Administration. When major flaws were discovered, Mayor Giuliani announced that he was reorganizing the CWA into a new Administration for Children's Services. And, to head it, he was naming Nicholas Scoppetta, a hard-charging former prosecutor. Moving quickly, Scoppetta hired new staff, improved training, and installed new computers. No effort was made, however, to address the problem of drug addiction among inner-city women—a major source of the city's child-abuse problem. And, as a result, the incidence of such abuse continued undiminished.

BY THE END OF 1995, the New York City Police Department had itself recognized the limits of its drug-fighting strategy. Amid signs that the city's drug trade was resurging, William Bratton asked John Timoney and Jack Maple to sit down once again and develop a new approach. With the precincts proving incapable of taking the enemy, they decided, it was time to launch a full frontal assault. The department would select several of the city's most drug-ridden districts and send in an occupying force of undercover cops. For months they would bivouac there, conducting buy-and-bust operations, raiding stash houses, padlocking bodegas. As Bratton described it in his book *Turnaround*, Operation Juggernaut was to rid the city of its drug problem once and for all:

> Prior to Juggernaut, the city's war on drugs had been our Vietnam; we were fighting a hit-and-run enemy and gone in and made a lot of contact when we could, but we'd never held the ground. We didn't have the tactics or the will to win. Juggernaut was the Normandy invasion. We were going to overwhelm our opponents, take the ground and never leave, and systematically take them out. The focus of our effort was going to be on the source of the problem: the drug dealers. We weren't going after the users. We would systematically take out the low-level street dealer, the midlevel operator, and high-level kingpin. We would attack them consistently on all fronts at all times. If you were a drug dealer, you were a marked man.

Normandy, in this case, was to be Brooklyn North, a broad swath of poverty encompassing such drug-plagued neighborhoods as Bushwick, Brownsville, and East New York. And D-Day was April 1, 1996. On it, the NYPD flooded the area with 1,000 of its finest undercover cops, their mission being to sweep the streets clean of dealers. Shortly after, a similar operation was launched in northern Manhattan.

As originally planned, these operations (renamed SatCom, for Strategic and Tactical Command) were to last six months. That was the amount of time it was thought necessary to dismantle the drug organizations in those neighborhoods. At the end of six months, however, the organizations were still there, and so the operations were extended. Every month or two, a new deadline would be set, but it, too, would be extended. In short, the city's drug dealers were proving far harder than the Germans to dislodge. And the reason, it seemed, was faulty intelligence about the enemy. Bratton's observation that the police were going to go after dealers, not users, suggested ignorance of a basic reality of the city's drug trade—that many of the city's dealers *were* users. And because those users were so numerous, the pool of potential sellers was virtually limitless. That's why the Sunshine Project failed. And that's why SatCom was encountering so much resistance. As 1996 came to a close, the operation was still in place.

With its phalanxes of undercover cops saturating drug-ridden neighborhoods, SatCom bore a strong resemblance to the TNT units that the department, under Bratton, had so derided. And, like TNT, SatCom was generating huge numbers of arrests. In 1996 the police would make a record 101,051 drug arrests, eclipsing the old mark of 94,887 set in 1989, at the height of the crack epidemic. And the city's jails were feeling the effect. "The operations in Brooklyn North and Manhattan North are really driving up our population," said Michael Jacobson, New York's commissioner of corrections. As the head of the city's jail system, Jacobson might be expected to applaud the NYPD's drug offensive. Instead, he was outspokenly critical. "Prison expenses are going through the roof," he grumbled. In 1980, he noted, his department spent about $150 million a year to house 6,000 to 7,000 inmates. In 1997, it was spending $800 million to house 18,000 to 21,000, of whom more than one-third were drug offenders. A pudgy, tousle-haired Giuliani appointee who had formerly worked in the city's budget office, Jacobson noted that these expenditures were part of "a zero-sum game. The money for corrections is coming out of other places, like health care and education." Because of all the drug arrests being made in the city, Jacobson said, "kids in New York schools have to attend classes with ninety other kids."

In a sense, then, the ongoing crisis in New York's school system was inseparable from Mayor Giuliani's drug policy. Cracking down on the city's drug dealers required a vast support network, including cops to arrest them, drivers to transport them, clerks to book them, jails to detain them, D.A.'s to prosecute them, legal-aid lawyers to defend them, juries to try them, judges to sentence them, bailiffs to guard them, interpreters to assist them, and, finally, prison cells to hold them. (By 1997, the relentless flow of drug offenders had driven the state's prison population to nearly 70,000—more than five times the number when the Rockefeller Laws were passed.) All of this was sucking up resources that could have otherwise been used to hire more teachers, build more schools, and buy more textbooks. And there was no end in sight. For, with its lopsided reliance on enforcement, the city was not beginning to get at the real root of the problem—the persistently high demand for drugs.

In most respects, "broken windows" was proving to be an effective policing strategy. The idea of cracking down on small offenses in order to prevent
larger ones was borne out by the city's sharply falling crime rates. By appre-
hending subway farebeaters, for instance, the police were able to keep robbers
and pickpockets out of the trains. And, once it became clear that jumping a
turnstile could result in an arrest, many stopped trying altogether; the threat
of apprehension was itself sufficient deterrent. Such was not the case with
drugs. Given the power of addiction, the normal rules of deterrence simply
did not apply. As Khamillo Parker put it, "If you've got a habit, you're going to
keep coming."

In October 1997, Mayor Giuliani, campaigning for a second term, declared in a speech that, if reelected, he would devote himself to confronting
"our biggest problem today, namely, drug abuse." Putting the cost of illegal
drugs to the city at more than $20 billion a year, Giuliani said that "we cannot
turn our back on this ever growing problem and we must resolve to challenge
ourselves to address it." Otherwise, he said, "we will only continue to bear the
burden of drugs, their attendant violence, their enormous cost to society and
the lost and wasted lives." So, after four years of arrests, dragnets, stings, and
investigations, drugs remained, by the mayor's own admission, New York's
number-one problem. There could be no more telling indictment of his own
drug policy.

19

Redemption

IN EARLY 1994, Yvonne Hamilton, having spent most of the last two years in drug treatment, left the Salvation Army center on 48th Street and moved in with her sister Joyce and her husband in their three-bedroom house in the Bronx. For the first time in years, Yvonne had a room to herself, complete with a twenty-five-inch TV set. Brimming with self-confidence, she turned her energies to her main goal—finding a job. Without one, she felt sure, her chances of staying sober were slim. And, compared to many recovering addicts, she had numerous advantages. For instance, her long record of work, beginning with the Job Corps and CETA and continuing on through to United Cerebral Palsy, had instilled in her such workplace values as punctuality and responsibility.

Even with such experience, though, Yvonne would discover how hard it is for recovering addicts to find work. From watching soaps on TV, she had gotten the idea that she would like to work in the health field. Doing some research, she found a community college in Yonkers that offered a course in becoming a paramedic, and she arranged an interview. Preparing for it, Yvonne worried about the eight-year gap in her résumé. In the recovery world, it is axiomatic that even the slightest reference to one's drug career—no matter how long ago —is an automatic job disqualifier; the stigma attached to addiction is simply too strong. So Yvonne carefully rehearsed a story about how she had been a cafeteria worker at New Hope Manor and an administrative assistant at the Salvation Army. Unfortunately, the nuns at New Hope had so inoculated her against lying that she involuntarily blurted out the truth about her past— immediately killing her chances of getting into the program. "I'm so disgusted with myself," she wailed afterward.

With that option closed, Yvonne turned to the help-wanted ads. Unfortunately, many of the jobs paid at or near minimum wage, ruling them out in Yvonne's mind. She wanted a *real* job, one that would provide both a living wage and an opportunity to use the skills she had picked up while in treatment. As the weeks passed, however, Yvonne kept lowering her sights, until she was inquiring about positions for cafeteria workers and home attendants (her mother's old job). The number of applicants was so great, however, that even these seemed beyond her reach. As summer approached, Yvonne, idle and moody, spent much of her time moping about the house and bickering with Joyce.

Then, in the summer, a cousin who lived in Spring Valley, about twenty miles north of the city, heard of Yvonne's plight and invited her to come stay with her. A part-time worker in a psychiatric hospital, Cousin Ellie lived in a rambling house with three other adults and six foster children, and Yvonne could help look after them. She jumped at the offer. For years, she had felt that her troubles in life stemmed from her being trapped in the ghetto; now she was going to be able to live among trees and breathe fresh air. To add to her expectation, she was able to pry Gerald loose from the woman who'd been caring for him and to take him along with her to Spring Valley.

Unfortunately, the town did not quite live up to its name. Though located just six miles west of the tony Hudson River town of Nyack, Spring Valley was a black minighetto, one of many depressed communities peppering the exurbs of New York. Its three-block Main Street was full of boarded-up storefronts, victims of the bustling strip malls that had sprung up in the area; the one movie theater in town showed porn. And, remarkably, drugs were no less available here than in East Harlem. As throughout the Hudson Valley, enterprising young dealers brought crack up from New York, selling $5 vials for $15 or $20. With a population of just 20,000, Spring Valley was able to support three crackhouses, and glowering young dealers would hang out at its rundown bus terminal, awaiting customers from nearby towns.

Yvonne was not tempted, however. Absorbed in her new caretaker duties, she generally stayed close to home, looking after the foster kids and her son. Gerald, now a strapping young boy, was proving to be a real handful, his behavior alternating between rowdy outbursts and dark, silent funks. "I think it was the drugs, or how I treated him when I was on drugs," Yvonne observed in a moment of self-reflection. Whichever the case, he needed close watching. Occasionally, Yvonne would slip out to a bar for a beer, but otherwise she remained abstemious.

Then, in early September, she got a call from 110th Street informing her that her sister Anne was dead. As much as Yvonne dreaded the prospect of returning to the old neighborhood, there was no one else to tend to the body, and so, with some money scraped together by Ellie, she reluctantly boarded a bus for the city. When she got to Clinton Building Number One, she learned that Anne had gone into a coma after shooting up in a drug den on the second floor. (She had moved there after the operation in 17E had been shut down.) Had the den mothers called for help immediately, Anne might have been saved, but business had been so good that they had held off for several hours, and by the time the paramedics arrived Anne was gone. Yvonne's anger deepened when she learned that the junkies had gone through her sister's pockets and stolen her money and ID. "How can you rob a dead person?" Yvonne asked. Deep down, of course, she knew that she had committed such deeds herself.

Seeing her distress, her old crack buddies pressed her to pick up a pipe. Yvonne had enough self-control to refuse, but, feeling sad and lonely, she bought a bottle of rum and took it to Central Park, where she proceeded to get plastered. After two days of tears, self-pity, and sleeping on park benches, Yvonne scrounged up some money for the bus ride home. Ellie, who had been relying on Yvonne to look after the kids, was livid, and it took all of Yvonne's persuasiveness to keep from being thrown out of the house. "All that work, and I go out and drink!" she cried after the incident. "It shows I'm still weak."

Then, in the spring of 1995, Yvonne got a break. Responding to a newspaper ad, she applied for a job at an Off-Track Betting site in nearby Nanuet. As part of the application, Yvonne had to be fingerprinted; to her amazement, none of her arrests turned up, and she got the job. The work—filing records and making payments to the sad sacks who patronized OTB—was not exciting, and the pay ($6 an hour) was meager, but, more than a year after leaving the Salvation Army, Yvonne finally had a job. With her new income, she was able to find an apartment of her own—the back half of a ramshackle bungalow owned by a Chinese man and his Haitian wife. With its thin walls, flimsy doors, and dingy kitchen, the apartment barely seemed worth the $650-a-month rent, but the living room and bedroom were sunny and spacious enough to accommodate the rest of Yvonne's brood: her lover, a fifty-year-old woman she'd met in Spring Valley; a young friend of the woman's; Gerald; a cat; and a ferret. At the age of forty, Yvonne was, for the first time in her life, struggling to maintain a stable, if somewhat irregular, household.

The pressures on her remained intense, however. The hours at OTB were sporadic, and she rarely took home more than $100 a week. As a single mother, she was eligible for $167 a month in welfare plus food stamps, but financially Yvonne was always in arrears, and she would wait until actual holes appeared in her shoes before shelling out the $15 for a new pair. Spring Valley itself was a fishbowl, and Yvonne—self-conscious about being with a woman—generally stayed home at night, reading the Bible and watching TV. Whenever she did venture out, she would be constantly reminded of the town's underside. On several occasions, she was accosted by a female crack dealer, who pestered her to buy something. Finally, Yvonne blew up. "If you don't stop bothering me," she snarled, "I'm going to get somebody to stick a pistol in you!" The woman did not approach her again.

In February 1996, Yvonne heard of a job opening at a local home for the disabled and went for an interview. The position—drawing up personal development plans for residents and monitoring their progress—entailed far more responsibility than she had ever had, but the administrators, impressed by her politeness and seriousness, hired her. The job paid $14 an hour, and Yvonne, working fifty hours a week, was at last earning a living wage. In the fall of 1996, she, Ellie, and several other cousins moved into a rambling five-bedroom house in Chestnut Ridge, a largely white community near Spring Valley. Yvonne had taken another step into the American mainstream.

Still, life was not easy. Now that she was a law-abiding citizen, she received a series of dunning notices—for back child support, outstanding loans, and other unsettled accounts. At one point, Ellie lost her job, and Yvonne had to assume more of the rent. Whenever she got ready to leave the house, Gerald —remembering all the times he'd been deserted as a child—would cling to her, and she would patiently have to reassure him of her return. Try as she might, Yvonne could not completely shake her past.

She remained stoical, however. Whatever trials she now faced, they seemed trivial compared to her past ones. And, whenever she felt her old urges kicking up, she would hear the voice of Sister Pat or Father Aquinas admonishing her about the importance of discipline and self-control, about the need not to give in to temptation. And she didn't. Six years after entering New Hope Manor, Yvonne Hamilton remained free of drugs.

THE VOICES whispering into Raphael Flores's ear were of a far different sort. The demons that had assailed him at Hot Line Cares were no less persistent in his room at the veterans residence on 119th Street. Often he would wake up in the middle of the night, sweating and shaking and terrified at his inability to dream. Desperate for relief, he would increase his dose of sleeping pills, only to become more despondent. Consumed by rage, Raphael would get into frequent spats with his fellow residents, including one fistfight. Sunk in self-pity, he would rail at how everyone else had gotten ahead while he—selflessly devoting himself to others—was alone and penniless.

For all his distemper, however, Raphael kept at his street work. Like the anonymous whiskey priest in Graham Greene's novel *The Power and the Glory,* he felt driven to continue his ministry despite all the fears that ate at him and all the doubts that sapped him. Bereft of close companionship, convinced of his failure as a father, shunned by those he had once inspired, and barred from his own center, Raphael saw his work with addicts as his one remaining salvation. In an odd way, his lack of access to Hot Line forced him to become even more innovative than usual. Wandering the streets of El Barrio, he was a one-man outreach team, approaching users and urging them to get help.

Visiting Sister Leontine's apartment on 111th Street, for instance, Raphael noticed a man who spent his days sitting on a cinder block in front of a tenement, sniffing from a can of carburetor fluid. Encrusted with dirt from head to foot, his face so blackened that he looked like a minstrel singer, the man, whose name ironically was Angel, seemed barely human, but Raphael could not pass without trying to engage him.

"I want to help you," he said gently one day, squatting in front of the man. Picking up one of the half-dozen canisters on the ground around him, he read the warning label: "Danger: Extremely Flammable."

"Angel, how long have you been sniffing this?" Raphael asked.

"A long time," Angel replied, his voice low and raspy. "I'm like a person from another world."

Getting down on his knees and gazing into his eyes, Raphael said, "I wish you didn't have to use this stuff. Will you let me get you in a hospital so that you can clean yourself up?"

"I don't want hospital!" Angel flared. "I don't want to clean myself. Ambulance come here—I beat them all up in the face!" And with that Angel stood up—he was tall and powerfully built—and tottered away.

Undeterred, Raphael returned the next day to continue the conversation, and the day after that, and once he felt he had Angel's confidence, he arranged for one of the city's mental-health outreach teams to come and evaluate him. Talking with Angel, they determined that he was a threat neither to himself nor to others and so could not be committed. Not a threat! The man was slowly poisoning himself, Raphael thought. It was yet another demonstration of the system's fundamental indifference.

He nonetheless continued to fight it. One day, while walking past the Aguilar Library, he was accosted by a sallow-looking dope peddler. "Hi," Raphael said with spontaneous charm. "I run a program. I can get you into a detox right away." "Yeah?" the man said, surprised. "Right away?" Confirming his offer, Raphael gave the man directions to Hot Line. "Tell them the chubby guy sent you," he said good-naturedly.

Unfortunately, it was not clear how much longer he would be able to direct people to Hot Line. For Martina's efforts to save the place were not faring well. Going over Hot Line's financial records, she found countless irregularities. And her fundraising initiatives always seemed to fall flat. Perplexed as to why, she pressed one of her contacts to level with her. In response, she received a blunt letter informing her that Hot Line had been placed on a secret list of organizations that, due to past financial mismanagement, were not to be funded. Hot Line, in effect, had been blacklisted. With that, Martina concluded that the place was beyond salvation, and she set March 1, 1994, as its closing date. With great regret, she called up the landlord to arrange a time to turn over the keys. Marvin, meanwhile, gathered up his meager belongings and disappeared into Brooklyn.

Hearing that the office was about to close, Raphael—as obstinate as ever—called up the landlord and persuaded him to give him the keys. Contacting

Con Ed and the phone company, he convinced them not to cut off their services. Showing up at the office, he found the place in total disarray, but, with the help of Ethel Curtis, who agreed to stay on, he hurriedly got things in order. In early May, Raphael reopened the office with a hundred-day deadline to arrange some funding.

Within days, the phone was again ringing and the addicts again streaming in. By early summer, Raphael was placing three people in treatment a day. On the fundraising front, however, he was doing no better than Martina, and by early August 1994 even he was having to face reality. As his self-imposed deadline neared, Raphael spent several nights sleeping in Hot Line's back room—a way of bidding farewell to the institution that had consumed most of his adult life. On August 12, he locked the door to Hot Line Cares for good.

Given Raphael's long-standing dependency on Hot Line, its collapse could have been expected to unhinge him further. Yet, in the weeks that followed, an odd thing happened. All the matters that had weighed on him—the constant worries about funding, the regrets about not being able to pay his staff, the endless exposure to people in pain—suddenly faded. For the first time in years, Raphael had no choice but to look after his own needs. Seeking to spend more time with his daughter, he began traveling regularly to Bridgeport; Monique was now pregnant, and the prospect of becoming a grandfather filled him with pleasure. Tending to his psychic wounds, Raphael began attending support groups (though for what he wouldn't say). After watching the movie *Sleepless in Seattle*, he bought the soundtrack and, back in his cubbyhole, would relax to the music of Louis Armstrong and Jimmy Durante; at the age of forty-seven, Raphael was discovering the joys of jazz. And, to his searches through the Concordance, he had added a new word: humility. "I'm trying to maintain my humbleness," he said, sitting in his room, his Bible open on the bed. Even the failure of Harold Camping's prophecy about 1994 did not rattle him. "It shook us all up," he said. "It was a wake-up call for a lot of us."

Desperate for a job, Raphael, after months of interviews, finally got one, as a detox counselor at St. Agnes Hospital in White Plains. After so many years of battling the system from outside, Raphael suddenly found himself inside. And there were things about it that he liked, such as the regular paycheck. But the frustrations were great, too. His main responsibility was working with the unit's Spanish-speaking patients, and every day he would lead them in a group session. Like most hospitals, though, St. Agnes made few efforts to refer clients to long-term programs, and Raphael reflexively began arranging hookups on his own. Throughout, he offered a series of suggestions about how the place could be improved. That did not endear him to his coworkers, and when the hospital decided to reduce its staff, Raphael was among the first to be let go.

In the months that followed, Raphael would land a series of jobs—as a group leader at a hospital in Queens, as a counselor in a detox unit in Yonkers, as an intake worker at a women's shelter in the Bronx. At each, though, he would see ways in which clients were being shortchanged. "We don't want to do anything we don't get paid for," one supervisor told him. Unable to accept such a philosophy, Raphael would invariably argue, and before long he would end up back on the street.

Such experiences made Raphael realize how much more work he needed on his humility. They also convinced him that he needed more training. And so, despite his age and his deep-seated fears about returning to school, he enrolled in a program at Long Island University to become a certified substance abuse counselor. Attending classes at the school's Brooklyn campus, Raphael studied addiction and relapse, psychology and epidemiology. After all the years of operating by instinct and improvisation, he was delighted to get some formal instruction. His professors, in turn, liked hearing about his street work. One, intrigued with Raphael's stories about Hot Line Cares, asked him to write a paper describing what he would do if he got a sudden windfall allowing him to reopen it. Raphael wrote down all the things he'd dreamed of for Hot Line—a full-time administrator, a team of youth volunteers, an outreach coordinator, a staff attorney, a psychologist, a proposal writer, even a lobbyist. If Hot Line reopened, he added with a flourish, the word "would spread in a heartbeat."

UNFORTUNATELY, HOT LINE'S return remained a possibility only on paper. In the meantime, Raphael sought to keep up its tradition on his rambles around the neighborhood. One afternoon, while hurrying along Third Avenue in search of a pay phone, he heard someone calling his name. Turning around, he saw a waiflike figure at the end of the block. Looking more closely, he saw it was Carol Ann Sanders. Raphael had run into Carol several times since her abrupt departure from St. Luke's two years earlier, but it had been many months since their last encounter. And he was struck by how much she had deteriorated. Her eyes had dark bags under them, and her hair, bleached a reddish blond, was greasy and knotted. She was also having trouble walking, because of a circulatory problem that had forced her to have an operation at St. Luke's the previous year. Collapsing into Raphael's arms, Carol told him how much pain she was in and how desperate she was to get help—so much so, in fact, that she had gone on her own to the detox unit at Metropolitan Hospital. No beds had been available, however, and she had been told to return the following Monday. Raphael immediately offered to help, and in the meantime he arranged for her to stay at Sister's.

On Sunday afternoon, Raphael stopped by the nun's apartment to discuss strategy with Carol. A cramped floor-through, the apartment was being renovated, and with the furniture having been moved out of the living room, Raphael and Carol had to sit on the floor, their backs propped up against the wall. Explaining her earlier decision to leave St. Luke's, Carol was candid. "I got rested and felt better and wanted to run some more," she said sheepishly.

This time was different, she said. Raphael was dubious. Carol had informed him that her junkie boyfriend was doing time in Rikers for ripping off a Barnes & Noble superstore, and Raphael suspected that she simply wanted a detox to tide her over. Still, he was willing to take a chance on her, and he had brought her a detox care package containing deodorant, socks, T-shirts, and a black sweatshirt.

As night approached, Carol grew restless. Dope was much harder to find than it had been two years earlier, but her habit would not let her rest. Because of the pain in her legs, she asked someone in the apartment to accompany her outside. Even with an arm to lean on, Carol had trouble walking, and she slowly hobbled down the three flights of stairs and onto the street. At one time, she could have simply walked to 110th Street and selected a pitcher from among the crowd there. Now she would have to locate one of the neighborhood's floating drug spots. Limping a block eastward on 111th Street, she came upon a young black man in a woolen maroon cap who was standing idly on the sidewalk. "You open?" she shouted from across the street. He gave a quick shake of the head, then turned away.

Discouraged, Carol trudged to the Thomas Jefferson Houses, a stolid housing project on Second Avenue. There, she approached a black youth standing by an entryway. "You a cop?" he rudely asked. Cursing him, Carol tottered back to Third, only to discover that another spot was closed. Finally, in the courtyard of the Johnson Houses on 112th Street, she spotted a short black man wearing wraparound sunglasses. "Hey, Shorty," she shouted, "remember me?" Shorty certainly did. A few months earlier, Carol had traded him a $500 Gucci necklace for three bags of dope. "How many you want?" he asked with a smile. Just one, Carol replied, and Shorty disappeared into a nearby stairwell. A few minutes later, he returned with a glassine envelope stamped "Fugitive," and Carol handed him ten bucks. Relieved, she limped back to Sister's. It had taken her nearly an hour to cop. "This isn't the spot anymore," Carol sighed, offering a grudging tribute to Rudy Giuliani's crackdown on the city's drug trade.

Unfortunately, the mayor had done nothing to make detox more available, and Carol and Raphael, arriving at Metropolitan at seven-twenty the following morning—twenty-five minutes before opening time—were dismayed to find two people ahead of them. According to the rules, they were supposed to wait outside, but with the temperature in the twenties and Carol barely able to stand, Raphael convinced the guard to let them into the lobby. Slipping into a worn plastic chair, Carol darkly eyed the competition—a pudgy Hispanic woman with inch-long white nails and a heavy onyx cross that brushed the top of her ample cleavage, and a husky black woman decked out in a black leather jacket, black jeans, and knee-high black leather boots.

When the woman at the front desk stepped up to her post, the other two women rushed up to get a pass; leaning on Raphael's arm, Carol lamely brought up the rear. "That black chick is trying to get ahead of everybody," she complained. "This system is really backwards," Raphael observed as he helped Carol up the stairs to the detox ward on the second floor. "You lose so many people this way." Fifteen minutes after they sat down, an intake worker asked the black woman to follow her through the door. The woman returned a short time later, a triumphant look on her face. "I got a bed!" she exulted. "Oh, *man!*" The intake worker announced that that was it for the day. "The rest of you have to come back tomorrow," she said emotionlessly. Carol looked at her in disbelief.

In a measure of how little things had changed in the city, Raphael suggested to Carol that they adopt the same course they had two years earlier when faced with a similar situation, which was to visit St. Luke's. Carol numbly agreed. Seeing her weakening condition, Raphael turned around and squatted down in front of her. "Put your arms around my neck," he commanded. Carol did, and Raphael, hoisting her on his back, bounded down the stairs, through the lobby, and out to First Avenue. He hailed a cab, which took them across town to St. Luke's. Again taking Carol on his back, Raphael led her up to the detox ward. After a short wait in the sitting room, Carol was summoned by an intake worker. While she was gone, Raphael began talking with a foul-smelling woman who was hunched over in a chair across from him. "I'm a counselor and can help get people into detox," Raphael explained, trying to connect. But the woman slumped down into her chair and made like she was asleep, and Raphael quickly backed off.

A half-hour later, Carol reappeared with the intake worker. Miraculously, a bed was about to become free, and she could be admitted that same day if her papers were in order. To see what she needed, Raphael led Carol back down to the Medicaid office on the ground floor. When the clerk punched her name into his computer, he found that the Medicaid she'd gotten at the time of her operation was still good. "An act of God!" Raphael declared. With a letter from the unit attesting to Carol's insured status, they went back to the detox ward, where she was certified for admission; now she had to go downstairs and across the street to the admissions office. By this point, Carol could barely stand, so Raphael hurried downstairs and, without asking anyone's permission, commandeered an empty wheelchair and brought it back to the ward. Missing one of its front wheels, the wheelchair wobbled badly, but Raphael nonetheless managed to maneuver Carol down to the ground floor, across the road, and into the admissions office. Looking pale and nervous, Carol began filling out the form Raphael had fetched for her.

As she did so, he noticed a young black man seated a few chairs away who was wearing an Army-green jacket and reading the *New York Times.* "You thinking of rehab?" Raphael asked.

"Yes, I want one," the man replied.

"What are you going in for?" Raphael continued.

"Heroin and alcohol," he said.

"I know a good program upstate," Raphael said. "I'll give you the number. You tell your counselor in detox, and they can start working on it right away."

By now, Carol had completed the form, and a short while later she was ready to go in. Raphael gave her a hug and promised to call the next day. Already, though, he was on to his next case.

CONCLUSION

20

A Way Out

IN BACKGROUND and temperament, it would be hard to find two individuals more dissimilar than Raphael Flores and Jerome Jaffe. The one—a hulking street worker with an outsized ego, mercurial temperament, and charismatic manner—was raised in a broken Puerto Rican family in the inner city. The other—a slightly built, self-effacing M.D. with a sardonic wit and searching mind—rose from a lower-middle-class Jewish family in Philadelphia to become one of the nation's leading psychopharmacologists. Yet, from such different starting points, the two men arrived at remarkably similar visions of how best to fight the nation's drug problem. And, as Raphael Flores's experiences in Spanish Harlem showed, what worked for Jerome Jaffe a quarter-century ago could prove just as effective today.

When Richard Nixon became president in 1969, the nation was in the grip of a serious heroin epidemic. In a few short years, his administration managed to bring it under control. It did so by recognizing, first of all, that the real problem facing the nation was not casual drug users but hard-core ones. The Nixon Administration further understood that many of those users wanted help, and that it was the government's responsibility to provide it, in the form of affordable, accessible, and effective treatment.

Today, the nation's drug problem is much larger and infinitely more complex. Overall, the United States now has an estimated *ten times* as many hard-core users as it did then. In the 1960s, the problem was limited largely to heroin; now, it includes cocaine, crack, methamphetamine, and angel dust. And today's addicts have many more problems than those of the past, from mental illness and homelessness to AIDS and tuberculosis.

Even so, the Nixon policy provides a model for how we might proceed today. Applying it, we would begin by scrapping the Office of National Drug

Control Policy—one of the most ineffectual bodies in Washington—and re-building it along the lines of the old Special Action Office for Drug Abuse Prevention. In accord with the Jaffe code, the office would be shorn of all supply-side duties and left to deal exclusively with demand-side ones. And, as during the Nixon years, the office would be placed in the hands of a specialist in addiction medicine. The four men who have headed ONDCP—William Bennett, Bob Martinez, Lee Brown, and Barry McCaffrey—have all lacked even rudimentary experience in the treatment, prevention, and epidemiology of drug abuse. And the results have been dire. If we want to make real inroads on the drug problem, we should entrust national policy to a C. Everett Koop–type figure, someone combining medical expertise with a commanding personal presence. And he should be backed by an Egil Krogh–like figure in the White House, someone who, invoking the authority of the president, could make sure the office's mission was carried out.

That mission, simply stated, should be the creation and maintenance of a comprehensive national treatment system for drug and alcohol abuse. Currently, the nation's treatment system can accommodate only half of the 3.6 million people believed to be in urgent need of help. According to ONDCP estimates, filling this gap would require spending an additional $3.4 billion a year at the federal level. Where to find such money in an era of small government? The 1999 federal drug budget came to just over $17 billion, of which $11.2 billion (66 percent) was for the supply side and $5.9 billion (34 percent) for the demand side. If the overall budget was held constant but the allocations for these two areas equalized, the demand side would receive an additional $2.65 billion—very close to the sum in question.

Now, as most students of drug policy are aware, the federal drug budget is largely a fiction, an amalgamation of the estimated expenditures of the fifty or so government agencies with a role in fighting drugs. Money taken from one agency does not automatically become available for use by another. Some have argued that, from a political standpoint, it would be easier to achieve an increase in treatment funding if the money did not come from law enforcement. Perhaps so. Nonetheless, the aggressive programs being pursued on the supply side have produced many unwelcome effects, from disrupted lives to strained relations with foreign governments to massive violations of civil liberties, and cutting them back could prove beneficial in its own right. Inviting targets include the $1.8 billion currently being spent on interdiction and the more than $500 million being spent on source-country programs—two areas that could be pared back without having much effect on the supply of drugs in the country. Also ripe for shrinkage is the DEA, whose budget ($1.2 billion in 1998) has soared in recent years without much to show for it. Most bloated of all is the U.S. Bureau of Prisons, which spends about $2 billion a year to house drug offenders. The premonition Jerome Jaffe had at the time of Nelson Rockefeller's harsh proposals, of billions of dollars being spent annually to warehouse small-time drug offenders, has become a grim reality. No effort at drug policy reform can hope to succeed without a thorough overhaul of the nation's drug-sentencing laws. A good starting point would be the decriminalization (not legalization) of marijuana possession, which would save some of the resources currently being squandered on pot arrests.

Even with a 50/50 split, the supply side would receive a larger share of the federal drug budget than it did under Nixon. In fact, a strong case could be made for returning to the 67/33 demand/supply split of that period. In today's political climate, however, simple parity is the best one can hope for.

Aside from making treatment more available, we must also make it more accessible. And, for a guide as to how to accomplish that, we might look to Jerome Jaffe's Illinois Drug Abuse Program. Thirty years after it was created, IDAP remains the most creative and comprehensive drug treatment system ever introduced in this country. Implementing a similar system in the nation's cities today could help significantly reduce the demand for drugs in them.

To take New York as an example, one would begin by setting up a central intake unit in each of the city's five boroughs. Manhattan, with its huge addict population, would ideally have two—one uptown, in Harlem, and the other downtown, on the Lower East Side. Appearing at these units, addicts would meet with a counselor to discuss the nature of their problem and the best way to address it; they would also receive a medical checkup to determine their physical condition. After deciding on the proper type of program, the counselor would consult a computerized directory of openings. Once a specific program was selected and the client accepted for admission, central intake would arrange transportation and assign an escort.

While clients were in treatment, the unit would monitor their progress to make sure they didn't get lost in the system. Clients ready to leave detox would be escorted back to central intake to discuss the next stage in the recovery process. For those encountering problems while in a program, central intake could intervene and arrange an alternative.

For any such system to work, treatment providers would have to become more flexible. The worlds of methadone maintenance and therapeutic communities are no less at odds today than they were back in the 1960s. Treatment providers must begin to accept the wisdom of Jerome Jaffe's principle of "different strokes for different folks," with its recognition that addicts have different needs and so require an array of programs. Once treatment providers do begin to cooperate, all types of creative arrangements become possible. For instance, one could imagine a modern-day version of IDAP's Tinley Park, with different treatment modes under one roof. It says a lot about the rigidities of the treatment world today that, in all of New York, there exists no program as sophisticated as this Jaffe brainchild of the late 1960s.

Detox similarly needs to be brought into the modern era. As Jaffe discovered in Chicago, there is no need, except in cases of medical emergency, to detox an addict in a hospital. The process could be performed just as effectively, and far more economically, in a nonmedical setting. If a client was detoxed in a residential center, he would, on being discharged, find himself already in a program—thus helping to avoid the revolving-door syndrome that today plagues so many detoxes.

Further emulating IDAP, treatment providers could engage in vigorous outreach. In Chicago, Patrick Hughes showed the value of sending teams of field-workers into copping zones. Raphael Flores gave his own demonstration of this in Spanish Harlem. Of course, outreach is not easy. It requires dedicated people willing to work in rough neighborhoods with an outcast population. Fortunately, a ready-made pool of such workers exists, in the form of recovering addicts. Their experiences with drugs make them instant experts in this field. Given the trouble many former users have in finding work, assigning them to outreach teams could accomplish two goals at once. Yvonne Hamilton, for instance, would have made a fine outreach worker on 110th Street. Needless to say, such workers would have to be watched closely to make sure they did not themselves slip back onto the street. For many, however, the opportunity to help others would constitute its own powerful form of therapy.

The idea of hiring recovering addicts to do outreach raises the broader issue of how to help such individuals resume a productive life. Clearly, finding a job is central to that process. Under the current system, however, treatment graduates are generally left to fend for themselves, and even someone as motivated as Yvonne Hamilton needed more than a year to find work. An IDAP-style system could help, for, with a central intake in place, a job-placement service could be attached to it, with counselors working to match graduates to jobs. Vocational-training programs could be linked as well. The prospect of obtaining such help at the end of the treatment process would no doubt convince many more to embark on it.

With an IDAP-type system in place, other units could be added as the need arose. Halfway houses could be set up to accommodate addicts as they prepared to enter treatment, and to receive them when they returned. As in Chicago, a medical section could be set up to deal with physical problems, a psychiatric section to address mental ones, and a pregnancy section to help deliver babies. Programs designed to treat alcoholism could also be integrated into the system, providing a seamless web of services for those abusing substances of any kind, illegal or not.

The potential for add-ons is limitless. One could imagine, for instance, creating mini–Hot Lines in the city's public-housing projects. At the Clinton Houses, the community center would be a logical site. Working with the project's residents, the unit could quickly learn who had drug and alcohol problems and figure out ways to combat them. It could work with the regulars in the project's drug dens, much as Raphael did with those in 17E. In particularly urgent cases, such as pregnant women using crack or addicted fathers beating their kids, these units could quickly intervene. By working closely with residents and gaining their trust, such on-site units would surely be more effective in preventing child abuse than New York's unwieldy child welfare bureaucracy.

Finally, a Hot Line–type unit could become a vehicle for engaging young people. In its heyday, Hot Line Cares was a magnet for the youths of Spanish Harlem. If similar units were set up in inner-city neighborhoods today, teenagers assigned to them could seek out and work with their troubled peers. This would provide a means of both keeping young people occupied after school as well as intervening with those headed on the downward slope to drug abuse.

How to prevent young people from using drugs is today a major preoccupation of policymakers and parents alike. To date, the nation's main weapon has been school-based programs designed to educate students about the hazards of drug use. Unfortunately, there is a growing body of research showing that these Just Say No–type programs by themselves do not work. For instance, the popular DARE program, which sends cops into schools to teach preteens about the perils of drugs, has been shown to have almost no impact on their future drug and alcohol use.

It's time to consider a new approach to prevention—one that, like the Jaffe code, would recognize that the main threat to young people is not the occasional, experimental use of drugs but their regular use. What the Nixon-appointed National Commission on Marihuana and Drug Abuse found in the early 1970s remains true today: Most students who experiment with pot will not develop problems with it or any other drug. Some will, however, and it is this group that should be the primary focus of prevention efforts. In addition to educating students about the hazards of drugs, we should set up early warning systems in our schools, in which teachers, counselors, and parents work together to detect students who are developing problems with drugs and to intervene with them at an early stage. And, to help youths who do get into trouble with drugs (or alcohol), we need to create more adolescent treatment centers—currently a major gap in the nation's treatment system.

Of course, a truly successful prevention campaign would require far more ambitious efforts than those described here. It would require making sure that young people—particularly those from disadvantaged backgrounds—have a genuine opportunity to lead fulfilling lives. That, in turn, would require providing them with good schools, decent housing, recreational programs, and meaningful job prospects—urgent priorities all. This, however, takes us far beyond the realm of drug policy. The public-health approach outlined here could not by itself eliminate the drug problem in the United States. It could, however, reduce that problem to a far more manageable scale.

Can it happen? As the careers of Jerome Jaffe and Raphael Flores show, challenging the prevailing wisdom on drugs can be a hazardous enterprise. Yet, as the failures of the drug war become more apparent, it might just become possible to usher in a new, more enlightened era of drug policy, one in which the nation's drug addicts are treated with the care and compassion they deserve.

Notes

A Note on Sources

THIS IS A WORK of both political and street reporting. In chronicling the activities of policymakers, I relied heavily on interviews with past and present officials, government reports, internal memos, congressional testimony, and newspaper articles. My single most important source was Dr. Jerome Jaffe, whom I interviewed dozens of times, both by telephone and in person. After being peppered with questions about what color shirt he was wearing on such-and-such a day thirty years ago, Jaffe decided to retrieve several boxes of documents that he had long ago placed in storage, and I was able to go through them in his townhouse in suburban Baltimore. They were rich in material on the early years of U.S. drug policy, and Jaffe—his memory thus jogged—was able to supply many missing details. What he wasn't able to remember, his wife Faith often could. These documents (referred to in the notes below as the Jaffe Papers) helped supplement those I found in the Nixon collection at the National Archives in College Park, Maryland (referred to as the Nixon Papers). Also valuable were documents that Edward Jay Epstein gathered while researching his book *Agency of Fear* (1977) and which he donated to the special collections department at Boston University's Mugar Memorial Library (the Epstein Papers). For the Carter years, I found many interesting documents at the Carter Library in Atlanta (the Carter Papers).

For data on the extent and nature of America's drug problem, I relied on a number of key sources. The National Household Survey on Drug Abuse (conducted by the U.S. Substance Abuse and Mental Health Services Administration) annually polls thousands of Americans about their drug-taking habits. The University of Michigan's Monitoring the Future study (also known as the National High School Senior Survey) annually questions eighth-, tenth-, and twelfth-graders about their drug use. Every year, the Drug Abuse Warning Network (DAWN) publishes a tally of drug-related visits to hospital emergency rooms. The National Narcotics Intelligence Consumers Committee issues an annual report (*The NNICC Report*) on the supply of illegal drugs in the United States. Data on crime are available in *Crime in the United States,* a yearly compilation of the FBI's Uniform Crime Reports. A good source of information on drug policy, budget, and trends is *The National Drug Control Strategy,* published annually since 1989 by the U.S. Office of National Drug Control Policy. For budget data prior to 1989, I have relied on *Treating Drug Problems,* edited by Dean Gerstein and Henrick Harwood, which on p. 217 offers a concise summary of federal expenditures on treatment, prevention, and criminal justice dating back to 1969. Among those who generously shared of their experiences in the national policy realm were Karst Besteman, Mathea

Falco, Philip Heymann, Mark Kleiman, Dr. Mitchell Rosenthal, and Dr. David Smith.

The street part of my research was, in many ways, far more difficult. Reporting on people immersed in the drug world presents problems of both access and ethics, and I wrestled with them during the four years I spent off and on in Spanish Harlem. In terms of access, I was helped immeasurably by Raphael Flores and his staff: Marvin Yates, Ethel Curtis, and Alain Bigot. My many visits to Hot Line Cares provided an excellent opportunity to meet drug users and learn about their lives. Most of them allowed me to sit in as they were counseled by Raphael and his staff; many agreed to talk about their lives in separate interviews.

Yvonne Hamilton by far shared the most. I met her in the summer of 1993, just after her return from New Hope Manor. Over the next year, I spoke with her regularly as she made her way through the Salvation Army program and then moved to the Bronx and, finally, Spring Valley. In addition to allowing me into her own life, Yvonne introduced me to some of her former cronies. I also met Yvonne's sister Anne, who was still deeply involved with drugs, and her sister Joyce, the schoolteacher. Together, they helped me piece together the saga of the Hamilton family. (Yvonne asked that I not use her real name in order to protect her family; "Yvonne Hamilton" was her street alias. I have also changed the names of some of the other users mentioned in the book, as indicated in the notes. In no case, however, have I changed any details regarding their lives.)

I also met many drug users on my visits to the Bronx-Harlem Needle Exchange, which set up shop every Tuesday afternoon at the corner of 110th Street and Park. Here, injecting-drug users would patiently line up to get clean needles —a wonderful opportunity for an inquiring reporter. In addition, I spent much time hanging out at 110th and Lexington, the center of the neighborhood's drug trade. Usually, there was enough commotion and foot traffic to allow me to stand around without attracting too much attention.

To check out what I was hearing on the street, I frequently spoke with police officers at the 23rd Precinct. When I found the cops and street people in agreement, I considered my information reliable. Generally, the police were very cooperative. Sergeant Steven Ringe, in particular, made himself available. Also helpful were Captain Ronald Welsh, Captain James Tuller, Captain Robert Curley, and Sergeant Ronald Mejia. In the Manhattan D.A.'s Office, Paul Shechtman provided much information and insight. I was particularly fortunate to stumble onto the Sunshine Project just as it was getting under way. Particularly helpful among neighborhood residents were Christiana Pinto, Sylvia Velazquez, Delbert Lewis, and Miriam Lopez-Falcon. For more general information on the New York drug world, I benefited from the insights of Bruce Johnson of the National Development and Research Institute; Richard Curtis of the John Jay School of Criminal Justice; John Galea of the New York State Office of Alcoholism and Substance Abuse Services, and Robert Silbering, special narcotics prosecutor for Manhattan.

IN THE COURSE of my research, questions about money frequently arose. In journalism, there are strict rules against paying sources for information. Anyone attempting to report on the drug world, however, quickly discovers that things aren't so easy. Early on, a recovering addict who had agreed to introduce me to a current user told me that most people involved with drugs, having few resources, expected to be compensated in some way for their cooperation. Actually, as my work progressed, I was struck by how many people did *not* ask for help. Some did, however, and I often found myself open to their requests. Journalism is an inherently exploitive enterprise, with reporters sucking information out of people without providing much in return. Such a relationship becomes particularly uncomfortable when one's sources have few assets aside from the facts of their lives. As long as I felt my subjects were not embellishing their stories in order to enhance their value, I did not mind helping out in small ways. Sometimes, that meant little more than buying them a hamburger or a pack of cigarettes; in other cases, it meant donating a few dollars. Once, when Yvonne's sister Anne asked for some help after having spoken with me for the better part of a morning, I gave her $10; her yelp of astonished pleasure indicated to me that I had overpaid.

Higher-ups in the drug trade, I found, were another matter. Highly mercenary, they will generally part with information only if well compensated. My interviews with Charlie, the Spanish Harlem drug lieutenant, cost me $50 a session; in all, we had four meetings, all but one held at a coffee shop near Columbia University. It was, I felt, a worthwhile investment; most of what he told me checked out with the 23rd Precinct.

In making such payments, my main worry was not getting tainted information, but affecting events. Since one of my main research aims was to see how the system dealt with people without means, I constantly faced situations where being generous could alter outcomes. When Yvonne began looking for work after leaving the Salvation Army, for instance, one of her biggest concerns was her missing teeth. "Who would want to hire someone with no teeth?" she would complain. Eventually, she went to a dentist to be fitted for some dentures, but she lacked the $200 to buy them. As a journalist, my inclination was to sit back and see what happened. But, having been helped so much by Yvonne, I felt it only right to help her in return, and so I gave her the $200. I also bought her occasional dinners and subway tokens, as well as movie passes to help her pass the time during her long months at the Salvation Army.

Other situations posed tougher choices. Accompanying Raphael on his rounds with Carol Ann Sanders, for example, I found myself at one point sitting in a coffee shop on 125th Street, listening to her tell Raphael that, if he didn't give her any money to buy some dope, she was going to head out into the street and turn a trick. Raphael didn't have any money to give; I did. Professionally, the correct course would have been to hang back and see what happened. Personally, though, I felt that I couldn't simply let Carol go off and put herself at risk, and so, when she went outside for a cigarette, I gave Raphael $5 to give her. In doing so, I had a nagging sense that I had somehow contaminated the petri dish. The next day, however, Raphael told me that, despite my contribution, Carol had gone off and turned a trick anyway. The incident, I think, shows just how unlikely it is that dispensing a few bucks here and there will change the ingrained habits of hard-core drug users.

INTRODUCTION: THE PROBLEM

9 Since 1981: *The National Drug Control Strategy, 1998: Budget Summary,* Office of National Drug Control Policy (ONDCP), p. 5.

9 In 1996, more than 1.5 million: *The National Drug Control Strategy, 1998,* ONDCP, p. 17.

9 The nation's state and federal prisons: *Correctional Populations in the United States, 1995,* U.S. Department of Justice, May 1997, pp. 10–11.

9 cocaine is cheaper: According to *The National Drug Control Strategy, 1998,*

the price per pure gram of cocaine declined from $162.17 in 1986 to $94.52 in 1996, while the purity of heroin went from 6.73 percent in 1981 to 41.48 percent in 1996. (p. 88)

9 the number of cocaine-related visits: *Year-End Preliminary Estimates from the 1996 Drug Abuse Warning Network,* U.S. Department of Health and Human Services, November 1997, p. 49.

10 a sharp rise in alcohol use: *Alcohol and Health,* 9th Special Report to the U.S. Congress, U.S. Department of Health and Human Services, June 1997, p. 4. See also Mark A. R. Kleiman, *Against Excess: A Drug Policy for Results* (Basic Books, 1992), p. 102. Prohibition, Kleiman writes, "seems, despite an enforcement effort that suffered from small resources, great incompetence, and systematic corruption, to have reduced the quantity of alcohol consumed, and the number of persons dying of chronic alcohol abuse, by between one-third and two-thirds."

10 doctors routinely began prescribing Valium: Robert Reinhold, "U.S. Wins Agreement on Warning to Doctors on Use of Tranquilizers," *New York Times,* July 11, 1980, p. A-1; Robert Reinhold, "Tranquilizer Prescriptions Drop Sharply; So Does Reported Incidence of Abuse," *New York Times,* September 9, 1980, p. C-1.

10 Drugs, the harm reductionists argue: For a good summary of this approach, see Ethan A. Nadlemann, "Commonsense Drug Policy," *Foreign Affairs,* January–February 1998, pp. 111–126.

10 Needle-exchange programs, for instance: See, for instance, "Review of University of California Report on Needle Exchange and Recommendations on Needle Exchange," memo prepared by the U.S. Centers for Disease Control and Prevention. "We believe," the memo states, "that the benefits of NEPs [needle-exchange programs] as a component of a comprehensive HIV prevention program for drug users exceed the theoretical risks of such programs. We conclude that the ban on Federal funding of NEPs should be lifted. . . ." (p. 2) The memo was part of a package of documents ("The Clinton Administration's Internal Reviews of Research on Needle Exchange Programs") released by the Drug Policy Foundation, March 7, 1995. See also *Needle Exchange Programs: Research Suggests Promise as an AIDS Prevention Strategy,* General Accounting Office (GAO/ HRD-93-60), March 1993.

11 apparent to anyone who visits: My assessment is based on regular visits I made to a program run by the Bronx-Harlem Needle Exchange at the corner of 110th Street and Park Avenue in Spanish Harlem.

11 In fact, teenage drug use: Monitoring the Future study, University of Michigan, results released December 18, 1997.

12 there are 3.6 million: Albert Woodward et al., "The Drug Abuse Treatment Gap: Recent Estimates," *Health Care Financing Review,* Spring 1997, pp. 5–17. The Office of National Drug Control Policy uses this same estimate. (Hard-core use is generally defined as cocaine use once or twice a week in every week during the past year, or heroin use on more than ten days during the past month.)

12 they consume about three-fourths: William Rhodes et al., *What America's Users Spend on Illegal Drugs, 1988–1995,* ONDCP, fall 1997, p. 6.

12 no great epidemic of chronic drug use: *National Household Survey on Drug Abuse: Population Estimates, 1996,* U.S. Department of Health and Human Services, July 1997, pp. 2, 29, 103. According to the survey, just 0.8 percent of the 18,000 people polled in 1996 had used cocaine in the past month, and a mere 0.2 percent had used heroin in the past year.

12 The research data consistently show: Woodward et al., "The Drug Abuse Treatment Gap"; on p. 15, the article states that "drug abusers who need special-

ized treatment" include "a disproportionate number of men, poor people, and people who report that they have committed crime, are not employed, have no health insurance, and receive welfare assistance." A similar assessment is offered by Dana Eser Hunt and William Rhodes in "Characteristics of Heavy Cocaine Users, Including Polydrug Use, Criminal Activity, and Health Risks," Abt Associates, Cambridge, Massachusetts, December 14, 1992, an unpublished paper commissioned by ONDCP. Interview with William Rhodes of Abt. In an intensive study of the hard-core users in one location (Cook County, Illinois), Abt found that about three-quarters were black. (*A Plan for Estimating the Number of "Hardcore" Drug Users in the United States,* ONDCP, fall 1997, p. iv)

According to the summer 1997 edition of ONDCP's *Pulse Check: National Trends in Drug Abuse,* "the majority of heroin abusers are within the traditional, older cohort of long-term users. . . . However, some areas report that there are more new, young heroin users. These new users include college students and suburban kids, but the majority are inner city youth." The spring 1996 issue of *Pulse Check* reports that heavy cocaine and crack use "is becoming more concentrated in a core of older, regular users. Several sources . . . characterize the population as older, established drug users who live mainly in inner city areas."

The links between poverty and drug addiction have been observed since at least the 1950s. In Isidor Chein et al., *The Road to H: Narcotics, Delinquency, and Social Policy* (Basic Books, 1964), a classic study of young heroin users in New York in the 1950s, the authors report that "drug use among juveniles is most frequently found in the most deprived areas of the city. . . . The areas of high incidence of drug use are characterized by the high incidence of impoverished families, great concentration of the most discriminated against and least urbanized ethnic groups, and high incidence of disrupted families, and other forms of human misery." (p. 10)

For a good summary of the research literature on the links between poverty and drug abuse, see Elliott Currie's *Reckoning,* esp. chap. 2, "Roots of the Drug Crisis," and chap. 3, "Lessons Ignored." "The link between drug abuse and deprivation is one of the strongest in forty years of careful research," Currie writes. (p. 77)

Part One: THE STREET, 1992

1: THE STREET WORKER

17 Lydia Botero: A pseudonym.

18 New York had just 500: Information provided by Richard Chady, public information officer, New York State Office of Alcoholism and Substance Abuse Services (OASAS).

18 the Beth Israel Medical Center: Interview with William Toler, chief physician assistant for the department of medicine and chemical dependency, Beth Israel.

21 On almost every social index: According to the 1992 *Annual Report on Social Indicators,* published by the New York City Department of City Planning, Manhattan's Community District 11, which encompasses Spanish Harlem, had a teen birth rate of 17.4 percent, an infant mortality rate of 15.0, and a public assistance rate of 28.9 percent. In Manhattan, only Community District 10, encompassing Central Harlem, ranked lower.

22 Every day, an estimated 5,000: Interview with Captain Ronald Welsh, Manhattan Narcotics Enforcement Unit, New York City Housing Police.

23 New York in the early 1990s: *Report and Recommendations to the Mayor on Drug Abuse in New York City* (the Katzenbach Report), May 1990, p. 25.

23 the city had some 55,000: Information provided by OASAS.

23 about 3,500 people: "Waiting List Survey," National Association of State Alcohol and Drug Abuse Directors, Washington, D.C., May 21, 1993.

23 drug treatment was the Balkans: *Report and Recommendations to the Mayor on Drug Abuse in New York City*, pp. 7, 27–28, 54. For a good description of the barriers that addicts face in trying to enter treatment, see Barry Bearak, "Road to Detox: Do Not Enter," *Los Angeles Times*, September 30, 1992, p. A-1, the last of a four-part series about a New York shooting gallery.

24 Carol Ann Sanders: A pseudonym.

27 hospitals had begun reducing: Information provided by OASAS; interview with John Coppola, executive director of the New York State Association of Alcoholism and Substance Abuse Providers.

28 (Medical studies have found): See Jerome Jaffe, ed., *Encyclopedia of Drugs and Alcohol* (Macmillan Library Reference USA, 1995), vol. 1, pp. 229–230.

28 detox by itself: Dean Gerstein and Henrick J. Harwood, eds., *Treating Drug Problems*, Institute of Medicine (National Academy Press, 1990), p. 176. "Consistently, *without subsequent treatment*, researchers have found no effects from detoxification that are discernibly superior to those achieved by untreated withdrawal in terms of reducing subsequent drug-taking behavior and especially relapse to dependence," the book notes.

28 only 14 percent of detox clients: Ibid.

28 In New York, hospitals are reimbursed: See Joseph Berger, "Cost-Cutting Plan Limits Choices for Revolving-Door Addicts," *New York Times*, June 17, 1997, p. B-1.

2: HARD CORE

29 Nancy Hamilton: This, and all other names in the Hamilton family, are pseudonyms.

32 From the start, crack found: For more on this, see my article "Crack's Destructive Sprint Across America," *New York Times Magazine*, October 1, 1989, pp. 38ff. See also "Crack Cocaine; Overview 1989," an unpublished report of the U.S. Drug Enforcement Administration, p. 13: "Although the problem has spread to rural and suburban areas, crack cocaine remains a predominantly inner-city, urban phenomenon that is mainly confined to minority sections."

32 Far more than heroin: Center on Addiction and Substance Abuse (CASA), "Substance Abuse and the American Woman," June 1996, pp. 38–39. "Some 40 percent of all crack addicts are women," this report states. "Experts attribute its popularity among women to its cheap price, their preference for smoking a drug rather than injecting one, and the sense of confidence that crack temporarily delivers." Black women, it notes, "are more than twice as likely as white women to be regular cocaine users . . . and are 14 times likelier to use crack cocaine during pregnancy."

32 The early tone was set by *Newsweek:* "Kids and Cocaine," March 17, 1986, pp. 58–65; "Crack and Crime," June 16, 1986, pp. 15–22; " 'Saying No,' " August 11, 1986, pp. 14–20.

32 (BEHIND GIRL'S CHAINING): *New York Times,* September 20, 1991, p. A-1.

33 "The Social Pharmacology of Smokeable Cocaine": John Morgan and Lynn Zimmer, "The Social Pharmacology of Smokeable Cocaine: Not All It's Cracked Up to Be," in Craig Reinarman and Harry G. Levine, eds., *Crack in America: Demon Drugs and Social Justice* (University of California Press, 1997), pp. 154–155.

33 Dan Baum, a former reporter: *Smoke and Mirrors: The War on Drugs and the Politics of Failure* (Little, Brown, 1996), p. 70.

37 "Today, many doubt": Morgan and Zimmer, "The Social Pharmacology of Smokeable Cocaine," p. 143.

37 *Cocaine Changes:* Dan Waldorf, Craig Reinarman, and Sheigla Murphy, *Cocaine Changes: The Experience of Using and Quitting* (Temple University Press, 1991), pp. 11, 107, 113–114, 116–118, 124, 139.

38 their reports offer a chilling look: The police reports were part of the management file on the apartment, which I was allowed to examine.

39 "Crack and Homicide in New York City": Paul J. Goldstein, et al., "Crack and Homicide in New York City," *Contemporary Drug Problems,* 16, no. 4 (Winter 1989), pp. 651–686. (This article is reprinted in Reinarman and Levine, *Crack in America,* pp. 113–130.)

39 Spunt concluded: Interview with Barry Spunt. See also Paul J. Goldstein, "Impact of Drug-Related Violence," *Public Health Reports* 102, no. 6 (November–December 1987), pp. 625–627.

39 As Goldstein noted in one study: "Drugs and Violent Crime," in N. A. Weiner and Marvin E. Wolfgang, eds., *Pathways to Criminal Violence* (Sage Publications, 1989), pp. 141ff.

40 the city had to go through a long series: Interview with Carol Fisler of the New York City Housing Authority.

41 George Soros's Lindesmith Center: Lindesmith Center, "Cocaine and Pregnancy," 1996.

41 The idea that babies exposed to crack: CASA, "Substance Abuse and the American Woman," pp. 84–87.

41 crack—more than almost any other factor—nullifies: Ibid., p. 91: "Perhaps more than any other drug, including heroin, crack cocaine becomes the primary 'relationship' in the addict's life at the expense of any instincts about her welfare and that of her children."

41 In New York, for instance, the introduction of crack: Data provided by New York City's Child Welfare Administration Office of Management Analysis. See also Peter Kerr, "Crack Addiction: The Tragic Toll on Women and Their Children," *New York Times,* February 9, 1987, p. B-1; and Gina Kolata, "In Cities, Poor Families Are Dying of Crack," *New York Times,* August 11, 1989, p. A-1.

42 Yvonne's neglect of Gerald: This is described in a Housing Police report in the management file on Apartment 4H.

43 New York State's drug laws: *The Nation's Toughest Drug Law: Evaluating the New York Experience* (The Association of the Bar of the City of New York, 1977), pp. 1–5. See also Human Rights Watch, "Cruel and Usual: Disproportionate Sentences for New York Drug Offenders," March 1997. "Sentences for drug offenders in New York state are among the most punitive in the country," this report states on p. 2. Interview with Paul Shechtman, formerly an aide to Manhattan District Attorney Robert Morgenthau.

43 a massive prison-building boom: Rex Smith, "New York's Prison Boom," *Newsday,* October 8, 1990, p. 6.

43 the number of inmates had kept pace: Statistics provided by the New York State Department of Correctional Services.

43 nearly one of every two new inmates: "Drug Offenders Committed to State Prison," New York State Department of Correctional Services, 1991, p. 1.

44 "To sentence a low-level guy": Interview with Judge Herbert Adlerberg. The actual cost of keeping an inmate in a New York State prison is about $25,000 a year.

45 two social workers sent a memo: This memo was in the management file of Apartment 17E.

3: PRIORITIES

49 Treatment Outcome Prospective Study: Robert L. Hubbard et al., *Drug Abuse Treatment: A National Study of Effectiveness* (University of North Carolina Press, 1989), pp. 7–10, 94, 102–104, 124–125, 128, 164.

49 An effort to fill this gap: C. Peter Rydell and Susan S. Everingham, *Controlling Cocaine: Supply Versus Demand Programs* (RAND, 1994), pp. xii–xix, 99–103. Interviews with Susan Everingham and Jonathan Caulkins of RAND.

50 Treatment is so effective: Gerstein and Harwood's *Treating Drug Problems* reports a similar effect for methadone. "Methadone maintenance," it states, "pays for itself on the day it is delivered, and posttreatment effects are an economic bonus." (p. 152)

51 A more recent study: "The National Treatment Improvement Evaluation Study, Preliminary Report: The Persistent Effects of Substance Abuse Treatment —One Year Later," U.S. Department of Health and Human Services, September 1996, pp. 1–2.

51 Every study of drug treatment: For a good summary of the research on the effectiveness of treatment, see Gerstein and Harwood, *Treating Drug Problems*, chap. 5, "The Effectiveness of Treatment," pp. 132–199.

51 Applying a common rule of thumb: Interview with John Coppola, New York State Association of Alcoholism and Substance Abuse Providers.

52 Charles Silberman spent a full day: Interview with Charles Silberman.

53 In 1989, the number of drug arrests: Cited in "Removing Drugs from Our Neighborhoods and Schools," speech by Rudolph Giuliani, October 1, 1997.

53 The group's report: *Report and Recommendations to the Mayor on Drug Abuse in New York City,* May 1990, pp. 2, 13, 25, 30, 31, 78.

54 DAVE, DO SOMETHING: *New York Post,* September 7, 1990, p. 1.

54 "Safe Streets, Safe City": "Safe Streets, Safe City: An Omnibus Criminal Justice Program for the City of New York," summary, New York City, Office of the Mayor, 1990. See also Ralph Blumenthal, "Dinkins Proposes Record Expansion of Police Forces," *New York Times,* October 3, 1991, p. A-1.

4: THE POLICE

55 "I can't tell you": Interview with Miriam Lopez-Falcon.

56 Among those she approached: Interview with Christiana Pinto.

56 Sylvia Velazquez: Interview with Sylvia Velazquez.

56 "We can build all the jails": Charles Rangel, statement before the Committee on Government Operations, U.S. House of Representatives, September 25, 1991.

56 He was particularly insistent: See, for instance, the Select Committee on Narcotics Abuse, *Annual Report for the Year 1989,* p. 90.

57 Rangel faithfully went along: See, for instance, Select Committee on Narcotics Abuse, *Annual Report for the Year 1990,* pp. 53–54, 128. The GAO report, *Methadone Maintenance—Some Treatment Programs Are Not Effective; Greater Federal Oversight Needed* (GAO/HRD-90-104), was released in March 1990.

57 On the subject of street-level: Interview with Charles Rangel.

57 Young Adam: See Todd S. Purdum, "Once Again, It's Rangel vs. Powell in Harlem," *New York Times,* August 9, 1994, p. A-1; interview with Adam Clayton Powell IV.

57 In June 1992, letters: Copies of these letters were provided by Charles Rangel's office.

58 Outwardly, Steve Ringe seemed: Interview with Steve Ringe.

59 the Two-Three was in the process: Ibid.

59 Community policing seemed: See *Policing New York City in the 1990s,* New York City Police Department, January 1991, pp. 53–54.

59 Taking over a force: Ruth Rendon, "After 5 Years, Houston's 1st Black Police Chief Is Still Firmly in Charge," *Los Angeles Times,* October 4, 1987, p. 1.

5: BUYERS AND SELLERS

65 Charlie: A pseudonym.

68 Dave: A pseudonym.

69 Luisa: A pseudonym.

72 an informed estimate comes from Walter Arsenault: Interview with Walter Arsenault.

6: EXPLOSION

73 police pressure was an important factor: See Gerstein and Harwood, *Treating Drug Problems,* p. 112: "Pressure from the criminal justice system is the strongest motivation reported for seeking public treatment."

73 he began making weekly visits: I went with Raphael to Rikers Island three times between August and October 1992.

76 she was in a place: After several tumultuous weeks at Hill House, Shondelle, alas, would jump out of a second-floor window and make her way to a local crackhouse, where she would be picked up by the police. Returning to New York, she would resume her freewheeling ways.

Part Two: WASHINGTON

7: APPRENTICESHIP

85 set up a Narcotic Advisory Council: Interview with James Moran, chief judge of the U.S. District Court for the Northern District of Illinois, formerly an Illinois state assemblyman who helped set up the Narcotic Advisory Council; "Report of the Illinois Narcotic Advisory Council to the Seventy-fifth General Assem-

bly," May 1967; "Narcotic Advisory Council State Activities," State of Illinois Department of Mental Health, January 31, 1966.

85 federal narcotics hospital in Lexington, Kentucky: David Courtwright, Herman Joseph, and Don DesJarlais, eds., *Addicts Who Survived: An Oral History of Narcotic Use in America, 1923–1965* (University of Tennessee Press, 1989), pp. 296–297; Raymond M. Glasscote et al., *The Treatment of Drug Abuse: Programs, Problems, Prospects* (Joint Information Service of the American Psychiatric Service and the National Association for Mental Health, 1972), p. 24.

86 Drug policy was the preserve: See Courtwright, Joseph, and DesJarlais, *Addicts Who Survived*, pp. 11–13, and David F. Musto, *The American Disease: Origins of Narcotic Control* (Oxford University Press, 1973), pp. 210–214. According to Musto, "These two federal statutes of 1951 and 1956 represent the high point of federal punitive action against narcotics." (p. 231) For a more extended discussion, see John C. McWilliams, *The Protectors: Harry J. Anslinger and the Federal Bureau of Narcotics, 1930–1962* (University of Delaware Press, 1990), pp. 14, 49–59.

86 After the election of John Kennedy: Musto, *The American Disease*, pp. 237–239.

86 For names, they turned: Interview with James Moran.

86 Jerry Jaffe was a specialist in psychopharmacology: Interview with Jerome Jaffe. Jaffe discusses his early career in a speech, "The Nathan B. Eddy Lecture: Science, Policy, Happenstance," 1984.

88 Then, in early 1965: Interview with Vincent Dole. See also Nat Hentoff's book about Marie Nyswander, *A Doctor Among the Addicts* (Rand McNally, 1968), pp. 13–15, 111–116. For an early report on Dole's findings, see Vincent P. Dole and Marie Nyswander, "A Medical Treatment for Diacetylmorphine (Heroin) Addiction," *Journal of the American Medical Association*, August 23, 1965, pp. 646–650.

89 On Staten Island: "Daytop Past & Present," *Daytopics*, 25th Anniversary Issue, pp. 4–8; Glasscote et al., *The Treatment of Drug Abuse*, pp. 83–101.

89 they became intensely competitive: Drug Abuse Council, *The Facts About "Drug Abuse"* (Free Press, 1980), p. 103.

90 "The eagerness with which": Jaffe's comment is contained in "The Nathan B. Eddy Lecture." His experience with Dr. Alfred Gilman is also described there.

91 The council's final report: "Report of the Illinois Narcotic Advisory Council," pp. 11, 21.

91 The Illinois Drug Abuse Program had begun: Information on IDAP came from interviews with Jerome and Faith Jaffe, Edward Senay, David Deitch, Arlene Lisner, Claude Rhodes, Patrick Hughes, and Jeanie Peake. Also, in April 1995, I visited old IDAP sites with Jaffe and Michael Darcy, a former Gateway resident who went on to become president of Gateway, which today has a multimillion-dollar budget and facilities in four states. The single best published description of IDAP is in Glasscote et al., *The Treatment of Drug Abuse*, pp. 127–151. See also Edward Senay, "Multimodality Programming in Illinois: Evolution of a Public Health Concept," in Joyce H. Lowinson and Pedro Ruiz, eds., *Substance Abuse: Clinical Problems and Perspectives* (Williams & Wilkins, 1981), pp. 396–401, and Tom Watts, "Methadone—Hope for Drug Addicts?" *Chicago Today*, November 16, 1980, p. 33.

92 a detox ward at Billings: Patrick Hughes et al., "Developing Inpatient Services for Community-Based Treatment of Narcotic Addiction," in *Archives of General Psychiatry*, September 1971, pp. 278–283.

92 Chicago's first therapeutic community: See Robert A. Kajdan and Edward C. Senay, "Modified Therapeutic Communities for Youth," *Journal of Psychedelic Drugs,* July–September 1976, pp. 206–214.

93 therapeutic community at Tinley Park: For a good description, see Glasscote et al., *The Treatment of Drug Abuse,* pp. 145–148. See also Jaffe, "The Nathan B. Eddy Lecture."

94 The number of clients with jobs: Glasscote et al., *The Treatment of Drug Abuse,* p. 142.

94 IDAP's work on the epidemiology: Interviews with Patrick Hughes and Claude Rhodes. Hughes's work is described in Patrick H. Hughes and Jerome H. Jaffe, "The Heroin Copping Area," in *Archives of General Psychiatry,* May 1971, pp. 394ff; Patrick H. Hughes, Edward C. Senay, and Richard Parker, "The Medical Management of a Heroin Epidemic," *Archives of General Psychiatry,* November 1972, pp. 585–591; and Patrick H. Hughes, *Behind the Wall of Respect: Community Experiments in Heroin Addiction Control* (University of Chicago, 1977).

96 a call from the White House: Interviews with Jaffe and Jeffrey Donfeld.

8: To the White House

97 If there was one word: Interview with Jeffrey Donfeld.

97 During the 1968 campaign: Speech delivered September 16, 1968, at the Anaheim Convention Center, transcript provided by the Richard Nixon Library.

98 Wilkinson would launch: Interview with Donfeld; memo from Bud Wilkinson, "A Preliminary Plan for Action," February 5, 1970, Epstein Papers.

98 the nation's governors: Carroll Kilpatrick, "Nixon Stresses Education in Drug Fight," *Washington Post,* December 4, 1969, p. 1.

98 researchers studying them: Richard Severo, "Methadone Is Credited with Improvement in Behavior," *New York Times,* May 27, 1970, p. 1.

98 In 1969, the federal drug budget: Strategy Council on Drug Abuse, *Federal Strategy for Drug Abuse and Drug Traffic Prevention, 1973,* 1973, pp. 76, 129–132. See also Domestic Council memo, "Drugs," July 15, 1970, Nixon Papers.

98 President Nixon nearly doubled: White House Fact Sheet, "Major Nixon Administration Actions in the Campaign Against Drug Abuse Since June 17, 1971," December 3, 1971, Nixon Papers.

98 At the time, most of the heroin: Alfred W. McCoy, *The Politics of Heroin: CIA Complicity in the Global Drug Trade* (Lawrence Hill, 1991), pp. 44–49, 63–64; "Booming Traffic in Drugs," *U.S. News & World Report,* December 7, 1970, pp. 40–44.

99 "I feel very strongly": Nixon memo to Kissinger et al., September 22, 1969, Nixon Papers.

99 Nixon had frequently raised the issue: Theodore White, *The Making of the President, 1968* (Atheneum, 1969), pp. 188–223.

99 At an early meeting: Epstein, *Agency of Fear,* pp. 64–65.

99 Nixon himself had singled out: "D.C. Should Not Stand for Disorder and Crime," statement of Richard Nixon, June 22, 1968, supplied by the Richard Nixon Library.

99 a presidential secretary: Leonard Downie, Jr., "President Pledges War on D.C. Crime," *Washington Post,* January 28, 1969, p. A-1.

99 Nixon announced a package: Robert L. Asher and Leonard Downie, "Nixon Details Plan to Make District Safe," *Washington Post,* February 1, 1969, p.

1; "Statement Outlining Actions and Recommendations for the District of Columbia," *Public Papers of the Presidents of the United States, 1969* (Government Printing Office, 1971), pp. 40–48.

100 Nixon would call up: Interview with John Ehrlichman; see also the transcript of an interview of Egil Krogh by Edward Jay Epstein, Epstein Papers.

100 he assembled about him: John Ehrlichman, *Witness to Power: The Nixon Years* (Simon & Schuster, 1982), pp. 82–84.

100 Krogh was the White House's Mr. Fix-it: Interview with Egil Krogh, Jr.; Craig Walters, "The Agony of Egil Krogh," *Washingtonian*, May 1974, pp. 60ff; J. Anthony Lukas, *Nightmare: The Underside of the Nixon Years* (Viking, 1976), pp. 73–74; Krogh-Epstein interview, Epstein Papers.

101 it was natural for him to look: Interview with Krogh; Krogh-Epstein interview, Epstein Papers.

101 he had gone to Paris: Interviews with Krogh and John Coleman, a DEA (then BNDD) agent who was stationed in Paris at the time; memo from Egil Krogh to Frank Cash, December 22, 1969, Nixon Papers.

101 treatment expert named Robert DuPont: Interviews with Krogh and Robert DuPont.

102 Of the two hundred interviewed: Interview with DuPont; Robert L. DuPont, "Heroin Addiction Treatment and Crime Reduction," *American Journal of Psychiatry*, January 1992, p. 857.

102 the NTA soon had more than 2,000 slots: "Facts About NTA," Government of the District of Columbia, December 3, 1970.

102 Donfeld summarized them: "Different Strokes for Different Folkes [*sic*]," June 19, 1970, Epstein Papers.

103 reports Krogh was getting: Krogh memo to Ehrlichman, "Status Report: D.C. Narcotics Program," September 14, 1970, Nixon Papers.

103 Ehrlichman felt far more constrained: Interview with John Ehrlichman.

103 Krogh convinced him: Interview with Krogh; memo from Krogh to Ehrlichman, untitled, October 29, 1970, Nixon Papers.

104 NIMH had shown little interest: Interviews with Jerome Jaffe and Krogh.

104 Moreover, NIMH: Drug Abuse Council, *The Facts About "Drug Abuse,"* p. 33.

104 Donfeld was sent to recruit him: The terms Jaffe agreed to are described in a November 4, 1970, memo, Jaffe Papers.

104 Ignoring the White House's request: Memo from Donfeld to Krogh, December 17, 1970, Epstein Papers.

104 the finished product: "Approaches to a National Policy and Program on Narcotics and Drug Abuse," pp. 3, 4, 63–64, 117, Jaffe Papers.

105 The Jaffe report: "Report of an Ad Hoc White House Committee on the Treatment and Prevention of Drug Addiction and Drug Abuse," pp. 4, 13, 22–25, 102–103, Jaffe Papers.

105 a two-paragraph note from Richard Nixon: January 6, 1971, Jaffe Papers.

105 Elvis Presley had suddenly appeared: Presley's handwritten note, plus other relevant documents, are among the Nixon Papers at the National Archives. Krogh describes his encounter with Presley in his own book, *The Day Elvis Met Nixon* (Pejama Press, 1994), a short, droll account of the event.

106 While the nation's crime rate: *Crime in the United States, 1970* (Government Printing Office, 1971), p. 65. See also Christopher Lydon, "F.B.I. Says Crime Rose 11% in 1970," *New York Times*, March 29, 1971, p. 1.

106 Washington's had fallen: *Crime in the United States, 1970,* p. 185. See also Paul W. Valentine and Alfred E. Lewis, "Major Crime in City Hits 5-Year Low," *Washington Post,* February 24, 1972, p. A-1.

106 In interviews, Chief Jerry Wilson: Bob Woodward and Claudia Levy, "Wilson Sees Crime Rate Here Declining All Year," *Washington Post,* April 18, 1972, p. C-1; Valentine and Lewis, "Major Crime in City Hits 5-Year Low," *Washington Post,* February 24, 1972, p. A-1. In "Cutting the Crime Rate: How Nation's Capital Does It," *U.S. News & World Report,* April 10, 1972, Wilson is quoted as saying that "it's definitely true that reducing dependence on drugs lessens reliance on crime to support a drug habit. There is no question that narcotics treatment and prevention programs are necessary to reduce street crimes." (p. 25)

106 the Narcotics Treatment Administration was treating: Robert L. DuPont, "Heroin Addiction Treatment and Crime Reduction," *American Journal of Psychiatry,* January 1972, p. 858.

106 he asked Donfeld to draft: "Domestic Council Summary Option Paper on a National Drug Program," March 19, 1971, Jaffe Papers.

106 Interestingly, John Mitchell: Interview with Krogh.

106 Elliot Richardson, the secretary of health: Memo to the president, "Domestic Council Decision Paper on Narcotic Addiction and Drug Abuse," March 19, 1971, Jaffe Papers.

106 Krogh arranged for a showdown: The agenda for the meeting is summarized in a White House memo, "Drug Initiatives," April 27, 1971, Epstein Papers; interview with Donfeld.

107 Vietnam had been flooded: "Armed Forces: As Common as Chewing Gum," *Time,* March 1, 1971, pp. 14–15; "South Viet Nam: Another Sort of H-Bomb," *Time,* April 19, 1971, pp. 21–22.

107 Steele, back from his trip: His visit to the White House is described in a memo from Max Friedersdorf to John Nidecker, April 29, 1971, Nixon Papers.

107 Krogh was not surprised: Interview with Krogh; Memo from Krogh to Ehrlichman, "Additional Funding for Narcotics Suppression—South Vietnam," November 6, 1970, Nixon Papers.

107 Jerome Jaffe in early May 1971: Interview with Jaffe. His thinking on Vietnam is described in "Looking Back Around the Corner," a speech published in *Problems of Drug Dependency, 1976,* National Academy of Sciences, and in "Footnotes in the Evolution of the American National Response: Some Little Known Aspects of the First American Strategy for Drug Abuse and Drug Traffic Prevention," *British Journal of Addiction,* June 1987, pp. 587–599.

108 Krogh sent a seven-page memo: "Drugs," May 14, 1971, Epstein Papers.

108 G.I. HEROIN ADDICTION: Alvin Shuster, *New York Times,* May 16, 1971, p. 1.

108 The White House's nervousness: Memo from Rumsfeld to Krogh, May 25, 1971, Nixon Papers.

109 Steele's report was blunt: "The World Heroin Problem: Report of Special Study Mission," May 1971. See also Felix Belair, Jr., "House Unit Cites Rise in G.I. Drug Use," *New York Times,* May 26, 1971, p. 14.

109 On May 26, he and Krogh: Memo from Dwight Chapin to H. R. Haldeman, May 26, 1971, Nixon Papers.

109 While Nixon had spoken: Interview with John Ehrlichman. An interesting look at Nixon's attitude toward drugs is provided in a May 26, 1971, entry in H. R. Haldeman's *Haldeman Diaries* (Putnam, 1994), p. 292: "He made the point earlier this morning that he wants to put out a statement on marijuana that's really

strong, as he said, one that tears the ass out of them. He also commented on the question of why all the Jews seem to be the ones that are for liberalizing the regulations on marijuana."

109 at the May 28 meeting: Krogh's agenda is outlined in a May 27, 1971, memo to Ehrlichman, Nixon Papers. In *Witness to Power,* Ehrlichman notes that drugs were one of the areas of domestic policy (along with abortion, race, aid to parochial schools, labor legislation, crime, welfare, and taxes) on which Nixon insisted on personally making all decisions. (p. 207)

110 Ehrlichman's shorthand notes: Nixon Papers.

110 even Nixon was aware: This is also apparent in a memo Nixon sent to Krogh on June 2, 1971, in which he asked Krogh to find the percentage of heroin addicts who started out on marijuana. "That clown Brown at the National Institute of Mental Health should even have this number," Nixon wrote. (Jaffe Papers)

110 A briefing had been scheduled: Jaffe describes this meeting in "Footnotes in the Evolution of the American National Response," p. 593.

111 According to Donfeld's notes: Memo for the president's file, July 2, 1971, Epstein Papers.

111 the French government had agreed: Interview with Krogh. The meeting of ambassadors at the White House is described in a memo from Krogh for the president's file, July 26, 1971, Jaffe Papers.

111 it seemed receptive to the idea: Epstein, *Agency of Fear,* p. 91.

112 Nixon escorted Jaffe to the press room: Nixon's statement is in "Remarks About an Intensified Program for Drug Abuse Prevention and Control," *Public Papers of the Presidents, 1971,* pp. 738–739.

9: THE GREAT EXPERIMENT

113 According to a June 1971 Gallup poll: "Poll Finds Drugs No. 3 Issue in U.S.," *New York Times,* June 17, 1971, p. 29.

113 nearly a hundred people were dying: "514 Addicts Died in City from Jan. 1 to June 17," *New York Times,* June 19, 1971, p. 40.

113 in Detroit seven people: "Heroin Shooting War," *Time,* June 21, 1971, p. 18; "The New Public Enemy No. 1," *Time,* June 28, 1971, p. 20.

113 "Each returned planeload": "The New Public Enemy No. 1," *Time,* June 28, 1971, p. 20.

113 Jaffe was clear about his priorities: At the June 17, 1971, press conference, Jaffe said, "Treatment ought to be available to all people who want it when they want it." See Av Westin and Stephanie Shaffer, *Heroes and Heroin: The Shocking Story of Drug Addiction in the Military* (Pocket Books, 1972), p. 190. The estimated number of heroin addicts is contained in *Drug Abuse Office, Control and Treatment Act of 1971,* a report of the Senate Committee on Labor and Public Welfare, November 24, 1971, pp. 2–3.

114 "It is plain that the shots": "NIMH Loses Control Over Drug Problems; Jaffe to Lead Attack Against 'Public Enemy #1,' " *Mental Health Scope,* Washington, D.C., Mid-June 1971, p. 1.

114 responsibility for the drug issue: *Annual Report,* 1973, SAODAP, p. 36.

114 At midnight on June 17: Memo from Melvin Laird to secretaries of the military departments, June 17, 1971, Nixon Papers. Laird's action on the Uniform Code of Military Justice is summarized in "Report to Congress on Section 501— Title V—Public Law 92-129," Department of Defense, Control of Drug and Alcohol Dependency, 1971, p. 2, Jaffe Papers.

114 With many questions remaining in the program: A good description of the early problems in the Vietnam program is contained in "A Bio-Behavioral and Public Health Approach to a Heroin Epidemic Among Military Personnel," a speech by Jerome Jaffe to the American Psychiatric Association, May 2, 1972, Jaffe Papers. For a thorough description of the Vietnam program, see Westin and Shaffer, *Heroes and Heroin.*

115 Krogh's trip went well: Interview with Egil Krogh.

115 a deal in which the Turks: John Herbers, "Nixon Says Turks Agree to Ban the Opium Poppy," *New York Times,* July 1, 1971, p. 1; Dana Adams Schmidt, "Poppy-Ban Cost to U.S. Disclosed," *New York Times,* November 21, 1971, p. 17; interview with Krogh.

115 When Jaffe and his party arrived: Interviews with Jerome Jaffe and Andrew Mecca, then administrative officer of the Vietnam drug program (later director of drug rehabilitation for the state of California). On reports of buying clean urine, see Westin and Shaffer, *Heroes and Heroin,* p. 206.

115 the FRAT machine: This is described in "Unmasking Addicts Among the Troops," *Medical World News,* July 16, 1971.

115 Of the 22,000 servicemen tested: John Herbers, "4.5% in G.I. Test Are Heroin Users," *New York Times,* July 18, 1971, p. 6.

115 stopped by the western White House: See Westin and Shaffer, *Heroes and Heroin,* pp. 223–228; interviews with Jaffe and Krogh.

116 Ehrlichman asked Krogh: Interviews with Krogh and John Ehrlichman.

116 he had a thousand details: Interview with Jaffe; "A Bio-Behavioral and Public Health Approach to a Heroin Epidemic Among Military Personnel," Jaffe Papers.

116 Krogh was leading: Interview with Krogh. A good account of Krogh's involvement with the Plumbers is in Lukas, *Nightmare,* pp. 68–108. See also "The 'Bag Job' at Dr. Fielding's," *Newsweek,* March 18, 1974, pp. 31–34, 39; and G. Gordon Liddy, *Will* (St. Martin's, 1980), pp. 199–205, 228, 234.

117 Jaffe was free to hire: Interviews with Jaffe and Paul Perito.

117 "On the day I was confirmed": Interview with Perito.

117 the legislation to authorize his office: Interviews with Jaffe, Krogh, and Perito. See also Dana Adams Schmidt, "New Drug Abuse Chief Is Told He Doesn't Have Enough Power," *New York Times,* June 29, 1971, p. 14; "White House and Senators Deadlocked Over Scope of Office on Drug Abuse," *New York Times,* November 1, 1971, p. 36; and memo from Paul Perito to Egil Krogh, "Unfortunate Developments in Senate Subcommittee Deliberations Concerning the Fate of President's Bill to Establish a Special Action Office for Drug Abuse Prevention," September 28, 1971, Jaffe Papers.

118 For example, Jonathan Cole: *Drug Abuse Prevention and Control,* Senate Committee on Government Operations, July 30, 1971, p. 442.

118 Daniel X. Freedman was even more outspoken: Interviews with Jaffe and Krogh. See also Lukas, *Nightmare,* p. 68.

118 On October 22, 1971, Jaffe: The memo, which is untitled, is in the Jaffe Papers.

118 Besteman had spent seven years: Interview with Karst Besteman.

119 Donfeld sent Jaffe a memo: "Targetting," December 3, 1971, Jaffe Papers.

119 At his office, he was receiving: Gleaned from Jaffe's daily schedules at SAODAP, Jaffe Papers.

119 PERLE MESTA HE'S NOT: *Signature,* February 1972, pp. 34–37.

119 PROGRESS SEEN IN DRIVE: *Washington Post,* February 2, 1972, p. A-17.

The monthly urine results are also summarized in a memo from Donfeld to Jaffe, "Vietnam Urinalysis Statistics," April 13, 1972, Jaffe Papers.

119 Congress voted unanimously: Dana Adams Schmidt, "Nixon Signs Law to Curb Drug Abuse," *New York Times,* March 22, 1972, p. 22.

119 federal spending on treatment: Gerstein and Harwood, *Treating Drug Problems,* p. 217.

120 The numbers ranged from 5: *Annual Report,* SAODAP, 1973, p. 18. See also Jaffe testimony in *Supplemental Appropriations Bill, 1973,* House Appropriations Committee, September 19, 1972, p. 1089. The buying up of waiting lists is described on p. 1090.

120 was operating thirty-seven methadone clinics: See testimony of Robert Newman, *Drug Addict Treatment and Rehabilitation Act of 1972,* Senate Committee on Labor and Public Welfare, May 24, 1972, pp. 87–93. See also Robert Newman, *Methadone Treatment in Narcotic Addiction: Program Management, Findings, and Prospects for the Future* (Academic Press, 1977), pp. 3–13, 95–100.

120 before long millions of dollars: Jaffe testimony, *Evaluating the Federal Effort to Control Drug Abuse,* Part I, House Government Operations Committee, May 1, 1973, p. 40; Francis X. Clines, "Anti-Drug Effort in City to Expand," *New York Times,* September 24, 1972, p. 56.

120 Haight-Ashbury Free Medical Clinic: Interviews with Jaffe and David Smith.

121 "He had no sense of time": Interview with Jim Gregg.

121 Methadone was the main flashpoint: Gary Hoenig, "The 'Cure' That Can Be a Killer," *New York Times,* October 1, 1972, p. IV-10; James M. Markham, "Methadone Found Rising as Killer," *New York Times,* March 14, 1972, p. 48; Karlyn Barker, "Methadone Overdose Deaths Rise Here," *Washington Post,* October 6, 1972, p. B-1.

121 the office created twice as many slots: *Annual Report,* 1973, SAODAP, p. 14; *Federal Strategy for Drug Abuse and Drug Traffic Prevention, 1973,* pp. 20, 145.

121 the office continued to be harassed: SAODAP's complaints are laid out in a seven-page SAODAP memo that is undated, untitled, and unattributed (a reflection of the subject's sensitivity), Jaffe Papers.

122 During a tennis match: See Mathea Falco and John Pekkanen, "The Abuse of Drug Abuse," *Washington Post,* September 8, 1974, p. B-1.

122 As in Chicago, Jaffe shrank: Information on the climate inside SAODAP came from interviews with Paul Perito, Jim Gregg, and Grasty Crewes, SAODAP's general counsel. The quote on Jaffe's paper backlog comes from his schedule for July 11, 1972, Jaffe Papers. SAODAP's internal problems are described in a memo from Perito to Jaffe, "Organizational, Personnel and/or Structural Situations," September 1, 1972, Jaffe Papers.

122 the White House commissioned: "Work Effort Analysis of the Special Action Office: Introduction and General Comments," pp. 3, 6, Jaffe Papers.

123 the White House set up an Office: Felix Belair, Jr., "President Opens Narcotics Drive," *New York Times,* January 29, 1972, p. 1. See also Drug Abuse Council, *The Facts About "Drug Abuse,"* pp. 39–40.

123 "The street pusher program": Memo from Ehrlichman to Nixon, "Urgent Additional Talking Points for Secretary Connally," February 8, 1972, Nixon Papers.

123 By late 1972, the number: *Federal Strategy for Drug Abuse and Drug Traffic Prevention, 1973,* p. 82.

123 "All indicators are": "Reduction in Client Waiting Time," SAODAP

memo, Jaffe Papers. See also "Metropolitan Briefs," *New York Times,* October 19, 1972, p. 51.

123 French agents destroyed: "Heroin Seizures by French Anti-Narcotics Agents," White House Fact Sheet, July 21, 1972, Nixon Papers.

123 the governments of Argentina, Brazil: "Programs Related to the State of the Union Message on Law Enforcement and Drug Abuse Prevention," White House Fact Sheet, March 14, 1973, Epstein Papers.

124 the government of Paraguay: "The U.S. Scores in the War on Drugs," *Newsweek,* August 28, 1972, p. 30.

124 "Our concentrated effort": "Heroin Shortage Situation Report," BNDD, Nixon Papers. See also Nicholas Gage, "East Coast Heroin Flow Is Reported Cut," *New York Times,* July 28, 1972, p. 4.

124 TURNAROUND ON DRUGS?: "Turnaround on Drugs?", *New York Times,* September 5, 1972, p. 36.

124 fewer arrestees were being picked up: "Cutting Addict Crime," *New York Times,* September 6, 1972, p. 44.

124 the city's crime rate dropped: Eric Pace, "Police Say Major Crimes Are Off 21.1% From '71," *New York Times,* July 11, 1972, p. 1.

124 "I, for one, feel": Chase is cited in Francis X. Clines, "Methadone Care Cutting Arrests," *New York Times,* September 3, 1972, p. 20.

124 the number of people dying: Robert DuPont, "Perspective on an Epidemic," paper prepared for the Washington Center for Metropolitan Studies, October 29, 1973.

124 And the city's crime rate: "A Turning Point in Fight Against Crime?" *U.S. News & World Report,* July 24, 1972, p. 83.

124 Seventy-two of the nation's: " '72 Progress in the Fight to Limit Crime," *U.S. News & World Report,* October 9, 1972, p. 65; "Street Crime: Who's Winning?" *Time,* October 23, 1972, pp. 55ff.

124 officials in both Washington and New York: See statement of Washington police chief Jerry Wilson in "Cutting the Crime Rate: How Nation's Capital Does It," *U.S. News & World Report,* April 10, 1972, p. 25. In New York, Police Commissioner Patrick Murphy cited the expansion in treatment, as well as improved work by the police and courts, in explaining the drop (David Burnham, "1972 Crime Total in City Fell 18% As Violence Rose," *New York Times,* March 7, 1973, p. 1). See also Dana Adams Schmidt, "Doctor Links Methadone Treatment to a Decline in Crime in the Capital," *New York Times,* March 13, 1972, p. 18, in which Robert DuPont argues that the crime rate had declined parallel with the expansion in drug treatment. Sanford Garelik, the president of the New York City Council, said that "concurrent with the decrease in these crimes [burglaries] is the sharp increase in the number of addicts under treatment or in custodial care in the New York City area." (*New York Times,* January 23, 1972, p. 58)

124 And he did just that: Carroll Kilpatrick, "Crime Tide Is Stemmed, Nixon Claims," *Washington Post,* October 16, 1972, p. 1; Robert B. Semple, Jr., "Nixon Says He Kept Vow to Check Rise in Crime," *New York Times,* October 16, 1972, p. 1.

125 *All* presidential appointees: Carroll Kirkpatrick, "Nixon Plans to Overhaul Staff, Cabinet," *Washington Post,* November 9, 1972, p. 1.

125 In a meeting with White House staff: Haldeman, *The Haldeman Diaries,* p. 532.

125 Nixon wanted to transfer some power: Theodore White, *Breach of Faith: The Fall of Richard Nixon* (Atheneum, 1975), pp. 171–175.

125 In mid-December 1972, Jaffe: Interviews with Jaffe and Roger Meyer; James M. Markham, "Uncertainty Marks Discussion of Authorities on Drug Addiction," *New York Times,* December 17, 1972, p. 48.

126 Matthew Dumont: His remarks are reprinted in Seymour Fisher and Alfred M. Freedman, eds., *Opiate Addiction: Origins and Treatment* (V. H. Winston & Sons, 1973), a compilation of papers delivered at the Puerto Rico meeting, pp. 163–169.

126 Rockefeller delivered his annual: Francis X. Clines, "Governor Asks Life Term for Hard-Drugs Pushers and for Violent Addicts," *New York Times,* January 4, 1973, pp. 1, 28. The *Times* editorial appeared on January 1, 1973, p. 40. The Lindsay analysis is cited in Max H. Siegel, "Lindsay Assails Governor's Plan to Combat Drugs," *New York Times,* January 10, 1973, p. 1.

127 Rockefeller was contemplating a run: "Rockefeller's 15 Years as Governor Reflect Achievement, Growth and Controversy," *New York Times,* December 12, 1973, p. 53.

127 To discuss the matter, Jaffe: Interview with Jaffe.

127 a White House summary of the meeting: Memo from Stefan Halper (a Jaffe aide) for the file, February 9, 1973, Jaffe Papers.

128 Polls taken in New York: James M. Markham, "Two Approaches That Don't Work," *New York Times,* March 11, 1973, p. IV-10.

128 Nixon asked Ehrlichman: Memo from Ehrlichman to the president, "Heroin Trafficking Legislation," March 8, 1973, Nixon Papers; "State of the Union Message to the Congress on Law Enforcement and Drug Abuse Prevention," March 14, 1973, *Public Papers of the Presidents, 1973,* pp. 192–202.

128 a March 9 memo: Memo from Jaffe to Ehrlichman, "Draft Bill to Amend the Controlled Substances Act," March 9, 1973, Nixon Papers.

128 Two weeks later, he announced: "Message to the Congress Transmitting Reorganization Plan 2 of 1973 Establishing the Drug Enforcement Administration," *Public Papers of the Presidents, 1973,* pp. 228–233.

128 the *Los Angeles Times* ran: Jack Nelson, March 28, 1973, p. 1.

128 In a memo to Ehrlichman's office: Memo from Geoffrey Shepard to Tod Hullin, March 28, 1973, Nixon Papers.

129 Jaffe wrote a letter: Interview with Jaffe. His resignation letter, dated March 29, 1973, is in the Jaffe Papers.

129 the FBI released its crime figures: *Crime in the United States, 1972,* pp. 218–220. See also Paul W. Valentine, "U.S. Crime Dips After 17-Year Rise," *Washington Post,* March 29, 1973, p. A-1; David Burnham, "1972 Crime Total in City Fell 18% as Violence Rose," *New York Times,* March 7, 1973, p. 1.

129 the number of narcotics-related deaths: "Narcotics-Related Deaths; Preliminary Data—Calendar Year 1973," SAODAP Fact Sheet, Jaffe Papers; James M. Markham, "Drugs Sampling Shows Deaths Dip," *New York Times,* February 13, 1973, p. 9.

129 the number of drug-related visits: DAWN Fact Sheet, SAODAP, Jaffe Papers.

129 the number of drug-related hepatitis cases: Press release, "Addicted Related Hepatitis Reaches a New Low," May 18, 1973, Health Services Administration, New York City.

129 just one heroin overdose death: Robert DuPont, "Perspective on an Epidemic," paper prepared for the Washington Center for Metropolitan Studies, October 29, 1973. See also Stuart Auerbach, "Drop in Heroin Use Cited," *Washington Post,* July 21, 1973, p. A-1.

129 And Washington's crime rate: Paul W. Valentine, "U.S. Crime Dips After 17-Year Rise," *Washington Post,* March 29, 1973, p. A-1.

129 the force had some 5,100 officers: "Cutting the Crime Rate: How Nation's Capital Does It," *U.S. News & World Report,* April 10, 1972, p. 24.

129 the number of heroin arrests in D.C.: Robert L. DuPont and Mark H. Greene, "The Decline of Heroin Addiction in the District of Columbia," unpublished paper.

129 Chief Jerry Wilson said: *Treatment and Rehabilitation of Narcotics Addicts,* House Judiciary Committee, May 24, 1972, pp. 767–769.

130 despite a sharp falloff in the number: Joseph A. Califano, Jr., *The 1982 Report on Drug Abuse and Alcoholism* (Warner Books, 1982), p. 86. See also Mark Moore, *Buy and Bust: The Effective Regulation of an Illicit Market in Heroin* (Lexington Books, 1977), pp. 192–195.

130 the number of federal and state inmates: *Sourcebook of Criminal Justice Statistics, 1974* (Government Printing Office, 1974), p. 434.

130 the spreading tentacles of Watergate: See Haldeman, *The Haldeman Diaries,* pp. 591–592, and Lukas, *Nightmare,* pp. 101, 306, 329–331.

130 two weeks later he was forced to resign: Linda Charlton, "Egil Krogh, Jr., A Watergate Casualty," *New York Times,* May 10, 1973, p. 37. See also "The Agony of Egil Krogh," *Washingtonian,* May 1974, pp. 60ff.

130 His sense of isolation deepened: Interviews with Jaffe and Peter Bourne, then SAODAP's assistant director.

130 setting up mechanisms: Jaffe's projects in this period are summarized in his testimony in *Evaluating the Federal Effort to Control Drug Abuse,* House Committee on Government Operations, May 1, 1973, pp. 3–4, 8–9. In New York, Jaffe noted, mobile intake units were being sent out into copping zones, with a car following so that those wanting treatment could be transported to a program without delay. Over a ten-week period, he said, the units had brought 4,000 people into treatment. (p. 25) See also *Annual Report,* 1973, SAODAP, pp. 18–20.

131 a letter of resignation: Jaffe Papers.

10: THE RETREAT

132 he went on the *Today* show: Transcript, "An Interview with Dr. Jerome Jaffe," August 8, 1973, Jaffe Papers.

132 Geoffrey Shepard of the domestic policy staff: Memo from Terrence O'Donnell to Geoffrey Shepard, "Proposal for Presidential Meeting with Dr. Jerome Jaffe," August 14, 1973, Nixon Papers.

133 Robert DuPont had helped convince: Interview with Robert DuPont; curriculum vitae.

134 a much-reduced operation: Interviews with DuPont and Karst Besteman.

134 DuPont was summoned to the White House: Interview with DuPont.

134 Heroin was hardly a new phenomenon: Elaine Shannon, *Desperados: Latin Drug Lords, U.S. Lawmen, and the War America Can't Win* (Viking, 1988), pp. 56–63.

134 The drought in the United States: "Top Source of Heroin Now Mexico," *Washington Post,* October 28, 1975, p. A-11.

135 the White House in April 1975: Interviews with DuPont and Richard Parsons.

135 *White Paper on Drug Abuse: White Paper on Drug Abuse,* A Report to

the President from the Domestic Council Drug Abuse Task Force, September 1975, pp. ix, 6, 11–12, 33, 68, 77.

135 the administration sent the Mexican government: "Ford Vows To Curb Heroin Trafficking," *Washington Post,* December 24, 1975, p. A-3; Shannon, *Desperados,* pp. 62–63.

135 In 1976, federal spending: Gerstein and Harwood, *Treating Drug Problems,* p. 217.

135 an estimated 25 to 30 million: *White Paper on Drug Abuse,* p. 25.

136 George Carlin cracked: Doug Hill and Jeff Weingrad, *Saturday Night* (Vintage, 1986), p. 172.

136 more than 400,000 people: In 1975, for instance, 416,000 people were arrested on marijuana charges (*Crime in the United States, 1975,* p. 179).

136 In Texas, pot possession: Fred P. Graham, "Efforts to Reduce the Harsh Penalties," *New York Times,* November 1, 1970, p. IV-4.

136 Keith Stroup: Interview with Stroup. See also Patrick Anderson, *High in America: The True Story Behind NORML and the Politics of Marijuana* (Viking, 1981), pp. 3–4, 14–15, 25–45. Anderson, a former Carter speechwriter, provides an entertaining account of the politics of marijuana during the Carter years. On Stroup, see also Paul Hendrickson, "The Mellowing of 'Mr. Marijuana,' " *Washington Post,* April 10, 1978, p. B-1.

136 But their final report: *Marihuana: A Signal of Misunderstanding,* First Report of the National Commission on Marihuana and Drug Abuse, GPO, March 1972, pp. 65–66, 136, 150–151, 159–160.

137 Stroup invited Bob DuPont: Interviews with Keith Stroup and DuPont. DuPont's speech is excerpted in the *Leaflet,* a publication of NORML, January 1975, p. 1. See also Anderson, *High in America,* p. 151.

137 In 1975, five more states: Anderson, *High in America,* p. 4.

137 at Bob DuPont's Narcotics Treatment Administration: Interview with DuPont.

137 Bourne, Carter told the press: *Public Papers of the Presidents, 1977,* bk. I, p. 290.

137 A graduate of Emory College: Information on Bourne's background comes from an interview with Bourne; curriculum vitae; Constance Holden, "Peter Bourne: Psychiatrist in the White House," *Science,* August 5, 1977, pp. 539–542; and Anderson, *High in America,* pp. 194–197.

138 a laudatory article in *Time* magazine: "Stress in Fight & Flight," *Time,* April 14, 1967, p. 57.

139 Bourne received a visit: Interviews with Egil Krogh and Peter Bourne.

139 In a gushing profile of Bourne: Stuart Auerbach, "There's More to Carter's 'Closest Friend' Than 'Flaky Accent,' " *Washington Post,* June 21, 1976, p. A-4.

139 That did not sit well: Laurence Stern, "Ironies of Political Process Catch Up with 2 Carter Aides," *Washington Post,* August 15, 1976, p. A-3.

139 Bourne complained in a memo: Memo from Bourne to Richard Harden, "Personnel List," February 17, 1977, supplied by Bourne.

139 Bourne began peppering the president: See, for instance, memo from Bourne to the president, "A World Health Initiative," February 4, 1977; memo from Mike Armacost to David Aaron, "Peter Bourne's Desire to Talk to Governments with Whom We Have No Formal Relations," May 3, 1977; and memo from Bourne to the president, "America Role in Space," September 15, 1977, all in the Carter Papers.

140 went to Mexico: Interviews with Bourne and Mathea Falco.

140 Bourne sent Carter a glowing report: Memo from Bourne to the president, "Mexican Narcotic Program," May 19, 1977, Carter Papers. See also James P. Sterba, "Open Border Strains U.S.-Mexico Relations," *New York Times,* April 3, 1977, p. 1.

140 The federal treatment budget: Karst Besteman, "Federal Leadership in Building the National Drug Treatment System," in *Treating Drug Problems,* vol. 2, Commissioned Papers on Historical, Institutional, and Economic Contexts of Drug Treatment, Institute of Medicine (National Academy Press, 1992), p. 79.

140 the city abruptly shut down: Gary Hoenig, "Drug Programs Aren't Working Out," *New York Times,* May 22, 1977, p. IV-6.

140 the Narcotics Treatment Administration: Alice Bonner, "City Drug Clinics To Be Reopened," *Washington Post,* July 17, 1976, p. 3; Alice Bonner, "Drug Center Reopens to Patient Overload," *Washington Post,* July 20, 1976, p. C-1.

140 Jaffe's beloved Illinois Drug Abuse Program: Interviews with Edward Senay, Jaffe's successor as IDAP's director, and Claude Rhodes.

141 he sent Hamilton Jordan a memo: Memo from Bourne to Jordan, February 2, 1977, Carter Papers; interviews with Bourne and Stroup; Anderson, *High in America,* pp. 197–199.

141 President Carter sent Bourne: Untitled memo, March 28, 1977, Carter Papers.

141 he now solicited his advice: Memo from Keith Stroup to Griffin Smith, "Suggestions for Section on Marijuana Policy," June 16, 1977, Carter Papers; Anderson, *High in America,* pp. 210–211.

141 "I am very concerned": Memo from Eizenstat to the president, "Message on Drug Abuse," July 7, 1977, Carter Papers.

141 Nonetheless, the final version: "Drug Abuse, Message to the Congress," August 2, 1977, *Public Papers of the Presidents, 1977,* bk. II, pp. 1400–1406.

142 CARTER SEEKS TO END: James T. Wooten, "Carter Seeks to End Marijuana Penalty for Small Amounts," *New York Times,* August 3, 1977, p. A-1.

11: THE COUNTERREVOLUTION

143 The spark came: Interview with Keith Schuchard. See also Peggy Mann, *Marijuana Alert* (McGraw-Hill, 1985), pp. 414–420; and Marsha Manatt (maiden name of Marsha Keith Schuchard), *Parents, Peers, and Pot* (U.S. Department of Health, Education, and Welfare, 1979), pp. 1–21.

144 an interview in *Science:* "Marihuana: A Conversation with NIDA's Robert L. DuPont," *Science,* May 14, 1976, pp. 647–649.

144 banged out an emotional letter: The letter from Schuchard to DuPont, dated March 17, 1977, was supplied by Schuchard.

144 DuPont was leery: Interview with Robert DuPont.

145 DuPont asked Schuchard: Letter from DuPont to Schuchard, June 16, 1977, supplied by Schuchard.

145 Rusche stopped by: Interview with Sue Rusche. See also Peggy Mann, *Marijuana Alert,* pp. 426–429.

145 Hoping to mobilize other parents: Interviews with Schuchard and Rusche.

146 Schuchard was disappointed: Interviews with Schuchard and Peter Bourne. Schuchard's reactions are described in a January 4, 1978, letter to Robert DuPont, supplied by Schuchard.

146 Seething, Schuchard fired off: Letter, January 4, 1978, supplied by Schuchard.

146 She sent another letter: Letter, February 28, 1978, Carter Papers.

147 the number of overdose deaths: *Heroin Indicators Trend Report—an Update, 1976–1978,* National Institute on Drug Abuse, 1979; "Drop in Heroin Deaths Laid to Poppy Destruction," *Washington Post,* February 11, 1978, p. B-5.

147 "The overall success": Bourne memo to Carter, "Monthly Drug Report #7," November 25, 1977, Carter Papers.

147 the bash that NORML was throwing: Anderson, *High in America,* pp. 10–24.

147 the ties between NORML and the Carter Administration: Ibid., p. 272.

147 The good feelings: Interviews with Bourne and Keith Stroup; Anderson, *High in America,* pp. 203–208, 249–252 (the "cultural genocide" quote is on p. 252); Jesse Kornbluth, "Poisonous Fallout from the War on Marijuana," *New York Times Magazine,* November 19, 1978, pp. 59ff; "NORML Head Keith Stroup Beats Administration Threat Effort," *New Times,* August 7, 1978, p. 16; memo from Bourne to Carter, "Paraquat," March 22, 1978, Carter Papers.

147 Gleaton, every spring, held a conference: Interview with Thomas Gleaton.

148 "many parents": Schuchard's speech, titled "The Family Versus the Drug Culture" and dated May 25, 1978, was on file at the offices of PRIDE in Atlanta.

148 One day in early July 1978: Anderson, *High in America,* pp. 274–287; Lawrence Meyer and Alfred E. Lewis, "Carter Aide Signed Fake Quaalude Prescription," *Washington Post,* July 19, 1978, p. A-1; Edward Walsh and Ronald Shaffer, "Carter Drug Adviser Put on Leave," *Washington Post,* July 20, 1978, p. A-1; James Wooten, "Carter's Top Drug Adviser Resigns in Conflict Over False Prescription," *New York Times,* July 21, 1978, p. A-1.

148 The same day the *Post* story appeared: Anderson, *High in America,* pp. 278–280; Ron Shaffer, "The Cocaine Incident," *Washington Post,* July 21, 1978, p. A-1.

149 In an emotional letter: Reprinted in the *Washington Post,* July 21, 1978, p. A-9.

149 A longtime member: Interview with Lee Dogoloff; curriculum vitae.

149 Gleaton and Schuchard had arranged: Interviews with Gleaton, Schuchard, and Dogoloff.

150 "the largest portion": *White Paper on Drug Abuse,* pp. 11–12.

150 in an annual survey of high school seniors: Lloyd D. Johnston, Patrick M. O'Malley, and Jerald G. Bachman, *National Survey Results on Drug Use from the Monitoring the Future Study, 1975–1993,* vol. 1, University of Michigan Institute for Social Research (U.S. Department of Health and Human Services, 1994), pp. 78–80 (henceforth referred to as *Monitoring the Future Study*).

151 While marijuana users: *Marihuana: A Signal of Misunderstanding,* p. 45.

151 parent groups were sprouting: Interviews with Gleaton, Schuchard, Rusche, Carla Lowe, Pat Barton, and Geraldine Silverman; see also Peggy Mann, *Marijuana Alert,* pp. 411–455.

151 "Reading, Writing, and Reefer": Interviews with Schuchard, DuPont, and Stroup.

152 Adolescent Drug Abuse Prevention Campaign: Memo from Dogoloff to Eizenstat, "Adolescent Drug Abuse Prevention Campaign," April 20, 1979, Carter Papers.

152 "reach consensus on a clear health statement": Memo summarizing principals' retreat, April 6, 1979, Carter Papers.

152 Schuchard had insisted on including: Interview with Schuchard. Her anger at changes made by NIDA are described in a letter to a NIDA official, dated November 28, 1979, supplied by Schuchard.

152 Even in its watered-down form: *Parents, Peers, and Pot* (Department of Health, Education, and Welfare, 1979), pp. 1–21, 24, 34–53.

153 Eventually, more than one million: Mann, *Marijuana Alert,* p. 421. See also Baum, *Smoke and Mirrors,* pp. 122–123.

153 In late 1979, Joyce Nalepka: Interview with Joyce Nalepka. See also Mann, *Marijuana Alert,* pp. 429–434.

153 The hearings themselves: *Health Consequences of Marihuana Use,* Senate Judiciary Committee, January 16–17, 1980. Nalepka's testimony is on pp. 201–202.

153 the movement's leaders decided: Interviews with Gleaton, Rusche, and Schuchard.

153 Among those named: "Seven Atlantans on Nat'l. Drug Free Youth Board," *Atlanta Daily World,* June 3, 1980, p. 3.

153 the nation was being hit: Stuart Auerbach, "New Heroin Connection," *Washington Post,* October 11, 1979, p. A-1; Nicholas Gage, "New Heroin Flow Helping Revive the French Connection," *New York Times,* January 12, 1980, p. 2.

154 Reflecting the sharp increase: Paul W. Valentine, "Glut of Heroin Triggers Surge in Drug Activity in the City," *Washington Post,* August 26, 1979, p. A-1; Jill Smolowe, "Rise in Drug Addicts Strains Program in New York State," *New York Times,* September 1, 1980, p. B-1.

154 "We may be at the edge": Memo from Dogoloff to Eizenstat, "Heroin from the Middle East and South Asia," February 13, 1980, Carter Papers; memo from Dogoloff to Eizenstat, "Drug Abuse Treatment," May 15, 1980, Carter Papers; interview with Dogoloff.

12: DISMANTLEMENT

155 Jerome Jaffe received an invitation: Memo from Richard H. Bucher to former SAODAP staff members, May 28, 1981, Jaffe Papers.

155 Jaffe was working as a professor: Interview with Jerome Jaffe.

155 "compulsive smoking syndrome": See Jane E. Brody, "Heavy Smoking Called Disorder," *New York Times,* June 5, 1975, p. 34.

156 Jaffe, who had taken inches: "JJ Notes for Comments on Occasion of SAODAP 10th Anniversary Dinner," June 17, 1981, Jaffe Papers.

156 ("the single biggest new health threat"): Robert DuPont, "A Fresh Perspective for the War on Drugs," *Washington Star,* July 2, 1981, p. A-18.

156 PRIDE conference: Thomas J. Gleaton, Keith Manatt Schuchard, and Helen W. Moore, eds., *P.R.I.D.E. Southeast Drug Conference Proceedings: 1980–1981,* National Parents Movement for Drug Free Youth (Georgia State University, 1982). Schuchard's comment is on p. 69.

157 Among those listening to Schuchard: Interview with Ann Wrobleski.

157 Mrs. Reagan needed a project: Ibid.

157 Mrs. Reagan had taken time: *New York Times,* October 24, 1980, p. 18.

157 She also heard from Patricia Burch: Interview with Patricia Burch.

158 Wrobleski had always thought: Interview with Wrobleski.

158 Sheila Tate, the first lady's: Interview with Sheila Tate.

158 Dr. Carlton Turner knew: Interview with Carlton Turner. For Turner's views, see his articles "Marijuana Research and Problems: An Overview," *Pharmacy International*, May 1980; and "The Marijuana Controversy," American Council on Marijuana, 1981. See also a curious interview with Turner in *High Times* (given before he joined the Reagan Administration), February 1982, pp. 35ff.

158 Raised by his mother: Interview with Carlton Turner; Jim Spencer, "The Drug Warrior: My Job Is to Free America of Addiction," *Chicago Tribune*, October 26, 1986, p. C-1.

159 At the 1980 Senate hearings: *Health Consequences of Marihuana Use*, Senate Judiciary Committee, January 16–17, 1980, pp. 102–110.

159 "He was such a combative person": Interview with Coy Waller.

159 "Some of the scientists": Interview with Sue Rusche.

159 PRIDE and the NFP: Interviews with Thomas Gleaton, Keith Schuchard, and Turner.

159 Three times, Turner was called: Interview with Turner.

160 Turner was summoned to the White House: Ibid.

160 federal drug policy needed a drastic overhaul: Ibid.

161 Under the direction of David Stockman: David Stockman, *The Triumph of Politics: How the Reagan Revolution Failed* (Harper & Row, 1986), pp. 141–142.

161 As a result, drug enforcement: Gerstein and Harwood, *Treating Drug Problems*, p. 217. This table also shows the sharp reduction in treatment funding.

161 a 43 percent reduction: Karst J. Besteman, "Federal Leadership in Building the National Drug Treatment System," in Gerstein and Harwood, *Treating Drug Problems*, vol. 2, pp. 80–81.

161 she had gone to London: Kitty Kelley, *Nancy Reagan: The Unauthorized Biography* (Simon & Schuster, 1991), pp. 346, 315. The Johnny Carson remark is on p. 319.

161 was replaced by James Rosebush: Interview with James Rosebush.

161 To develop a strategy: Interviews with Turner, Wrobleski, Tate, and Rosebush.

162 One of many "tough love" programs: For a good description of the Straight program, see Dan Baum, *Smoke and Mirrors*, pp. 157–161. See also Eve Zibart, "Controversy Over Drug Program Extends to New Va. Clinic," *Washington Post*, January 2, 1983, p. C-1.

162 arriving at the hall: Interviews with Turner, Wrobleski, and Tate. See also James S. Rosebush, *First Lady, Public Wife: A Behind-the-Scenes History of the Evolving Role of First Ladies in American Political Life* (Madison Books, 1987), p. 44; and Enid Nemy, "Mrs. Reagan, in Florida, Sees Efforts to Fight Drug Abuse," *New York Times*, February 16, 1982, p. B-10.

162 the entourage flew to Dallas: Donnie Radcliffe, "The Texas Mission; Nancy Reagan Carries Her Drug War to Dallas," *Washington Post*, February 17, 1982, p. C-1; Enid Nemy, "Mrs. Reagan Deplores a Drug 'Epidemic,' " *New York Times*, February 17, 1982, p. C-1; Enid Nemy, "First Lady Finds a Cause," *New York Times*, February 19, 1982, p. B-5.

162 "After months of publicity": Donnie Radcliffe, "Polishing the Image; Nancy Reagan Finds Media Success on the Road," *Washington Post*, February 19, 1982, p. D-1.

163 At the conference: Interviews with Wrobleski, Turner, and Gleaton; *National Drug Conference Highlights, 1982* (PRIDE, 1982), pp. 1–2; Rosebush, *First Lady, Public Wife*, p. 44.

163 she was due to visit Central High School: Interviews with Turner and Wrobleski. See also Clara Germani, "First Lady Takes Her Anti-Drug Campaign on the Road," *Christian Science Monitor,* September 30, 1982, p. 6.

163 Carlton Turner coached her: Interview with Turner.

163 Appearing on a radio talk show: Donnie Radcliffe, "Nancy Reagan on the Road in Iowa; Protests & Pie for the 'Feature Act,'" *Washington Post,* August 6, 1982, p. D-1.

163 Straight, for instance: Zibart, "Controversy Over Drug Program Extends to New Va. Clinic."

164 Carlton Turner did exempt one area: Interview with Turner.

164 In 1981, the DEA was eradicating marijuana: Mann, *Marijuana Alert,* p. 313.

164 the U.S. Forest Service: Ibid., p. 314.

164 Turner began pressuring Colombia: Interview with Turner.

164 The immediate crisis: Jo Thomas, "Violence and Graft Increase in Florida Along with Its $7 Billion Flow of Drugs," *New York Times,* March 5, 1981, p. A-16; Guy Gugliotta and Jeff Leen, *Kings of Cocaine: An Astonishing True Story of Murder, Money, and Corruption* (Simon & Schuster, 1989), pp. 11–13, 19, 107; Paul Eddy, Hugo Sabogal, and Sara Walden, *The Cocaine Wars* (Norton, 1988), pp. 59–68.

164 Carlton Turner went to southern Florida: Interview with Turner.

164 "mother ships": See Eddy, Sabogal, and Walden, *The Cocaine Wars,* p. 116.

164 Turner helped put together: Interview with Turner; Gugliotta and Leen, *Kings of Cocaine,* pp. 69–70; Eddy, Sabogal, and Walden, *The Cocaine Wars,* pp. 96–97.

164 the mother ships were simply putting: Interview with John Coleman, agent, DEA.

165 In one startling incident: Gugliotta and Leen, *Kings of Cocaine,* pp. 71–73.

165 a kilogram went for $60,000: "Cocaine: Middle Class High," *Time,* July 6, 1981, p. 59.

165 Not until the mid-1980s: Interview with John Lawn, former administrator, DEA.

165 U.S. drug agents: Joel Brinkley, "4-Year Fight in Florida 'Just Can't Stop Drugs,'" *New York Times,* September 4, 1986, p. A-1; Bill Curry, "Illicit Drugs Pour in via 'Crazy Colombians,'" *Washington Post,* August 13, 1979, p. A-1.

13: STORM WARNINGS

166 cocaine was so scarce: Ann Crittenden and Michael Ruby, "Cocaine: The Champagne of Drugs," *New York Times Magazine,* September 1, 1974, pp. 14ff.

166 In the summer of 1981: "Cocaine: Middle Class High," *Time,* July 6, 1981, pp. 56ff.

166 The 1975 *White Paper on Drug Abuse: White Paper on Drug Abuse,* A Report to the President from the Domestic Council Drug Abuse Task Force, September 1975, pp. 25, 33.

166 As late as 1980: "Drug Dependence: Nonnarcotic Agents," in Harold Kaplan, Alfred Freedman, and Benjamin Sadock, eds., *Comprehensive Textbook of Psychiatry,* 3rd ed., vol. 2 (Williams & Wilkins, 1980), pp. 1621–1622.

167 Richard Pryor made headlines: "When Cocaine Can Kill," *Newsweek,* June 23, 1980, p. 30.

167 Two years later, John Belushi: Bob Woodward, *Wired: The Short Life and Fast Times of John Belushi* (Simon & Schuster, 1984), pp. 372–374.

167 NBC anchorwoman Jessica Savitch: "Tragic Sign-Off for a Golden Girl," *Time,* November 7, 1983, p. 100.

167 pro athletes like Steve Howe: Pete Axthelm, "Cocaine Crisis in the NFL," *Newsweek,* July 25, 1983, p. 52; Ronald Sullivan, "N.F.L. Says Players' Cocaine Use Could Threaten Integrity of Game," *New York Times,* June 27, 1982, p. 1.

167 Across the country, private hospitals: "Kicking the Cocaine Habit," *Newsweek,* January 24, 1983, p. 50; "Getting Straight," *Newsweek,* June 4, 1984, pp. 62ff.

167 Even more enterprising: Alfonso A. Narvaez, "Cocaine Hotline Draws a Thousand Calls a Day," *New York Times,* June 1, 1983, p. B-2; "Strung Out and Calling It Quits," *Time,* May 23, 1983, p. 24; Neal Karlen, "Hot-Lining for Help," *Newsweek,* June 4, 1984, p. 64.

167 A two-tier treatment system: For a good description of this phenomenon, see Gerstein and Harwood, *Treating Drug Problems,* chap. 6, "Two Tiers: Public and Private Supply," pp. 200–219.

168 Among the most persistent: Interview with Karst Besteman.

168 Things were far worse: The survey results appear in *Alcohol, Drug Abuse, and Mental Health Administration,* House Appropriations Committee, pt. 10, May 10, 1984, pp. 701–718.

168 Testifying before the House: *Drug Abuse Treatment and Prevention— 1984,* House Select Committee on Narcotics Abuse and Control, June 26, 1984, pp. 74–75.

169 Besteman was hardly the only: The same hearing at which Besteman testified featured similar warnings from other treatment specialists, including Robert Newman and Mitchell Rosenthal.

169 the University of Michigan's annual survey: *Monitoring the Future Study,* pp. 78–80.

169 A survey of five hundred: Richard D. Lyons, "Cocaine Survey Points to Widespread Anguish," *New York Times,* January 3, 1984, p. C-1.

169 "Without question": Jane E. Brody, "Personal Health," *New York Times,* May 23, 1984, p. C-6.

169 The administration's own: *1984 National Strategy for Prevention of Drug Abuse and Drug Trafficking,* Drug Abuse Policy Office, The White House, 1984, pp. 22–23.

169 "If people can afford to go out": Interview with Carlton Turner.

169 Pat Burch represented the polite one: Interview with Patricia Burch and Susan Silverman, a fellow NFP board member.

170 she could have two thousand telegrams: Interview with Carolyn Burns, NFP staff member.

170 The "shock troops": Interview with Thomas Gleaton.

170 Moulton came to wield enormous influence: Interview with Otto Moulton. See also Mann, *Marijuana Alert,* pp. 434–436.

171 Nancy Reagan's office: Interviews with Moulton and Ann Wrobleski.

171 Moulton scoured the publications: In one telling incident, Moulton convinced NIDA director William Pollin to send a letter to school librarians asking them to remove sixty-four NIDA titles deemed obsolete—a move that prompted accusations of censorship. See "Fed Dope Bureau Censors Drug Info," *High Times,* April 1984, p. 19.

171 Over the years, he compiled a list: Interview with Moulton.

171 Dr. David Smith's experience: Interview with David Smith.

171 in a monograph for NIDA: Smith's comment is cited in Edgar H. Adams and Jack Durell, "Cocaine: A Growing Public Health Problem," in John Grabowski, *Cocaine: Pharmacology, Effects, and Treatment of Abuse,* NIDA Research Monograph no. 50, 1984, p. 9.

171 In early 1983: Letter from Otto Moulton to John J. Bellizi, executive director of the International Narcotic Enforcement Officers Association, April 7, 1983, on file at the library of National Families in Action in Atlanta.

172 "I am confused": Letter from Otto Moulton to Robert DuPont, September 27, 1982. DuPont reply to Moulton, October 13, 1982. Subsequent Moulton letter to DuPont, April 7, 1983. Second DuPont reply, April 28, 1983. All are on file at the National Families in Action library.

172 along with a brief note: Turner letter to Moulton, June 8, 1983, on file at the National Families in Action library.

173 Moulton tried to get the administration: Interview with Smith.

173 they eventually convinced Nancy Reagan: Interviews with NFP executives.

173 "The NFP was a Republican organization": Interview with Gleaton.

173 "a lot of the parent groups wouldn't affiliate": Interview with Tom Adams.

174 Nancy Reagan arrived: Interviews with Adams and Wrobleski. See also Frank Thorsberg, UPI dispatch, July 4, 1984.

174 Frye presented Mrs. Reagan: D'Vera Cohn, UPI dispatch, February 23, 1985.

174 Just Say No gained national attention: Interview with Adams.

174 "Mrs. Reagan never understood": Ibid.

175 Adams asked some friends at NBC: Ibid.

175 The speech was a "fiasco": Interview with Turner.

175 The summit was attended: Adela Gooch, "First Ladies Come Together to Fight Drug Abuse," Reuters dispatch, October 21, 1985; Betty Cuniberti, "Drug Abuse Worldwide, Nancy Reagan Tells Forum," *Los Angeles Times,* October 22, 1985, p. 4; Donnie Radcliffe, "Surprise for Nancy Reagan: A Nicaraguan Appeal at Drug Abuse Talks," *Washington Post,* October 21, 1985, p. B-1.

175 she had surpassed the president: Fred Barnes, "Nancy's Total Makeover: How White House Beauticians Gave the First Lady a New Look," *New Republic,* September 16, 1985, pp. 16ff.

175 CO-STARRING AT THE WHITE HOUSE: *Time,* January 14, 1985, pp. 25ff.

175 "Even while Mrs. Reagan's critics": Quoted in "Nancy's Total Makeover," *New Republic,* September 16, 1985.

14: THE DELUGE

177 the paper ran a front-page article: Jane Gross, "A New, Purified Form of Cocaine Causes Alarm as Abuse Increases," *New York Times,* November 29, 1985, p. 1. (On November 25, 1984, the *Los Angeles Times* had mentioned the appearance of cocaine "rock" in the city's ghettos, but the report did not attract much attention.)

177 "To understand how crack": Gary Webb, "Dark Alliance: The Story Behind the Crack Explosion," *San Jose Mercury News,* August 18–20, 1996, p. 1.

178 the cocaine trade had become: *The NNICC Report, 1985–1986,* National Narcotics Intelligence Consumers Committee, June 1987, pp. 26, 31. "Colombian

organizations," it stated, "remained in control of illicit cocaine traffic at the whole-sale level from conversion and packaging, to transportation and at least through the first level of wholesale distribution in the United States." (p. 31)

178 In New York City: See my article "Crack's Destructive Sprint Across America," *New York Times Magazine,* October 1, 1989, pp. 38ff. See also Terry Williams, *The Cocaine Kids* (Addison-Wesley, 1989), pp. 22–25, 39–43, 51–53.

178 From the start, crack flourished: See my "Crack's Destructive Sprint Across America." For a description of parallel developments in Detroit, see William M. Adler, *Land of Opportunity: One Family's Quest for the American Dream in the Age of Crack* (Atlantic Monthly Press, 1995), pp. 116–117, 135–136, 140–141.

179 DRUG TREATMENT IN CITY: Peter Kerr, "Drug Treatment in City Is Strained by Crack, a Potent New Cocaine," *New York Times,* May 16, 1986, p. A-1.

179 Jaffe was back in Washington: Interview with Jerome Jaffe.

180 In 1986, the federal treatment budget: Gerstein and Harwood, *Treating Drug Problems,* p. 217.

180 One of the volumes: Miriam Cohen, *Marijuana: Its Effects on Mind and Body,* The Encyclopedia of Psychoactive Drugs (Chelsea House, 1985), p. 8.

181 The parent groups exploded: Otto Moulton's complaints are outlined in a Committees of Correspondence fact sheet, "Critique: Encyclopedia of Psychoac-tive Drugs: Marijuana," November 1985.

181 Jaffe appeared before the subcommittee: *Reauthorization of the National Institute on Alcohol Abuse and Alcoholism and the National Institute on Drug Abuse,* Senate Committee on Labor and Human Resources, February 20, 1986, pp. 70–71.

181 Two days earlier, Len Bias: Roy S. Johnson, "All-America Basketball Star, Celtic Choice, Dies Suddenly," *New York Times,* June 20, 1986, p. A-1; "Examiner Confirms Cocaine Killed Bias," *New York Times,* June 25, 1986, p. D-25.

182 The three networks: *Television News Index and Abstracts,* Vanderbilt Television News Archive, 1986, pp. 1088–1368. See also Jimmie L. Reeves and Richard Campbell, *Cracked Coverage: Television News, the Anti-Cocaine Crusade, and the Reagan Legacy* (Duke University Press, 1994), pp. 265–266.

182 The "lesson of Len Bias's death": " 'Cocaine Is a Loaded Gun,' " *News-week,* July 7, 1986, p. 26.

182 DRUGS: THE ENEMY WITHIN: "Drugs: The Enemy Within," *Time,* Sep-tember 15, 1986.

182 the sudden spread of crack: See my "Crack's Destructive Sprint Across America." See also *The NNICC Report, 1988,* April 1989, p. 37; *Drug Trafficking: A Report to the President of the United States,* U.S. Department of Justice, August 3, 1989, pp. 7–9, 27–30, 33–40; and William E. Schmidt, "Police Say Use of Crack Is Moving to Small Towns and Rural Areas," *New York Times,* September 10, 1986, p. A-1.

182 So did the demand for treatment: *The NNICC Report, 1988,* pp. 36–37; "Drug Rehab: The Addict Glut," *Newsweek,* August 25, 1986, p. 34.

182 At a July 15 hearing: *The Crack Cocaine Crisis,* joint hearing before the House Select Committee on Narcotics Abuse and Control and the Select Commit-tee on Children, Youth, and Families, July 15, 1986, pp. 30, 38, 41–43.

182 Operation Blast Furnace: Elaine Shannon, *Desperados,* pp. 355–357; Joel Brinkley, "U.S. Sends Troops to Aid Bolivians in Cocaine Raids," *New York Times,* July 16, 1986, p. A-1.

183 House Speaker Thomas P. O'Neill announced: Reginald Stuart, "O'Neill Proposes Congress Mount Attack on Drugs," *New York Times,* July 24, 1986, p. A-1.

183 The job of developing: Interview with Turner. See also Bernard Weinraub, "White House Says Reagan Plans New Campaign Against Drug Use," *New York Times,* July 29, 1986, p. A-1.

183 Already, an estimated one-fourth: Kenneth B. Noble, "Should Employers Be Able to Test for Drug Use?" *New York Times,* April 17, 1986, p. B-7; Robert Lindsey, "Worker Drug Test Provoking Debate," *New York Times,* May 3, 1986, p. 1. For a good overview of the use of drug testing as government policy, see J. Michael Walsh and Jeanne G. Trumble, "The Politics of Drug Testing," in Robert H. Coombs and Louis Jolyon West, eds., *Drug Testing: Issues and Options* (Oxford University Press, 1991), pp. 22–47.

183 Cough syrup containing codeine: Jerome H. Jaffe, ed., *Encyclopedia of Drugs and Alcohol,* vol. 1, pp. 415–419.

183 Turner drafted an executive order: Interview with Carlton Turner; Bernard Weinraub, "Reagan Seeks Drug Tests for Key U.S. Employees," *New York Times,* August 5, 1986, p. A-24.

184 candidates were challenging their opponents: "Jar Wars: Candidates Make Drugs an Issue," *Newsweek,* September 29, 1986, p. 21.

184 preparing huge omnibus drug bills: "Drug Control: Highlights of P.L. 99-570, Anti Drug Abuse Act of 1986," Congressional Research Service, Library of Congress, October 31, 1986. See also Gerald M. Boyd, "Reagan Signs Anti-Drug Measure; Hopes for 'Drug-Free Generation,' " *New York Times,* October 28, 1986, p. B-19; and Julie Rovner, "Massive Anti-Drug Measure Ready for Reagan's Signature," *Congressional Quarterly,* October 25, 1986, pp. 2699–2707.

184 Since 1970, the federal government: *Mandatory Minimum Penalties in the Federal Criminal Justice System,* U.S. Sentencing Commission, August 1991, p. 6.

184 approved a series of whopping new sentences: *Cocaine and Federal Sentencing Policy,* U.S. Sentencing Commission, February 1995, p. 1.

184 When a *Newsweek* reporter called: Interview with Turner.

185 REAGAN AIDE: "Reagan Aide: Pot Can Make You Gay," *Newsweek,* October 27, 1986, p. 95.

185 Turner's comments drew ridicule: Elizabeth Kastor, "Reagan Aide Takes Issue with Newsweek Story," *Washington Post,* October 22, 1986, p. C-1.

185 Turner stepped down: Interview with Turner.

185 the parent movement itself was imploding: Interviews with Pat Burch, Susan Silverman, Joyce Nalepka, Sue Rusche, and Thomas Gleaton.

185 "Crack was an easy scapegoat": Interview with Keith Schuchard.

185 Schuster was well known: Interview with Charles Schuster.

186 the rate of HIV transmission: Lawrence K. Altman, "Spread of AIDS Virus Is Unabated Among Intravenous Drug Takers," *New York Times,* June 4, 1987, p. A-1.

187 the Reagan cutbacks had caused: See Ball and Ross, *The Effectiveness of Methadone Maintenance Treatment* (Springer Verlag, 1991), p. 2: "Although the programs that developed from the Dole-Nyswander model were generally underfunded, during the 1980s even this level of financial support was reduced. As a consequence, programs were forced to curtail treatment and rehabilitative services, staff turnover was high, and the quality of care declined. At the same time, many programs were beset with community opposition, lack of administrative support, and general public apathy or hostility."

187 the president's own AIDS commission: *Report of the Presidential Commission on the Human Immunodeficiency Virus Epidemic,* June 24, 1988, pp. 95–96, 171; Sandra Boodman, "Reagan Turns Aside AIDS Panel Report," *Washington Post,* August 3, 1988, p. A-1.

187 ($500,000 donated by the sultan of Brunei): Donnie Radcliffe, "Washington Ways," *Washington Post,* October 2, 1984, p. E-1.

187 the first lady quietly transferred: Interview with Tom Adams.

187 At a rally at the Universal Amphitheatre: Penelope McMillan, "6,000 Echo First Lady's 'Just Say No,' " *Los Angeles Times,* May 14, 1987, p. II-6.

188 growing commercialization of Just Say No: Interview with Adams.

188 it made clear in a letter to Adams: Cited in Tom Adams, *Grass Roots: How Ordinary People Are Changing America* (Citadel Press, 1991), pp. 244–246.

188 After a March 1987 meeting: Ibid., pp. 250–253; interview with Adams.

189 Just Say No had become: See Irvin Molotsky, "Ex-Aides to Drug Drive Say Company Exploits It," *New York Times,* August 13, 1988, p. 6.

189 "She'd go to these rap sessions": Interview with Donnie Radcliffe.

189 33.7 percent of American high school seniors: *Monitoring the Future Study,* pp. 78–80.

189 the Reagan years were marked: See National Household Survey figures cited in *National Drug Control Strategy,* the White House, February 1995, p. 139. The estimated number of occasional cocaine users declined from 8.1 million in 1985 to 5.8 million in 1988.

190 the government's Drug Abuse Warning Network: *The NNICC Report, 1988,* pp. 32–33; "Cocaine Assessment," Unified Intelligence Division, DEA, October 1992, appendix B.

190 the number of annual cocaine-related deaths: *The NNICC Report, 1988,* p. 33.

190 Nor had heroin gone away: Ibid., pp. 65–66.

15: THE PHILOSOPHER-CZAR

191 According to one poll: Robin Toner, "Optimistic Mood Greets 41st President," *New York Times,* January 20, 1989, p. A-1.

191 the murder rate jumped: *Crime in the United States, 1988* (Government Printing Office, 1989), p. 79; Richard Berke, "Capital Offers a Ripe Market to Drug Dealers," *New York Times,* March 28, 1989, p. A-1.

191 George Bush promised a new one: "Inaugural Address," *Public Papers of the Presidents, 1989,* bk. I, p. 3.

191 a new Office of National Drug Control Policy: William J. Bennett, *The De-Valuing of America: The Fight for Our Culture and Our Children* (Summit, 1992), pp. 97–98.

191 Burch was a close friend of George Bush: Interview with Patricia Burch; Bennett, *The De-Valuing of America,* p. 96.

192 Bennett was interested: Ibid., p. 95.

192 Meeting with George Bush: Ibid., p. 97.

192 Education had been his lifelong concern: Ibid., pp. 100–103.

192 using U.S. military planes: Ibid., p. 102.

192 he quickly sought to catch up: Ibid., pp. 104, 109, 111.

193 Jaffe agreed to come to Washington: Interview with Jerome Jaffe.

193 Dr. Herbert D. Kleber: Interview with Kleber; curriculum vitae; Herbert Kleber, "The Drug Dependence Unit of the Connecticut Mental Health Center," in J. G. Cull and R. E. Hardy, eds., *Organization and Administration of Drug Abuse Treatment Programs* (Charles C. Thomas, 1974), pp. 51–60.

193 Bennett was stocking his personal staff: Interviews with Kleber, Stanley Morris, Reggie Walton, and other ONDCP staff members. For more on this, see

my article, "The Two William Bennetts," *New York Review of Books,* March 1, 1990, pp. 29–33.

194 "I think I was the only person": Interview with Frank Kalder.

194 "Bennett filled his personal staff": Interview with Morris.

194 But John Walters became taken: Interview with John Walters and Morris.

194 "Andean Initiative": *United States Anti-Narcotics Activities in the Andean Region,* Report of the House Committee on Government Operations, November 30, 1990, pp. 10–17. See also Bernard E. Trainor, "Military's Widening Role in the Anti-Drug Effort," *New York Times,* August 27, 1989, p. 1.

195 Herbert Kleber was having similar frustrations: Interviews with Kleber and Linda Lewis, one of his deputies.

195 "Let's face it": "The Role of Treatment in a War on Drugs: Some Preliminary Thoughts," speech by Bennett to the Alcohol and Drug Abuse Prevention Task Force Conference, San Diego, California, June 6, 1989.

195 Those beliefs, in fact: My account of Bennett's intellectual development relies heavily on his book *The De-Valuing of America,* as well as on John Judis, "Mister Ed," *New Republic,* April 27, 1987, pp. 16–19; Rowland Evans and Robert Novak, "Bill Bennett: Secretary *for* Education," *Reader's Digest,* March 1988, pp. 104–109; Bruce Babbitt, "The Billy Pulpit," *Washington Monthly,* August 1988, pp. 45–48; Tom Morgenthau and Mark Miller, "The Drug Warrior," *Newsweek,* April 10, 1989, pp. 20–24; Paul M. Barrett, "Behind Antidrug Plan Is the '60s Odyssey of 'Czar' Bill Bennett," *Wall Street Journal,* September 6, 1989, p. A-1; and Fred Bruning, "William Bennett's Crusade," *Newsday Magazine,* September 10, 1989, pp. 11ff.

197 "not, ironically, through intellect": Bennett, *The De-Valuing of America,* p. 27.

198 "Somewhere along the way": Ibid., pp. 94–95.

198 In his maiden speech: "Drugs: Consequences and Confrontation," address, May 3, 1989.

198 According to the University: *Monitoring the Future Study,* pp. 78–80.

198 the typical profile of callers: Mark S. Gold, "Dramatic Increase in Cocaine Use," *Alcoholism and Addiction Magazine,* October 1988, p. 8. A survey of callers to the hot line in 1987, Gold wrote, "suggested that cocaine abusers as a group are younger, poorer, have less education and are more likely to be unemployed than in 1983 or 1985."

199 A 1988 report: Community Epidemiology Work Group, *Epidemiologic Trends in Drug Abuse,* U.S. Department of Health and Human Services, December 1988, pp. 29–32.

199 THE AMERICAN DRUG PROBLEM: Peter Kerr, "The American Drug Problem Takes on Two Faces," *New York Times,* July 19, 1988, p. IV-5.

199 "TWO-TIER" DRUG CULTURE: Michael Isikoff, " 'Two-Tier' Drug Culture Seen Emerging," *Washington Post,* January 3, 1989, p. A-3.

199 "Our office was created": Interview with Bruce Carnes.

199 "Bruce would say": Interview with Kalder.

199 "We had to fight": Interview with Lewis.

200 the tenth floor was eagerly awaiting: Interviews with Carnes, Kalder, David Tell, and John Carnevale. For survey results, see Michael Isikoff, "Drug Abuse Said to Decline," *Washington Post,* August 1, 1989, p. A-1, and Bennett, *The De-Valuing of America,* pp. 122–123. Bennett's comment—that "this substantial falloff in the overall number of drug users was great news and gave a great lift" —differs with the recollection of ONDCP staff members.

200 "like a punch to the stomach": Interview with Kalder.

200 "He panicked": Interview with Tell.

200 The result was a grand muddle: *National Drug Control Strategy*, The White House, September 1989, pp. 2, 4–5, 11, 17, 24, 30, 39, 41, 111–123.

202 Bennett decided to hit the road: Bennett, *The De-Valuing of America*, p. 127.

202 Bennett visited Women Inc.: I was present for Bennett's visit. See my article "The Two William Bennetts," *New York Review of Books*, March 1, 1990, pp. 29–33.

205 Kleber would continue his tutorials: Interview with Kleber.

205 a white paper on treatment: *Understanding Drug Treatment*, An Office of National Drug Control Policy White Paper, June 1990.

205 He became so distracted: Interviews with Kalder, Carnes, Walters, Kleber, and Tell.

205 he decided to call it quits: Neil A. Lewis, "Bennett to Resign as Chief of U.S. Anti-Drug Effort," *New York Times*, November 8, 1990, p. A-26.

205 THE SKIPPER QUITS: A. M. Rosenthal, *New York Times*, November 9, 1990, p. A-35.

205 John Walters and Bruce Carnes: Interviews with Walters, Carnes, Kalder, and Lewis. See Gordon Witkin, "The Bad-News Drug Czar," *U.S. News & World Report*, February 10, 1992, p. 33; and Michael Isikoff, "Martinez Suffers Setbacks in Post as Anti-Drug Chief," *Washington Post*, February 24, 1992, p. A-1.

205 Kleber in mid-1991 sent Martinez a memo: Memo from Herbert D. Kleber to Bob Martinez, "Strategy IV: A New Presidential Initiative," undated.

206 "An utter non-starter": Interview with Carnes.

206 the purge of the professionals: Interviews with Kleber, Lewis, Walton, and Morris.

206 ONDCP would become a dumping ground: See Sean Holton, "Drug War: Patronage Is Prolific," *Orlando Sentinel*, June 28, 1992, p. A-1. The article estimated that more than 40 percent of ONDCP's employees were political appointees—a higher proportion than for any other U.S. government agency.

206 Richard "Digger" Phelps: "Ex-Notre Dame Coach to Get Drug Policy Job," *Washington Post*, March 6, 1992, p. A-21.

206 John Carnevale, a senior budget analyst: Interview with Carnevale.

206 a four-page internal memo: "Cocaine Supply: Source Country and Interdiction Issues," Executive Summary, ONDCP, May 1, 1992.

16: AN OFFICER AND A GENERAL

208 Clinton had had to face: David Maraniss, *First in His Class: A Biography of Bill Clinton* (Simon & Schuster, 1995), pp. 419–423.

208 "If drugs were legal": See transcript of presidential debate printed in the *New York Times*, October 12, 1992, p. A-14.

208 "Thousands of addicts": Bill Clinton and Al Gore, *Putting People First* (Times Books, 1992), pp. 72–73.

209 crime had gone down: George James, "Crime Down in New York for 2d Year in Row," *New York Times*, March 19, 1993, p. A-1.

209 One of the first African-Americans: Alan Bernstein, "Brown's Strengths and Weaknesses Documented in a Long Career of Service," *Houston Chronicle*, November 23, 1997, p. A-1.

209 In a statement to Congress in 1991: Statement submitted to the House

Committee on Government Operations, Subcommittee on Legislation and National Security, September 25, 1991.

209 Brown's own trials as an African-American: Interview with Brown; curriculum vitae; M. A. Farber, "Leading the Hunt in Atlanta's Murders," *New York Times Magazine*, May 3, 1981, pp. 63ff; William K. Stevens, "Houston's Mayor and Police at Odds," *New York Times*, March 16, 1982, p. A-1; Dan Balz and Art Harris, "Atlanta's Troubleshooter Is Installed as Houston Chief to Clean Up Police," *Washington Post*, April 20, 1982, p. A-7; Ruth Rendon, "After 5 Years, Houston's 1st Black Police Chief Is Still Firmly in Charge," *Los Angeles Times*, October 4, 1987, p. 1; Mitch Gelman, "For Brown, It's Long Way from Okla.," *Newsday*, December 19, 1989, p. 4; Mitch Gelman, " 'Storefronts' Battle Houston Crime," *Newsday*, December 20, 1989, p. 28; George James, "Brown's Gospel: Community Policing," *New York Times*, August 14, 1991, p. B-1; Joseph Treaster, "Police in New York Shift Drug Battle Away from Street," *New York Times*, August 3, 1992, p. A-1; Dave Von Drehle, "N.Y. Police Commissioner Resigns," *Washington Post*, August 4, 1992, p. A-3.

210 An investigation into the incident: " 'Mayoral Control' Exercised Too Late," *Newsday*, July 21, 1993, p. 80.

210 the White House had pared: Michael Isikoff, "Under Clinton, Drug Policy Office's Hot Streak Melts Down," *Washington Post*, February 10, 1993, p. A-14.

210 Brown sat for a detailed briefing: Interviews with Brown and John Carnevale.

211 According to a study: Douglas C. McDonald, Patricia Cole, and Sharon Teitelbaum, "Does the Supply of Drug Treatment Services in the Public System Meet the Demand for Them? An Assessment of National Survey Data," Abt Associates, July 1992 (unpublished), p. 23.

211 After polling various experts: Interview with Carnevale.

211 increase of $355 million: *National Drug Control Strategy, Budget Summary*, The White House, February 1994, pp. 4–5.

211 the Pentagon's antinarcotics budget: Ibid., p. 23.

211 the United States had remained awash: See "Drug Control: Heavy Investment in Military Surveillance Is Not Paying Off," GAO (GAO/NSIAD-93-220), September 1993, a sharp critique of the Defense Department's role in the antidrug area. The report states that, despite DoD expenditures of nearly $976 million on drug surveillance, "cocaine production has increased, the estimated flow into the United States is essentially undiminished, and cocaine remains affordable and available on American streets. Any shifts in smuggling tactics or increases in either heroin traffic from Asia or drugs from other countries will probably further reduce the contribution that military surveillance can make to the war on drugs." (p. 35) See also James Brooke, "U.S. Aid Hasn't Stopped Drug Flow from South America, Experts Say," *New York Times*, November 21, 1993, p. 10; and Don Podesta and Douglas Farah, "Drug Policy in Andes Called Failure," *Washington Post*, March 27, 1993, p. A-1.

211 Cañas described these shortcomings: Interview with Richard Cañas.

212 a "controlled shift": Interview with Cañas. See also Michael Isikoff, "U.S. Considers Shift in Drug War," *Washington Post*, September 16, 1993, p. A-1.

212 more than $200 million: *National Drug Control Strategy, Budget Summary*, February 1994, p. 8.

212 1994 *National Drug Control Strategy:* Ibid., pp. 1–4.

212 It had a tradition of chopping treatment requests: Interview with John

Carnevale. For an example occurring shortly before Brown took office, see Michael Isikoff, "Clinton's Drug Program Request Trimmed $231 Million by House," *Washington Post,* July 2, 1993, p. A-9.

212 And that, Lee Brown felt sure: Interviews with Brown and Carnevale.

213 the University of Michigan released: Monitoring the Future study, summary of results released December 18, 1997.

213 McMahon was intensely loyal: Interview with ONDCP staff members.

213 the issue was being tracked: Interview with Liz Bernstein, an aide in the White House communications office.

213 "We have the unenviable role": Quoted in Joseph Treaster, "Study Finds Marijuana Use Is Up in High Schools," *New York Times,* February 1, 1994, p. A-1.

213 STUDY FINDS MARIJUANA USE IS UP: Ibid.

213 he got it that same day: Interviews with James Burke and Joseph Califano.

214 Burke had secured: Interview with Burke.

214 Califano could not have started CASA: Joseph A. Califano, Jr., *Radical Surgery: What's Next for America's Health Care* (Times Books, 1994), pp. xiii–xiv.

214 CASA, in turn, produced a study: See, for example, Center on Addiction and Substance Abuse, "Cigarettes, Alcohol, Marijuana: Gateways to Illicit Drug Use," October 1994.

214 Burke did most of the talking: Interviews with Burke, Califano, and Brown.

214 had promised to put 100,000 new cops: Clinton and Gore, *Putting People First,* p. 72.

215 "Crime is this year's anti-incumbent issue": William Schneider, "Crime Pays for the Politicians," *Washington Post,* November 7, 1993, p. C-1.

215 the nation's crime rate had fallen: Stephen Braun and Judy Pasternak, "A Nation with Peril on Its Mind," *Los Angeles Times,* February 13, 1994, p. A-1.

215 the networks were airing stories: Ellen Edwards, "Networks Make Crime Top Story," *Washington Post,* March 3, 1994, p. C-1.

215 panicked legislators in the House and Senate: See, for example, Helen Dewar, "Senate Doubles Crime Bill," *Washington Post,* November 5, 1993, p, A-1.

215 In his State of the Union address: "Remarks Before a Joint Session of the Congress on the State of the Union," *Public Papers of the Presidents, 1994,* bk. I, p. 133.

215 The task of selecting a site: Interview with Liz Bernstein.

216 And so, on the morning: I was present for the event at the Prince George's County Correctional Center.

216 In his speech, the president: "Remarks at Prince George's County Correctional Center in Upper Marlboro, Maryland," *Public Papers of the Presidents, 1994,* bk. I, pp. 210–214.

216 "I tell you": *Treasury, Postal Service, and General Government Appropriations, FY 1995,* Senate Appropriations Committee, February 23, 1994, pp. 29–31.

216 he visited the District of Columbia General Hospital: I was present for this event.

217 Brown expanded on the point: "Remarks of Dr. Lee Brown," Grand Rounds, D.C. General Hospital, March 16, 1994.

217 Brown's name would barely appear: The *Post's* index for 1994 contains just one entry for Brown for the entire year (a June 17 story about his views on Burma).

217 the administration remained silent: Interviews with Bernstein and Carnevale.

218 handed over a secret list: Interview with Senate Appropriations Committee staff member.

218 Congress would approve only $57 million: Interviews with Carnevale and Bernstein. See also the budget table on p. 319 of *The National Drug Control Strategy, 1996: Program, Resources, and Evaluation,* ONDCP.

218 A thirty-four-year-old political operative: Interview with Rahm Emanuel. See also Naftali Bendavid, "Crime Agenda Has His Political Stamp," *Legal Times,* March 25, 1996; and Elisabeth Bumiller, "The Brothers Emanuel," *New York Times Magazine,* June 15, 1997, pp. 23–27.

218 the drug office contacted Lloyd Johnston: Interviews with ONDCP staff members.

218 As the report on the meeting noted: *Increase in Use of Selected Drugs: Monitoring the Future Study of 8th-, 10th-, and 12th-Graders,* Preliminary Report, prepared by Richard Clayton and the Ann Arbor Group, June 6, 1994, pp. 1–16. The survey figures listed in the report come from the Monitoring the Future study.

219 The health risks from this: See, for example, Brooke A. Masters and Lisa Leff, "The Drug of Choice: Schools Call Alcohol Top Problem," *Washington Post,* March 31, 1991, p. A-1, and Center on Addiction and Substance Abuse, "Rethinking Rites of Passage: Substance Abuse on America's Campuses," June 1994. On p. 2, the report states that "abusive drinking" constitutes "the biggest substance abuse problem facing colleges and universities today."

219 the alcohol industry was a major backer: For instance, both Anheuser-Busch and Edgar Bronfman, Jr., an executive of the Seagram Company, were major contributors to the Democratic Party. For more, see my article, "Strong Stuff," *New York Times Magazine,* March 22, 1998, pp. 39–40.

219 "We were trying to focus": Interview with Charlotte Hayes.

219 an action plan was ready: "Adolescent Drug Prevention: Policy Recommendations," revised draft, submitted to ONDCP by CSR, Incorporated, July 27, 1994.

219 Signaling the change, the drug czar: The details of Brown's travels are drawn from ONDCP press releases, which the drug office regularly faxed to reporters in an effort to drum up interest in his activities. Brown's statement on marijuana is taken from a September 18, 1995, release titled "White House Drug Czar, Kentucky Governor, and Governor's Marijuana Task Force Eradicate Marijuana Crops; Implements Administration's Marijuana Initiative." See also Rene Sanchez, "Clinton Drug Chief Targets Marijuana," *Washington Post,* July 18, 1995, p. A-3; and "National Marijuana Conference to Study Dangers of Pot," *Morning Edition,* National Public Radio, July 20, 1995.

220 "The Yankees have struck out": "White House Drug Czar Calls 'Striiike!' on Yankees for Strawberry; Worst Possible Message to Youth of America," ONDCP press release, June 20, 1995.

220 Eventually, the Yankee boss: Interview with Brown.

220 Brown had considerably more success: See Jack Curry, "Yankees Criticized for Signing Strawberry," *New York Times,* June 21, 1995, p. B-11. Brown appeared on *Nightline* on June 22, 1995.

220 By the time he stepped down: One of Brown's main reasons for resigning was his interest in running for mayor of Houston, and in November 1997 he was elected to that post.

220 only 35 percent of the federal drug budget: *The National Drug Control Strategy, 1996: Program, Resources, and Evaluation,* pp. 298, 312–319.

Actually, even the 35 percent figure was artificially inflated as a result of some dubious accounting decisions made in calculating the national drug budget. Of the

$2.7 billion supposedly spent on drug treatment in 1995, for instance, $962 million came from the Department of Veterans Affairs. While some of that money did go for the treatment of addicted veterans, most went for the general medical care of veterans diagnosed as having a drug problem. If one looks solely at the federal block grant for drug treatment—the main source of treatment funding for the general addict population—total treatment expenditures in 1995 came to just $942 million, or 7 percent of the total drug budget. In 1974, by contrast, treatment accounted for 41 percent of the budget. See Patrick Murphy, "Keeping Score: The Frailties of the Federal Drug Budget," RAND Drug Policy Research Center Issue Paper, January 1994, pp. 3–4; and Gerstein and Harwood, *Treating Drug Problems,* p. 217.

221 The task of replacing Brown: Interview with Rahm Emanuel.

221 Barry R. McCaffrey was one: Biography, Barry R. McCaffrey, U.S. Southern Command, provided by ONDCP.

221 His father—Lieutenant General: James Kitfield, *Prodigal Soldiers* (Simon & Schuster, 1995), pp. 33, 101.

221 McCaffrey was an early proponent: Ibid., p. 132.

221 an award from the NAACP: McCaffrey biography.

221 While at SouthCom, he had overseen: Barry McCaffrey, Testimony before the House Committee on Government Reform and Oversight, Subcommittee on National Security, International Affairs, and Criminal Justice, October 1, 1996, statement provided by ONDCP, pp. 3–4.

221 "there's been no diminishment": Remarks by General Barry McCaffrey at the Heritage Foundation, January 11, 1996, Federal News Service. See also R. Jeffrey Smith, "Cocaine Flow Not Slowed, General Says," *Washington Post,* January 12, 1996, p. A-23.

222 a reception hosted by Tipper Gore: Interview with Ellen Weber, codirector of the Legal Action Center in Washington, who attended the event.

222 "Our treatment and education programs": *Nomination of Barry McCaffrey to Be Director of the National Drug Control Policy,* Senate Judiciary Committee, February 27, 1996, pp. 62, 29. See also Christopher Wren, "New Drug Czar Is Seeking Ways to Bolster His Hand," *New York Times,* March 17, 1996, p. 18, which quotes McCaffrey as saying that while law enforcement was very important, "that's not how we're going to solve the problem. We need treatment, prevention."

222 McCaffrey had wrangled: Ann Devroy, "About-Face: Clinton to Restore Staff He Cut from Anti-Drug Office," *Washington Post,* March 6, 1996, p. A-15.

222 "to disrupt the cocaine airbridge": Letter from Barry McCaffrey to members of the House Appropriations Committee, Subcommittee on Foreign Operations, Export Financing, and Related Programs, May 21, 1996, provided by ONDCP. Appropriations documents accompanying the letter lay out the sums to be spent.

222 McCaffrey had obtained: Devroy, "About-Face."

222 He chose to bring all 30: *The National Drug Control Strategy, 1998: Budget Summary,* p. 145.

222 a new Office of Strategic Planning: Ibid.; interview with Pancho Kinney.

222 The crucial job of drafting: Interview with Kinney.

222 McCaffrey instituted: See *Performance Measures of Effectiveness: A System for Assessing the Performance of the National Drug Control Strategy,* ONDCP, January 26, 1998.

222 McCaffrey insisted that the Pentagon: Interview with Barry McCaffrey. See also Bradley Graham, "Drug Control Chief Won't Let Pentagon Just Say No," *Washington Post,* November 24, 1997, p. A-17.

223 In December 1996: Sam Dillon, "U.S. Ex-General Lavish in Praising Mexican Allies in Drug War," *New York Times,* December 12, 1996, p. A-19.

223 "a guy of absolute, unquestioned integrity": Julia Preston, "A General in Mexico's Drug War Is Dismissed on Narcotics Charges," *New York Times,* February 19, 1997, p. A-1.

223 McCaffrey spent a full week: Interview with Kinney.

223 "our current interdiction efforts": Memo from Pancho Kinney to Barry McCaffrey, "November 12 Southwest Border Interagency Meeting," October 28, 1997, ONDCP. This memo contains the figures on the number of trucks inspected for drugs.

223 there had accumulated a vast storehouse: Probably the most widely cited of these studies was Peter Reuter, Gordon Crawford, and Jonathan Cave, *Sealing the Borders: The Effects of Increased Military Participation in Drug Interdiction* (RAND Corporation, 1988). It concluded that a major increase in interdiction efforts, while perhaps producing more seizures, would have little effect on the amount of cocaine consumed in the United States.

223 ways to escalate the drug war in Mexico: See *Report to Congress,* vol. 1, "United States and Mexico Counterdrug Cooperation," ONDCP, September 1997, esp. pp. 18–23. The description of the new X-ray technology is in a Customs Service supplement to that report, p. 14. See also Neil A. Lewis, "U.S. to Wage a High-Tech War on Drugs at the Mexican Border," *New York Times,* September 17, 1997, p. A-5.

223 "If you want to stop drug abuse": Interview with McCaffrey.

224 McCaffrey's 1999 budget: *The National Drug Control Strategy, 1998: Budget Summary,* ONDCP, p. 69.

224 Jerome Jaffe was working: Interview with Jerome Jaffe.

224 study after study had confirmed: See Gerstein and Harwood, *Treating Drug Problems,* p. 136. Noting that methadone has been the subject of "literally hundreds of studies," the book states that, from them, "strong evidence has accumulated about the safety and effectiveness of methadone." See also Ball and Ross, *The Effectiveness of Methadone Maintenance Treatment,* pp. 239–244, and Mark Kleiman, *Against Excess,* pp. 184–185. "Perhaps the best-established fact in the drug treatment literature," Kleiman writes, "is that methadone works. Methadone clients use substantially less heroin and commit substantially fewer crimes than they would if they were not on methadone, and methadone maintenance has the highest retention rates among all treatment modalities."

225 frozen at 115,000 slots: *The National Drug Control Strategy, 1998,* ONDCP, p. 40.

225 As a result, most cities: Christopher Wren, "Ex-Addicts Find Methadone More Elusive Than Heroin," *New York Times,* February 2, 1997, p. 12. The eight states without clinics were Idaho, Mississippi, Montana, New Hampshire, North Dakota, South Dakota, Vermont, and West Virginia.

225 the intricate web of federal regulations: see *Methadone Treatment Manual,* U.S. Department of Justice, June 1973.

225 Jaffe had also inserted a provision: Ibid., pp. 22, 55.

Part Three: The Street, 1993–1997

17: RISE AND FALL

229 An elderly, gray-haired Puerto Rican immigrant: Interview with Anna McLaughlin.

229 And the treatment world: Center on Addiction and Substance Abuse, "Substance Abuse and the American Woman," June 1996, pp. 11–12, 105–106, 112–116; Julia Clarke and Jill Kirschenbaum, "Sobering Truths," *City Limits,* May 1994, pp. 8–12; Currie, *Reckoning,* pp. 269–278.

230 Yvonne's year at New Hope: The description of Yvonne's time at New Hope is based on her own recollections, as well as on a visit I made to the facility in May 1994, about a year after she had left. On my visit, I interviewed both Sister Pat Conway and Father Aquinas, as well as several residents. In piecing together the story of Yvonne's stay at New Hope, I was greatly aided by having access to her various writing assignments and letters, which she provided me.

231 New Hope featured a ladderlike approach: The New Hope program is described in several brochures, including "New Hope Manor: A Residential Substance Abuse Treatment Center for Young Women."

235 Over and over, studies have found: See Hubbard et al., *Drug Abuse Treatment,* pp. 94–95, 103–105, 125, and Gerstein and Harwood, *Treating Drug Problems,* p. 135.

235 Unfortunately, most of the residents: Like many facilities, New Hope Manor does not keep formal figures on its dropout rates (or at least does not make them public); the rates mentioned here were pieced together from interviews with Sister Pat, Father Aquinas, Yvonne, and other program residents.

235 they have high dropout rates: Benjamin F. Lewis and Roy Ross, "Retention in Therapeutic Communities: Challenges for the Nineties," in F. M. Tims, G. De Leon, and N. Jainchill, eds., *Therapeutic Community: Advances in Research and Application,* NIDA Research Monograph no. 144, p. 103; George De Leon, "Retention in Drug-Free Therapeutic Communities," in Roy Pickens, Carl Lukefeld, and Charles Schuster, eds., *Improving Drug Abuse Treatment,* NIDA Research Monograph no. 106, p. 227.

236 Synanon practiced a strict form: See Lewis Yablonsky, *The Tunnel Back: Synanon* (Macmillan, 1965); *The Facts About "Drug Abuse,"* pp. 99–100.

236 (In the late 1970s, it was investigated): Robert Lindsey, "A Changed Synanon the Subject of Inquiry," *New York Times,* December 10, 1978, p. 1.

236 TCs have eliminated some: For a balanced discussion of therapeutic communities' benefits and drawbacks, see Gerstein and Harwood, *Treating Drug Problems,* pp. 154–167, 188–189. For a highly favorable description of TCs, see Sally Satel, "Yes, Drug Treatment Can Work," *City Journal,* Summer 1995, pp. 46–54.

236 they tend to stay for long periods: Jennifer Trone and Douglas Young, *Bridging Drug Treatment and Criminal Justice,* Vera Institute of Justice, 1996. In a study of treatment-alternative-to-prison programs in New York, the authors found that 75 percent of the people mandated to residential programs remained six months or longer—a higher rate than for most voluntary enrollees. (p. 14) See also Gerstein and Harwood, *Treating Drug Problems:* "Contrary to earlier fears among clinicians, criminal justice pressure does not necessarily vitiate treatment effectiveness and probably improves retention." (p. 11)

236 "I'll never forget": Interview with Rhonda Ferdinand. The Brooklyn dis-

trict attorney's office reports that half of all defendants turn down the offer of treatment as an alternative to prison, and that of these, 19 percent said they simply did not want residential drug treatment. (*Drug Treatment Alternatives-to-Prison,* Kings County District Attorney, Sixth Annual Report, November 1996.)

236 "TCs are hostile and barbaric": Interview with Stephan Sorrell. At the time I interviewed him, Sorrell (who has since passed away) was running a methadone program in New York, in addition to sitting on Daytop's board.

237 Women have an especially hard time: Lewis and Ross, "Retention in Therapeutic Communities," p. 105. "With respect to gender differences in TC retention," the authors note, "it is clear that there are universally lower retention rates for women. Males stay in treatment significantly longer than females." See also Clarke and Kirschenbaum, "Sobering Truths," pp. 8–12.

237 "Most programs are heavily confrontational": Interview with Father Aquinas.

238 112 adult rehabilitation centers: Interview with John Cheydleur, program development officer of the Salvation Army's Eastern Territory ARCs. Also helpful was a Salvation Army brochure, *What Everyone Should Know About Adult Rehabilitation Centers.*

239 overcome by cravings for the drug: For more on the cravings addicts feel while in treatment, see Lewis and Ross, "Retention in Therapeutic Communities," p. 105.

239 The lack of counseling: This is based on interviews with Yvonne and several other ARC residents and confirmed by an ARC counselor, who in an interview described her sense of being overwhelmed by the size of her caseload and confounded by the types of problems her clients faced. (The counselor requested anonymity.)

241 Yvonne's assessment is disputed: Interview with John Cheydleur. For a highly favorable view of the Salvation Army's work with addicts and the poor, see Sallie Tisdale, "Good Soldiers," *New Republic,* January 3, 1994, pp. 22–27.

242 Martina was well acquainted: Interview with Martina Coriano.

244 "Raphael became overextended": Interview with Jerry Frohnhoefer.

244 a potent stew of medications: The details about this were provided by Raphael Flores.

18: THE MAYOR

246 "If there's one problem": "Drug Abuse in New York City," speech delivered October 18, 1993.

246 neither Dinkins nor his police commissioner: Interview with Lee Brown.

246 the city had created about 10,000: Figures provided by the New York State Office of Alcoholism and Substance Abuse Services (OASAS).

247 a 1982 *Atlantic Monthly* article: James Q. Wilson and George L. Kelling, "Broken Windows," *Atlantic Monthly,* March 1982, pp. 29–38.

247 Bratton enlisted two of his top aides: Interview with John Timoney.

247 seemed worthy of the Keystone Kops: Interview with Timoney. For a critique of TNT sponsored in part by the NYPD, see Michele Sviridoff et al., "The Neighborhood Effects of Street-Level Drug Enforcement: Tactical Narcotics Teams in New York," Vera Institute of Justice, August 1992.

247 under the community policing regimen: In its efforts to discredit community policing, the police department leaked several memos summarizing the short-

comings of the program. For a summary, see John Marzulli, "Community Cops Program a Bust," *New York Daily News,* January 24, 1994, pp. 4–5; and Alan Finder, "Community Police Officers Cited on Hours and Training," *New York Times,* January 26, 1994, p. B-3.

248 use of the term was forbidden: Interview with Timoney.

248 Instead, they were going to earn: Interview with Timoney. "Police Strategy No. 3: Driving Drug Dealers Out of New York," Mayor of the City of New York, April 6, 1994. See also Clifford Krauss, "Giuliani Sets New Policy to Spur Drug Arrests by Officers on Beats," *New York Times,* April 7, 1994, p. A-1.

248 Sergeant Steve Ringe was wary: Interview with Steve Ringe.

249 Bratton's efforts to streamline: Interviews with Timoney and Ringe. See also James Lardner, "The C.E.O. Cop," *New Yorker,* February 6, 1995, pp. 45–57; Craig Horowitz, "The End of Crime as We Know It," *New York,* August 14, 1995, pp. 20ff; and William Bratton, *Turnaround: How America's Top Cop Reversed the Crime Epidemic* (Random House, 1998), pp. 233–239.

250 THE END OF CRIME: *New York,* August 14, 1995.

251 Luisa: A pseudonym.

251 Bettina: A pseudonym.

251 78,977 cocaine and heroin arrests: Blanche Frank and John Galea, "Current Drug Use Trends in New York City," New York State OASAS, June 1997.

251 the federal government's Drug Abuse Warning Network: Ibid.

252 agents were able to buy cocaine: Ibid.

252 The data for heroin: Ibid.

252 the reason could be found in Colombia: "New York Drug Trends," internal DEA report, October 1995. See also Christopher S. Wren, "Colombians Enter the Heroin Market," *New York Times,* February 11, 1996, p. 51.

252 "The drug trade is going": Interview with John Galea.

252 "The sellers": Interview with Bruce Johnson. Information on the changing nature of the street-level drug trade was also provided by Richard Curtis of the John Jay College of Criminal Justice in New York City.

252 Khamillo Parker: His real name. I interviewed him on numerous occasions between the fall of 1995 and the summer of 1997, when he suddenly disappeared from the streets.

253 The number of buyers: On the continuing high level of demand for drugs in the city, see Frank and Galea, "Current Drug Use Trends in New York City," New York State OASAS, June 1996 and December 1996.

254 As for new treatment slots: Information supplied by New York State OASAS.

254 treatment waiting lists: "Estimated Number of Individuals Needing Treatment," National Association of State Alcohol and Drug Abuse Directors, August 30, 1997.

254 the Family Rehabilitation Program: "Family Rehabilitation Program: Preliminary Outcome Data and Projected Impact of Proposed Cuts," National Development and Research Institute, November 21, 1994. Interview with Steven Magura of NDRI.

254 the case of Elisa Izquierdo: Lizette Alvarez, "A Mother's Tale: Drugs, Despair and Violence," *New York Times,* November 27, 1995, p. B-1.

255 When major flaws were discovered: Lizette Alvarez, "Report in Wake of Girl's Death Finds Failures in Child Agency," *New York Times,* April 9, 1996, p. A-1.

255 a new Administration for Children's Services: See Dale Russakoff, "The Protectors," *New Yorker,* April 27, 1997, pp. 58–71.

255 the New York City Police Department: Interview with Timoney.

255 As Bratton described it: Bratton, *Turnaround*, p. 275. See also an article Bratton wrote for the *New York Times* op-ed page, "How to Win the War Against Crime," April 5, 1996, p. A-27. In it, he called the new drug operation the "largest, most comprehensive antidrug initiative ever undertaken by an urban police department," the goal of which was "to permanently eradicate drug sales in northern Brooklyn."

255 the NYPD flooded the area: Dan Morrison, "New War on Drugs," *Newsday*, May 6, 1996, p. A-5; Clifford Krauss, "Brooklyn Drug Sweeps Begin to Make Inroads," *New York Times,* May 10, 1996, p. B-3; Alice McQuillan, "Rudy Pledges 20M Drug War," *New York Daily News,* April 4, 1996, p. 8.

256 and so the operations were extended: Interview with Timoney.

256 a record 101,051 drug arrests: "Removing Drugs from Our Neighborhoods and Schools," speech by Rudolph Giuliani, October 1, 1997.

256 "The operations in Brooklyn North": Interview with Michael Jacobson.

257 In October 1997, Mayor Giuliani: "Removing Drugs from Our Neighborhoods and Schools," October 1, 1997.

19: REDEMPTION

259 Unfortunately, the town: This is based on a visit I made to see Yvonne in Spring Valley in November 1995.

260 Yvonne scrounged up some money for the bus ride home: Yvonne asked me to help her with the bus fare, which I did.

265 she asked someone in the apartment to accompany her: I was that person.

Conclusion

20: A WAY OUT

272 Currently, the nation's treatment system: *The National Drug Control Strategy, 1998,* p. 86. See also Woodward et al., "The Drug Abuse Treatment Gap: Recent Estimates," *Health Care Financing Review,* Spring 1997, p. 12.

272 an additional $3.4 billion a year: Memo from John Carnevale to Richard Turman, "Treatment Gap," ONDCP, October 23, 1997.

272 The 1999 federal drug budget: *The National Drug Control Strategy, 1998, Budget Summary,* p. 16.

272 the federal drug budget is largely a fiction: See Patrick Murphy, "Keeping Score: The Frailties of the Federal Drug Budget," RAND Drug Policy Research Center Issue Paper, January 1994.

272 Some have argued: See, for instance, Peter Reuter, "Rebalancing the Drug Control Budget: A Shadow Play," *Drug Policy Analysis Bulletin,* Federation of American Scientists, January 1997, pp. 2–3.

273 to detox an addict in a hospital: Already, in some cities (Chicago, for instance), detox is performed primarily in nonmedical settings. See Gerstein and Harwood, *Treating Drug Problems,* p. 176: "On technical grounds, detoxification of most illicit drugs in most cases can occur as safely and effectively on an ambulatory basis as in a bedded setting."

274 Yvonne Hamilton, for instance: On several occasions, Yvonne expressed her interest in doing such work.

275 the popular DARE program: See *Alcohol and Health,* 9th Special Report to the U.S. Congress, U.S. Department of Health and Human Services, June 1997, p. 303. According to "two well-controlled studies," this report noted, DARE, while positively affecting youths' attitudes about substances, "had little overall effect on alcohol use." See also Mathea Falco, *The Making of a Drug-Free America: Programs That Work* (Times Books, 1992), p. 43: "Studies have shown that DARE does not reduce tobacco, alcohol, or drug use." For a good summary of the research on drug prevention, see Institute of Medicine, *Pathways of Addiction: Opportunities in Drug Abuse Research* (National Academy Press, 1996), pp. 139–154.

Select Bibliography

Adams, Tom. *Grass Roots: How Ordinary People Are Changing America*. Citadel Press, 1991.

Adler, William M. *Land of Opportunity: One Family's Quest for the American Dream in the Age of Crack*. Atlantic Monthly, 1995.

Anderson, Patrick. *High in America: The True Story Behind NORML and the Politics of Marijuana*. Viking, 1981.

Association of the Bar of the City of New York and the Drug Abuse Council. *The Nation's Toughest Drug Law: Evaluating the New York Experience*, 1977.

Ball, John C., and Alan Ross. *The Effectiveness of Methadone Maintenance Treatment*. Springer Verlag, 1991.

Baum, Dan. *Smoke and Mirrors: The War on Drugs and the Politics of Failure*. Little, Brown, 1996.

Bennett, William J. *The De-Valuing of America: The Fight for Our Culture and Our Children*. Summit, 1992.

Bourgois, Philippe. *In Search of Respect: Selling Crack in El Barrio*. Cambridge University Press, 1995.

Bratton, William. *Turnaround: How America's Top Cop Reversed the Crime Epidemic*. Random House, 1998.

Brecher, Edward M. *Licit and Illicit Drugs*. Little, Brown, 1972.

Califano, Joseph A., Jr. *The 1982 Report on Drug Abuse and Alcoholism*. Warner, 1982.

Center on Addiction and Substance Abuse. "Substance Abuse and the American Woman." June 1996.

Chein, Isidor, et al. *The Road to H: Narcotics, Delinquency, and Social Policy*. Basic Books, 1964.

Clinton, Bill, and Al Gore. *Putting People First: How We Can All Change America*. Times Books, 1992.

Courtwright, David; Herman Joseph; and Don DesJarlais. *Addicts Who Survived: An Oral History of Narcotic Use in America, 1923–1965*. University of Tennessee Press, 1989.

Currie, Elliott. *Reckoning: Drugs, the Cities, and the American Future*. Hill & Wang, 1993.

Drug Abuse Council. *The Facts About "Drug Abuse."* Free Press, 1980.

Duke, Steven B., and Albert C. Gross. *America's Longest War: Rethinking Our Tragic Crusade Against Drugs*. Putnam, 1993.

Eddy, Paul; Hugo Sabogal; and Sara Walden. *The Cocaine Wars*. Norton, 1988.

Ehrlichman, John. *Witness to Power: The Nixon Years*. Simon & Schuster, 1982.

Epstein, Edward Jay. *Agency of Fear: Opiates and Political Power in America.* Rev. ed. Verso, 1990.

Falco, Mathea. *The Making of a Drug-Free America: Programs That Work.* Times Books, 1992.

Gerstein, Dean R., and Henrick J. Harwood, eds. *Treating Drug Problems,* vol. 1, A Study of the Evolution, Effectiveness, and Financing of Public and Private Drug Treatment Systems, Committee for the Substance Abuse Coverage Study, Division of Health Care Services, Institute of Medicine. National Academy Press, 1990.

————. *Treating Drug Problems,* vol. 2, Commissioned Papers on Historical, Institutional and Economic Contexts of Drug Treatment. National Academy Press, 1992.

Glasscote, Raymond M., et al. *The Treatment of Drug Abuse: Programs, Problems, Prospects.* Joint Information Service of the American Psychiatric Service and the National Association for Mental Health, 1972.

Gugliotta, Guy, and Jeff Leen. *Kings of Cocaine: An Astonishing True Story of Murder, Money, and Corruption.* Simon & Schuster, 1989.

Haldeman, H. R. *The Haldeman Diaries.* Putnam, 1994.

Hentoff, Nat. *A Doctor Among the Addicts.* Rand McNally, 1968.

Hubbard, Robert L., et al. *Drug Abuse Treatment: A National Study of Effectiveness.* University of North Carolina Press, 1989.

Hughes, Patrick. *Behind the Wall of Respect: Community Experiments in Heroin Addiction Control.* University of Chicago Press, 1977.

Jaffe, Jerome, ed. *Encyclopedia of Drugs and Alcohol.* Macmillan Library Reference USA, 1995.

Johnston, Lloyd D.; Patrick M. O'Malley; and Jerald G. Bachman. *National Survey Results on Drug Use from the Monitoring the Future Study, 1975–1993,* vol. 1, Secondary School Students, University of Michigan Institute for Social Research, U.S. Department of Health and Human Services, 1994.

Kelley, Kitty. *Nancy Reagan: The Unauthorized Biography.* Simon & Schuster, 1991.

Kitfield, James. *Prodigal Soldiers: How the Generation of Officers Born in Vietnam Revolutionized the American Style of War.* Simon & Schuster, 1995.

Kleiman, Mark A. R. *Against Excess: A Drug Policy for Results.* Basic Books, 1992.

Krogh, Egil. *The Day Elvis Met Nixon.* Pejama Press, 1994.

Liddy, G. Gordon. *Will.* St. Martin's, 1980.

Lukas, J. Anthony. *Nightmare: The Underside of the Nixon Years.* Viking, 1976.

Manatt, Marsha. *Parents, Peers, and Pot.* National Institute on Drug Abuse, Department of Health, Education, and Welfare, 1979.

Mann, Peggy. *Marijuana Alert.* McGraw-Hill, 1985.

Maraniss, David. *First in His Class: A Biography of Bill Clinton.* Simon & Schuster, 1995.

McCoy, Alfred W. *The Politics of Heroin: CIA Complicity in the Global Drug Trade.* Lawrence Hill, 1991.

McWilliams, John C. *The Protectors: Harry J. Anslinger and the Federal Bureau of Narcotics, 1930–1962.* University of Delaware Press, 1990.

Moore, Mark Harrison. *Buy and Bust: The Effective Regulation of an Illicit Market in Heroin.* Lexington Books, 1977.

Musto, David F. *The American Disease: Origins of Narcotic Control.* Oxford University Press, 1973.

National Commission on Marihuana and Drug Abuse. *Marihuana: A Signal of Misunderstanding.* Government Printing Office, March 1972.

Newman, Robert G. *Methadone Treatment in Narcotic Addiction: Program Management, Findings, and Prospects for the Future.* Academic Press, 1977.

Reeves, Jimmie L., and Richard Campbell. *Cracked Coverage: Television News, the Anti-Cocaine Crusade, and the Reagan Legacy.* Duke University Press, 1994.

Reinarman, Craig, and Harry G. Levine, eds. *Crack in America: Demon Drugs and Social Justice.* University of California Press, 1997.

Report and Recommendations to the Mayor on Drug Abuse in New York City (Katzenbach Report). Mayor's Office, May 1990.

Reuter, Peter; Gordon Crawford; and Jonathan Cave. *Sealing the Borders: The Effects of Increased Military Participation in Drug Interdiction.* RAND Corporation, 1988.

Rhodes, William, et al. *What America's Users Spend on Illegal Drugs, 1988–1995.* Office of National Drug Control Policy, Fall 1997.

Rosebush, James S. *First Lady, Public Wife: A Behind-the-Scenes History of the Evolving Role of First Ladies in American Political Life.* Madison Books, 1987.

Rydell, C. Peter, and Susan S. Everingham. *Controlling Cocaine: Supply Versus Demand Programs.* RAND Corporation, 1994.

Shannon, Elaine. *Desperados: Latin Drug Lords, U.S. Lawmen, and the War America Can't Win.* Viking, 1988.

Simon, David, and Edward Burns. *The Corner: A Year in the Life of an Inner-City Neighborhood.* Broadway Books, 1997.

Sviridoff, Michele, et al. "The Neighborhood Effects of Street-Level Drug Enforcement: Tactical Narcotics Teams in New York." Vera Institute of Justice, August 1992.

United States Sentencing Commission. *Cocaine and Federal Sentencing Policy.* Special Report to the Congress, February 1995.

———. *Mandatory Minimum Penalties in the Federal Criminal Justice System.* Special Report to the Congress, August 1991.

Waldorf, Dan; Craig Reinarman; and Sheigla Murphy. *Cocaine Changes: The Experience of Using and Quitting.* Temple University, 1991.

Westin, Av, and Stephanie Shaffer. *Heroes and Heroin: The Shocking Story of Drug Addiction in the Military.* Pocket Books, 1972.

White, Theodore. *The Making of the President, 1968.* Atheneum, 1969.

———. *Breach of Faith: The Fall of Richard Nixon.* Atheneum, 1975.

Williams, Terry. *The Cocaine Kids: The Inside Story of a Teenage Drug Ring.* Addison-Wesley, 1989.

Yablonsky, Lewis. *The Tunnel Back: Synanon.* Macmillan, 1965.

Acknowledgments

When, back in 1988, the *New York Review of Books* sent me to Colombia to write about the Latin American cocaine trade, I had little notion that the issue of drugs would engross me for most of the next ten years. But Robert Silvers, the *New York Review*'s editor, urged me to keep writing about the subject, and before long I found myself fully absorbed. Without his encouragement and suggestions, I doubt that this project would ever have gotten off the ground.

Early on, I was fortunate to receive the backing of the Alicia Patterson Foundation, which provided me the freedom to explore my new preoccupation. Jim Silberman, then the head of Summit Books, saw in my articles the potential of a book and signed me up to do one. As I plunged ahead, my research took many unexpected turns, and that I was able to follow them fully was due largely to the MacArthur Foundation, whose largess provided me that greatest of book-writing luxuries, time.

My research benefited greatly from the assistance of John Carnevale, who shared insights he'd gleaned over his many years of work at the Office of National Drug Control Policy. The manuscript was greatly improved by careful readings (in all or part) by Larry Zuckerman, Patti Cohen, Nancy Hass, Linda Ricci, Paul Samuels, Mimi Doretti, Chuck Sabel, and David Gelber. I am particularly indebted to Carol Bergman, who, drawing on her long years of work in Washington on drugs and criminal justice, supplied information, served as a sounding board, and, when necessary, argued with me, all of which forced me to refine and clarify my views. I'd also like to thank Spencer Klaw, for all he taught me about writing, and Aryeh Neier, for his general support over the years. Thanks, too, to friends Jocelyn Baltzell, Philip Weiss, and Helen Winternitz for their moral support, and to Danica Gallagher for her pointers on how New York City works.

My agent, Kathy Robbins, read innumerable drafts of the book, and her suggestions played an important part in molding it; her assistant, David Halpern, offered encouragement at key moments. At Simon & Schuster, Alice Mayhew, deploying her unique editorial talents, helped shape a long and unwieldy manuscript; her assistant, Roger Labrie, was forever ready to help with matters large and small.

Finally, I want to thank Raphael Flores, who allowed me to accompany him on his daily rounds, and Jerome Jaffe, who fielded my endless requests for information with unflagging patience and good humor. Without their generosity in sharing their experiences and insights, this book could not have been written.

Index

McMahon, Ricia, 213, 215
Madison, James, 192
Madison Center, 192
malt liquor, 31, 45, 48
Manhattan D.A.'s office, 61, 62
  Homicide Investigations Unit of, 72
Manhattan North Narcotics, 59–60, 61, 67
Mann, Peggy, 153
Maple, Jack, 247, 255
Marcos, Imelda, 175
marijuana, 32, 35, 86, 109, 135–37
  active ingredients of, 159
  arrests for possession of, 136
  "blunts," 45
  Clinton Administration's media campaign
    against, 219–20
  crack mixed with, 76
  decriminalization of, 136–37, 141–42,
    145, 153, 158, 172, 189, 273
  federal government's supply of, 158, 159,
    160
  as "gateway" drug, 150, 151, 153
  high school seniors' surveyed use of, 11,
    150–51, 169, 183, 189, 213, 217, 218–
    219
  homosexuality and, 184–85
  law abuse potential of, 135
  paraquat sprayed on, 140, 147
  popularity of, 113, 135–36, 145
  possible beneficial effects of, 186
  smuggling of, 164–65
  see also parent anti-marijuana movement
Marijuana Conference, 219
Martinez, Bob, 205, 272
Mathias, Charles, 153, 159
Medicaid, 18, 19, 21, 24, 25–26, 30, 76
Medicare, 161
Meese, Edwin, 159
Mejia, Ronald, 61, 67, 68
methadone, 10–11, 22, 24, 27, 88, 126
  addictiveness of, 88, 98, 103
  black market in, 121
  origin of, 87
  overdoses of, 121, 124, 129
methadone-maintenance programs, 23, 49,
  56–57, 91–93, 98, 102, 110, 111, 120,
  127, 224–26, 252–53, 273
  effectiveness of, 88, 101, 103, 105, 106,
    111
  origin of, 87, 88–89
  see also treatment, drug; treatment
    centers
Metropolitan Hospital, 41, 64, 77, 238, 243,
  264
Metsky, Ellen, 148
Mexico, 9, 134–35, 153, 164, 178
  paraquat used in, 140
  U.S. anti-drug efforts and, 9, 134–35,
    140, 146–47, 184, 223–24

Meyer, Roger, 126, 155
Miami, Fla., 164, 179, 182, 192
Michigan, University of, 186
  drug use surveys of, 11, 150, 169, 183,
    189, 213, 214, 217, 218–19
Minnick, Walter, 125
Mitchell, John, 99, 106, 114
Monitoring the Future drug-use surveys,
  11
Morgan, John, 33, 37
Moriarty, Erin, 55
morphine, 88, 132
Morris, Stanley, 192–93, 194–95, 206
Moulton, Connie, 171
Moulton, Otto, 170–73, 181, 186
Mundo, Joseph, 215, 216
Murillo, Rosario María, 175
Murphy, Morgan, 107, 115
Murphy, Sheigla, 37
Muskie, Edmund, 117
Musto, David, 199

NA (Narcotics Anonymous), 12
Nadelmann, Ethan, 32
Nader, Ralph, 136
Nalepka, Joyce, 153, 157, 185
Narcotic Advisory Council, 85, 86, 90–91
Narcotics Anonymous (NA), 12
narcotics antagonists, 89–90
Narcotics Treatment Administration (NTA),
  102, 106, 133, 137, 140, 149
National Commission on Marihuana and
  Drug Abuse, 136, 151, 275
National Drug Control Strategy, 200–201,
  212
National Drug Policy Board, 192
National Endowment for the Humanities
  (NEH), 192, 197
National Federation of Parents for
  Drug-Free Youth (NFP), 153, 156,
  157, 159, 169–73, 184, 185, 186, 187
National Household Survey on Drug Abuse,
  12, 200, 206
National Humanities Center, 197
National Institute of Mental Health
  (NIMH), 86, 98, 104–5, 110, 117–18,
  122
National Institute on Drug Abuse (NIDA),
  49, 119, 144, 145, 149, 168, 171, 173,
  174, 177, 181, 182, 185
  Addiction Research Center of, 179, 186,
    193
  establishment of, 134
  National Household Surveys on Drug
    Abuse of, 200, 206
  Parents, Peers, and Pot handbook of,
    152–53
National Institutes of Health (NIH), 101–2,
  134

About the Author

Michael Massing is a contributing editor of the *Columbia Journalism Review* and a frequent contributor to the *New York Review of Books.* Named a Mac-Arthur Fellow in 1992, he has been reporting on the drug world for the last ten years. His articles have appeared in the *New York Times*, the *New Yorker*, the *Atlantic Monthly*, and many other publications. He lives in New York.